Emerging Concepts in Neuro-Oncology

Emerging Concepts in Neuro-Oncology

Editor: Mariana Garland

AMERICAN
MEDICAL PUBLISHERS
www.americanmedicalpublishers.com

AMERICAN
MEDICAL PUBLISHERS
www.americanmedicalpublishers.com

Cataloging-in-publication Data

Emerging concepts in neuro-oncology / edited by Mariana Garland.
p. cm.
Includes bibliographical references and index.
ISBN 979-8-88740-089-1
1. Nervous system--Tumors. 2. Brain--Tumors. 3. Brain--Cancer.
4. Central nervous system--Tumors. 5. Nervous system--Cancer.
I. Garland, Mariana.
RC280.N4 E44 2023
616.993 83--dc23

American Medical Publishers,
41 Flatbush Avenue,
1st Floor, New York,
NY 11217, USA

ISBN 979-8-88740-089-1 (Hardback)

Contents

Preface

The study of the brain and spinal cord neoplasms (tumors) is known as neuro-oncology. These tumors are dangerous and may prove to be fatal. Astrocytoma, glioma, glioblastoma multiforme, ependymoma, pontine glioma, and brain stem cancers are a few types of central nervous system cancers. Diagnostic imaging of the brain and spinal cord, lumbar puncture and cerebrospinal fluid analysis, and pathologic diagnosis are the standard diagnosis methods of the diseases. Radiotherapy, chemotherapy, corticosteroids, and neurosurgical interventions are standard treatment methods within this field. Advancements in imaging technologies such as computed tomography (CT), magnetic resonance imaging (MRI), and positron emission tomography (PET) have helped in ensuring accurate diagnosis, treatment planning, response assessment, prognosis, and surveillance of the highly complex CNS malignancies. The book consists of contributions made by international experts. The various studies that are constantly contributing towards advancing technologies and the evolution of neuro-oncology are examined in detail within this book. Scientists and students actively engaged in this field will find it full of crucial and unexplored concepts.

Various studies have approached the subject by analyzing it with a single perspective, but the present book provides diverse methodologies and techniques to address this field. This book contains theories and applications needed for understanding the subject from different perspectives. The aim is to keep the readers informed about the progresses in the field; therefore, the contributions were carefully examined to compile novel researches by specialists from across the globe.

Indeed, the job of the editor is the most crucial and challenging in compiling all chapters into a single book. In the end, I would extend my sincere thanks to the chapter authors for their profound work. I am also thankful for the support provided by my family and colleagues during the compilation of this book.

Editor

1

Novel Endocrine Targets for GBM Therapy

Judith Marcela Dueñas-Jiménez,
Irene Aguilar-García,
María de la Luz Galván-Ramírez,
Sergio Horacio Dueñas-Jiménez,
Jorge David Rivas-Carrillo, Anne Santerre and
Erika Priscilla Domínguez-Rangel

Abstract

Astrocytomas are brain tumors from glial cells, and they are classified by the World Health Organization (WHO) as astrocytoma, grade I or benign; astrocytoma, grade II or malignant; anaplastic astrocytoma, grade III; and glioblastoma multiforme or grade IV. The high-grade gliomas have an incidence of 6.03/100,000. The frequency of GBM is higher in men than in woman by a 50%. The survival of patients with GBM varied between 14 and 18 months, and less than 10% patients survive for 5 years. The main treatments for GBM consist of surgical tumor resection, radiotherapy, and chemotherapy. These tumors present different endocrine characteristics, such as expression of aromatase enzyme, estrogen, progesterone, as well as testosterone receptors. In addition, patients with GBM produce estradiol in high concentrations when compared to those with low-grade astrocytomas. The highest mRNA expression of ERα and aromatase in GBM patients had been postulated as prognostic biomarkers. The aromatase inhibitors had been used in the treatment of breast cancer in postmenopausal women with satisfactory results. At present time, several research groups are interested in testing these inhibitors for treating GBM.

Keywords: glioblastoma, endocrine characteristics, estradiol receptor, aromatase, aromatase inhibitors

1. Introduction

Glioblastoma multiforme (GBM) tumor occurs either as a primary tumor when it is formed de novo or a secondary tumor when the tumor progresses from grade II or III to grade IV. GBM is a diffuse and infiltrative tumor with a high mitotic activity, nuclear atypia, pleomorphism, and necrosis. GBM is the most frequently occurring brain tumor (12–15%) and represents 50–60% of all astrocytomas. There are two variants of glioblastoma: Glioblastoma of giant cells and gliosarcoma. GBM affects the cerebral hemispheres, mostly the white substance of the cerebral hemispheres. GBM primary has a bad prognostic due to its molecular heterogeneity. On the basis of its transcriptional subtype, GBM primary is also classified as neural, classical, and mesenchymal as well as proneural for GBM secondary. In GBM primary occurs the amplification of epidermal growth factor (EGF), and the *PTEN* gene is mutated in 45% of GBM primary cases, whereas in GBM secondary, the EGF amplification does not occur. The chromosome alteration in GBM involves a loss of the chromosome 10. The treatment for this kind of tumor after a safe surgical process also involves radiotherapy (RT) and the pharmacological treatment using the alkylating agent Temozolamide (TMZ), and different combinations of this agent with antitumor drugs such as the Bevacizumab. In spite of these treatments, there is a short survival period for GBM patients (14–18 months), which promotes the development of different clinical trials (II or III) to provide the patient a treatment with a better outcome. These new approaches are based on the molecular aspects of GBM to make the treatments more individualized.. This chapter describes the main GBM endocrine and molecular characteristics now known and makes a proposal on future treatments for GBM patients on the basis of these molecular characteristics.

2. Epidemiology

The incidence can change by age; in adults, for example, gliomas are the most frequent primary central nervous system tumors recurring in 70% of the patients. The average age of patients with GBM primary is 62 years, while for secondary GBM patients, it is approximately 45 years. The ethnicity and geographical localization are also of great importance in their epidemiology [1]. These tumors represent about 31% of newly diagnosed tumors in the United States and 81% of malignant tumors of the brain. The incidence of brain cancer in Europe is of 5.5/100,000 individuals, and the minor incidence is in sub-Saharan Africa with 0.8/100,000 individuals [2]. High-grade gliomas, anaplastic astrocytoma (AA) and GBM, have an incidence of 6.03/100,000 [3,4]. It has been shown that the incidence of GBM with respect to gender and ethnicity was different. The white people had the highest incidence of 2.5/100,000, Latin white people 1.8/100,000, and black people 1.5/100,000 [5].

3. Molecular characteristics of GBM

The current molecular characterization of GBM has allowed different classifications of the tumor subtypes and revealed intracellular pathways that might contribute to the development of new and effective therapeutic targets. The new molecular classification can distinguish individual somatic mutations within the same tumor grade, since tumors are highly variable from patient to patient [6,7]. Thus, using molecular markers facilitate study of heterogeneity of glioma, and subsequently its diagnosis and treatment.

Intensive molecular analyses have revealed a variety of deregulated genetic pathways involved in the DNA damage and repair, apoptosis, cell migration, angiogenesis, and in the cell cycle. Molecular analyses show that they arise from different genomic alterations, which may influence the response to therapy. The Cancer Genome Atlas (TCGA) Research Network (2008) has established a comprehensive catalog of genomic abnormalities driving tumor genesis, thus subclassifying glioblastoma into at least four molecular subtypes, featuring distinct genetic, epigenetic, and transcriptional alterations [6,8]. Tumor variants are classified based on somatic mutations as: isocitrate dehydrogenase (IDH) and Tumor Protein (TP53). Glioblastoma is also classified based on it′s transcriptional signature as: classical, mesenchymal, neural or proneural. Classification is also given by variations in the number of gene copies, by mutations in Epidermal Growth Factor Receptor (EGFR) or by DNA hypermethylation of promotor-associated CpG islands [9].

The majority of glioblastoma cases are primary brain tumors that grow rapidly without major clinical or histological evidence of a less malignant precursor lesion. These tumors mainly affect the elderly and are genetically characterized by loss of heterozygosity (LOH) on 10q, EGFR amplification, p16INK4a deletion, and fosfatidilinositol-3,4,5-trisfosfato 3-fosfatasa (*PTEN*) mutations [10,11]. Secondary glioblastoma tumors develop through progression from low-grade diffuse astrocytoma or AA and are pronounced in younger patients [12]. The disruption of tumor-suppressor gene *TP53* is implicated in the progression of many types of human malignancies; adult glioblastoma patients with *TP53* mutation may have a more severe consequence than those without *TP53* mutations [10]. It has also been shown that *TP53* mutations, but not *p53* expression, correlate with a more aggressive form of the disease. Studies have also reported that glioblastoma with *TP53* mutations are more frequent in women than in men, and may occur in younger patients [13]. In addition, some studies suggest that *TP53* mutations may occur in patients of any age group. In contrast, EGFR amplification preferentially occurs in older patients. Thus, multiple genes are involved in the initiation of the disease, and variability occurs in different age and sex groups in the progression of GBM. It is of interest that after careful analysis of age and disease progression, no significant difference in survival was observed in patients with primary and secondary glioblastoma. During the progression of glioblastoma, additional mutations and genetic alterations accumulate, which may alter disease severity and patient survival.

GBM primary and secondary can also differ significantly, depending on their pattern of promoter methylation and in the expression of profiles at the RNA and protein levels. LOH on 10q is shown to be most frequent in both primary and secondary glioblastomas [14]. *TP53* mutations are detected early in the pathway, and frequent genetic alterations can lead to secondary glioblastoma. In 77 Japanese patients with GBM primary, 22% had *TP53* mutations, 21% *PTEN* mutations, 32% *EGFR* amplification, 42% *p16 INK4a* homozygous deletion, and 69% LOH on chromosome 10q in those patients [15]. The frequencies of these genetic alterations at the population level were similar to those reported in Europe. This study noted a positive association between *EGFR* amplification and *p16 INK4a* deletion.

4. Glioblastoma multiforme risk factors

GBM is the most aggressive form of malignant glioma. Several syndromes are associated with the increased incidence of GBM, such as Lynch syndrome, Li–Fraumeni syndrome, melanoma–neural system tumor syndrome, Ollier disease, and Maffucci syndrome [16]. A small proportion (5–10%) of patients has a family history of glioma. Genes too exist that are involved in gliomagenesis and participate in glioma growth, such as telomerase reverse transcriptase (TERT) [17], *EGFR* [18,19], coiled-coil domain containing protein 26 (*CCDC26*) [20],Cyclin-dependent Kinase inhibitor 2B [17], *TP53* [21,22,23], and the regulator of telomere elongation helicase 1 (*RTEL1*) [24,25].

5. Endocrine characteristics of GBM

5.1. Estrogen receptors

GBM exhibits different endocrine characteristics. GBM expresses high levels of estrogen receptor alpha (mRNA ERα) and low levels of estrogen receptor beta (ERß); expression of mRNA ERα is positively correlated to the survival of GBM patients and could be used as a prognostic factor [26]. In contrast, the low expression of ERß in GBM has been related to a worse prognosis for survival and could be used as a biomarker for prognosis too [27,28]. Furthermore, activation of the signaling pathways induced by ERβ suppresses glioma growth in a model in vivo [29].

The coactivator family of estrogen receptors (SRC) is composed of three members, SRC-1, SRC-2, and SRC-3 [30,31]. SRC-1 increases the transcriptional activity of ER [32,33]; it also participates in the tumor progression and survival of several lines of human cancer [34,35]. SRC-2 is localized in different regions of the brain and mediates a variety of steroids-dependent functions [36,37]. SRC-3 is overexpressed in different types of cancer (breast, ovary, prostate, stomach, endometrium, esophagus, and pancreas) [38,39,40,41]. In astrocytoma cell lines, SRC1 and SRC-3 have been detected [42]. 17-/i> estradiol induces the growth of several cell lines of human astrocytoma through the ERα, and its interaction with SRC-1 and SRC3 suggests that ERα has an important role in the growth of astrocytoma [43].

5.2. Progesterone receptors in GBM

Progesterone receptors (PRs) are expressed in 100% of high-grade astrocytomas. The predominant isoform expression of PR in GBM is PRB. In astrocytomas, the molecular mechanisms involved in the differential expression of PR isoforms are unknown. It is important to know what PR isoform is expressed in the brain tumor, because progesterone can exert different cell functions depending on the expression pattern of PR isoforms [44,45].

In several cell contexts, human PRB functions as a transcriptional activator of progesterone-responsive genes, whereas PRA acts a repressor of transcriptional steroid hormone receptors inclusive PRB [46]; PR expression assessed by immunohistochemistry directly correlates with the histological grades of astrocytomas; these results suggest that PR-positive tumors possess a high proliferative potential [47]. However, no conclusive data exists about the PR as a marker of prognosis.

Progesterone significantly decreases GBM tumor growth and promotes the survival time in approximately 60% of mice. Synergistic effects of progesterone and Temozolomide (TMZ) have been observed in the glioblastoma cell lines U87MG and U118MG. A significant decrease in PCNA (a marker of cell proliferation) expression in both U87MG and U118 cell lines was observed by the effect of progesterone alone (80 μM) or by the combination of 80 μM progesterone and 100 μM TMZ, when compared to control, and this has a significantly statistic outcome than that with TMZ alone. Cell survival was reduced in 58%, with the combined treatment of progesterone and TMZ (P 80 μM + TMZ 100 μM after) when compared to that with MTZ alone. Further, progesterone inhibited O-6-methylguanine-DNA-methyltransferase (MGMT) expression as well as the EGFR/PI3K/AkT/mTOR signaling pathway, which is highly active in GBM. Progesterone + TMZ also inhibited the cell migration, suggesting that the combination therapy could contain the spread of tumor in vivo [48].

5.3. Androgen receptor in GBM

The androgen receptor (AR) is present in astrocytomas of low and high grades, with a higher expression in AA compared to astrocytomas grade I, II, and GBM. AR expression no affect the survival time of GBM patients [49,50] described a higher expression of AR in GBM tumors in women and men compared to periphery normal brain tissue.

5.4. Aromatase

Aromatase is an enzyme encoded by *CYP19* gene localized in chromosome 15q 21.2. It converts androgens in estrogens; this enzyme is expressed mainly in ovary, testis, placenta, brain, lung, stomach, and adipose tissue [51]. Aromatase is composed of 503 amino acids and is the major source for estrogen production in postmenopausal women. The aromatase works in three steps; first, the C19 methyl group of androgenic substrate is oxidized to formic acid in concomitant aromatization of ring A to the characteristic phenolic ring A of estrogen [52].

Aromatase expression in GBM tumor is negatively correlated to the survival of GBM patients and has been proposed as a possible prognosis biomarker for astrocytomas [29].

17–ß estradiol levels in GBM tumor are highest, compared to low-grade astrocytomas (I, II) or astrocytoma anaplastic (grade III). The concentration of 17–ß estradiol in GBM seems to be directly involved in the tumor growth.

6. GBM treatment

GBM tumors show a large number of aberrations with a pronounced mitotic activity, neoangiogenesis, and necrosis. Its proliferative rate is three to five times more than the proliferative rate in AA [53].

On the basis of a recent GBM classification as proneural, neural, classical, and mesenchymal, diverse types of treatments must be created to make a molecular personalized therapy [6] (**Table 1**). Performing molecular assays is complex, as their cost may be an obstacle for a routine use.

Treatment	Overall survival (OS)	Progression-free survival (PFS)	Side effects	Author
TMZ/RT	14.6 months	6.9 months	Myelosuppression	Stupp (2005)
RT	12.1 months	5.0 months	Skin reactions, cardiac complications	Stupp (2005)
Bev/TMZ /RT	20.5 months	10.7 months	Myelosuppression, arterial thromboembolism, gastrointestinal perforation	Gilbert (2014) Chinot (2014)
Bev	15.7	10.6	Arterial thromboembolism, arterial gastrointestinal perforation	
Cilengitide/RT	26.3 months	13.5 months		Stupp (2014)
Nimotuz umab/RT	22.3 months	7.7 months	Headache, nausea, vomiting, anemia, myalgia	Westphal (2015)
Nimustine	28.4 months	18.9 months	Chest pain and cianosis peribucal	Kim (2011)
Enzastaurin	17.1 months	9 months	Lymphopenia	Wick (2013)
Tipifarnib	80.3 weeks	18.1 weeks	Headache, nausea, vomiting	Ducassou (2013)
Everolimus	13.9 months	11.3 months	Anemia, higher levels of cholesterol in the blood, low phosphorus	Hainsworth (2012)

Table 1. Effects on survival of different treatments for GBM patients and their side effects.

The standard treatment for GBM patients includes brain radiation, a maximal surgery and .chemotherapy with the alkylating agent TMZ.

A larger number of new drugs and virus-based therapy are being evaluated in phase II and III trials as well.

In a phase III trial including recently diagnosed GBM patients, the median overall survival (OS) for GBM patients was 14.6 months with chemotherapy and RT, and 12.1 months with RT alone with a median follow-up of 28 months [63].

In phase III of another study, 978 patients received standard radiation and TMZ with or without Bevacizumab, an angiogenesis inhibitor used at 10 mg/kg, every 2 weeks with a median follow-up of 20.5 months. The OS between bevacizumab group and placebo group was no different, and side effects such as hypertension, thromboembolic events, intestinal perforation, and neutropenia were more common in the bevacizumab group. The progression-free survival (PFS) was significantly improved in the experimental arm (10.7 vs 7.3 months, $P = 0.007$) [64]. In another phase (III) trial with 458 patients, newly diagnosed GBM received radiation and TMZ with or without bevacizumab (10 mg/kg each for 2 weeks and TMZ for six cycles). With bevacizumab monotherapy (15 mg/kg), the median of PFS was of 10.6 months in the bevacizumab group as compared to 6.2 months in the placebo group.

6.1. Aromatase inhibitors (AIs)

The conversion of androstenedione and testosterone to estrogens can be blocked by the aromatase inhibitors; these pharmacological agents have a high specific activity to reduce, importantly, estrogen production. The AIs are classified in two types: I.—steroid inhibitors and II.—nonsteroid inhibitors; they are reactive species that bind covalently and irreversibly or noncovalently and reversibly to aromatase, respectively. The latter class interacts with the heme cofactor by employing its azole moiety. Third generation inhibitors are composed of triazole derivatives: anastrozole, letrozole, and the steroidal examestane. These inhibitors provided greater clinical benefits with a robust aromatase inhibition of 98% or more. The aromatase inhibitors have been successfully used for the treatment of estrogen receptor-positive breast cancer in postmenopausal women [65]. Letrozole has a more potent inhibitory effect on estrogen synthesis than anastrozole [66]. Letrozole has been tested in a GBM model using Sprague–Dawley rats orthotopically implanted with C6 cells. Imaging analysis employing μPET/CT showed an important reduction in the volume of tumor (>75%) after 8 days of letrozole treatment (4 mg/kg/day) [67].

The AIs, namely 3b-hydroxyandrost-4-en-17-one (1), androst-4-en-17-one (12), 4a,5a-epoxy androstan-17-one (13a), and 5a-androst-2-en-17-one (16), induced an antiproliferative effect on MCF7 breast cancer cells, and this effect was due to a cell cycle arrest and cell death by apoptosis [68]. Table 1 shows different treatments for GBM and their effect on OS. It also exhibits the progression-free survival, with the side effects observed in these studies.

6.2. Hormone release growth hormone (GHRH) inhibitors

GHRH inhibitors had been used for the treatment of various cancers or disorders that express growth hormone (GH) or GHRH production. GHRH antagonists suppress GH or insulin-like growth factor (IGF-1) in transgenic mice overexpressing the *GHRH* gene; GHRH antagonists can inhibit the rat pituitary tumor cells overexpressing the GHRH receptors (p-GHRH-R). These antagonists also inhibit GH secretion [70]. There is evidence that GHRH antagonists are well tolerated in humans; however, more phase I–III clinical trials are necessary to probe the efficiency of these antagonists [71]. GHRH antagonists inhibit cancers that depend on IGF-1 as a growth factor [72–74]. GHRH antagonists can also inhibit various autocrine factors such as GHRH, GH, or VEGF by binding to the tumoral GHRH receptors, resulting in a tumor growth suppression [75,76]. In addition, GHRH antagonists could provoke tumor cell death by active cell pathways producing apoptosis [77,78].

The presence of the GHRH-R variant SV1 differs from the pGHRH by a short segment of the extracellular ligand-binding domain of the receptor protein in normal tissue and in various neoplastic tumors, lymphomas, small-cell lung carcinomas, pancreatic cancer, glioblastomas, and prostate cancer [79–81]. In several experimentally formed tumors, GHRH antagonist inhibits the growth and metastasis of cells expressing these receptor types. This inhibition occurs by binding to the full length of the GHRH-R or SV1 [79,80,82]. Kovácks et al., 2010 observed a strong GH release inhibition by the JV-1-63, reducing tumor growth (46%) of DBTRG-05 glioblastomas. Their experiments were conducted on nude mice. JV-1-63 antagonists caused an upregulation of mRNA expression of pGHRHR and downregulation of SV1 expression in vitro [82].

The use of aromatase and GHRH inhibitors could have a clinical use in patients with GBM once adequate phase II or III clinical trials are made.

Author details

Judith Marcela Dueñas-Jiménez[1*], Irene Aguilar-García[1], María de la Luz Galván-Ramírez[1], Sergio Horacio Dueñas-Jiménez[1], Jorge David Rivas-Carrillo[1], Anne Santerre[2] and Erika Priscilla Domínguez-Rangel[1]

*Address all correspondence to: judithmarceladuenas@gmail.com

1 University Center for Health Sciences, University of Guadalajara, Guadalajara, Jalisco, México

2 University Center for Biological and Agricultural Sciences, University of Guadalajara, Guadalajara, Jalisco, México

References

[1] Hou LC, Veeravagu A, Hsu AR. Tse VC recurrent glioblastoma multiforme: a review of natural history and management options. Neurosurg Focus 2006; 20(4):E5.

[2] Rosen ST. Cancer Treatment and Research, vol. 163. Duarte, CA, 2015; pp. 1–14. DOI: 10.1007/978-3-319-12048-5

[3] Dolececk TA, Propp J, Stroup N, Kruch C. CBTRUS statistical report: primary brain and central nervous system tumors diagnosed in the United States in 2005–2009. Neuro Oncol 2009; 15(Suppl 5): 1–49. DOI: 10.1093/neuonc/nos218

[4] Wen P, Kesari S. Malignant gliomas in adults. N Engl J Med 2008; 359: 492–507. DOI: 10.1056/NEJMra0708126

[5] Chakrabarti I, Cockburn M, Cozen W, Wang Y-P, Preston-Martin S. A. population-based description of glioblastoma multiforme in Los Angeles County, 1974–1999. Cancer 2008; 104(12): 2798–2806. DOI: 10.1002/cncr.21539

[6] Verhaak RG, Hoadley KA, Purdom E, Wang V, Qi Y, Wilkerson MD, et al. Integrated genomic analysis identifies clinically relevant subtypes of glioblastoma characterized by abnormalities in PDGFRA, IDH1, EGFR, and NF1. Cancer Cell 2010; 17(1): 98–110. DOI: 10.1016/j.ccr.2009.12.020

[7] Dunn G, Rinne M, Wykosky J, Genovese G, Quayle S, Dunn I, et al. Emerging insights into the molecular and cellular basis of glioblastoma. Genes Dev 2012; 26(8): 756–784. DOI: 10.1101/gad.187922.112

[8] Noushmehr H, Weisenberger DJ, Diefes K, Phillips HS, Pujara K, Berman BP, et al. Identification of a CpG island methylator phenotype that defines a distinct subgroup of glioma. Cancer Cell 2010; 17(5): 510–522. DOI: 10.1016/j.ccr.2010.03.017

[9] Brennan CW, Verhaak RGW, McKenna A, Campos B, Noushmehr H, Salama SR, et al. The somatic genomic landscape of glioblastoma. Cell 2013; 155(2): 462–477. DOI: 10.1016/j.cell.2013.09.034.

[10] Huang PH, Mukasa A, Bonavia R, Flynn RA, Brewer ZE, Cavenee WK, Furnari FB, White FM. Quantitative analysis of EGFRvIII cellular signalling networks reveals a combinatorial therapeutic strategy for glioblastoma. Proc Natl Acad Sci U S A 2007; 104: 12867–12872. DOI: 10.1073/pnas.0705158104

[11] Khasraw M, Lassman AB Advances in the treatment of malignant gliomas. Curr Oncol Rep 2010; 12(1): 26–33. DOI: 10.1007/s11912-009-0077-4.

[12] Ohgaki H, Kleihues P. Genetic pathways to primary and secondary glioblastoma. Am J Pathol 2007; 170(5): 1145–1453. DOI: 10.2353/ajpath.2007.070011

[13] Zawlik I, Kita D, Vaccaella S, Mittelbronn M, Franceschi S, Ohgaki H. Common polymorphisms in the MDM and TP53 genes and the relationship outcomes in glioblastomas. Brain Pathol 2009; 19(2): 188–194. DOI: 10.1111/j.1750-3639.2008.00170.x.

[14] Nagajaran R, Costello J. Molecular epigenetics and genetics in neuro–oncology. Neurotherapeutics 200; 6(3): 436–446. DOI: 10.1016/j.nurt.2009.04.002.

[15] Fukushima T, Favereaux A, Huang H, Shimizu T, Yonekawa Y, Nakazato Y, Ohagki H. Genetic alterations in primary glioblastomas in Japan. J Neuropathol Exp Neurol 2006; 65(1):12–18. DOI: http://dx.doi.org/10.1097/01.jnen.0000196132.66464.96

[16] Temel JS, Greer JA, Muzikansky A et al. Early palliative care for patients with metastatic non-small-cell lung cancer. N Engl J Med 2010; 363(8):733–742. DOI: 10.1056/NEJMoa1000678.

[17] Rajaraman P, Melin BS, Wang Z, McKean–Cowdin R, Michaud DS, Wang SS, et al. Genome – wide association study of glioma and meta – analysis. Hum Genet 2010; 131(12): 1877–1888. DOI: 10.1007/s00439-012-1212-0

[18] Walsh KM, Anderson E, Hansen HM, Decker PA, Kosel ML, Kollmeyer T, et al. Analysis of 60 reported glioma risk SNPs replicates published GWAS findings but fails to replicate associations from published candidate–gene studies. Genet Epidemiol 2013; 37(2): 222–228. DOI: 10.1002/gepi.21707

[19] Sanson M, Hosking FJ, Shete S, Zelenika D, Dobbins SE, Ma Y et al. Chromosome 7p11.2 (EGFR) variation influences glioma risk. Hum Mol Genet 2011; 20(14): 2897–2904. DOI: 10.1093/hmg/ddr192

[20] Jenkins RB, Wresnch MR, Johnson D, Fridley BL, Decker PA, Xiao Y, et al. Cancer genetics. Cancer Genet 2011; 204(1): 13–18. DOI: 10.1016/j.cancergencyto.2010.10.002

[21] Enciso–Mora V; Hosking FJ, Di Stefano AL, Zelenika D, Shete S, Broderick P, et al. Low penetrance susceptibility to glioma is caused by the variant rs 783782222. Br J Cancer 2013; 108(10): 2178–2185. DOI: 10.1038/bjc.2013.155

[22] Stacey SN, Sulem P, Jonasdottir A, Masson G, Gudmunson J, Gudbartsson DF et al. A germiline in the TP53 polyadenylation signal confers susceptibility. Nat Genet 2011; 43(11): 1098–1103. DOI: 10.1038/ng.926.

[23] Egan KM, Nabors LB, Olson JJ, Monteiro AN, Browning JE, Madden MH, et al. Rre TP53 genetic variant associated with glioma risk and outcome. J Med Genet 2012; 49(7): 420–421. DOI: 10.1136/jmedgenet-2012-100941

[24] Shete S, Hosking FJ, Robertson LB, Sanson M, Malmer B, et al. Genome - wide association study indentifies five susceptibility loci for glioma. Nat Genet 2009; 41(8): 899–904. DOI: 10.1038/ng.407

[25] Wrensch M, Kenkins RB, Chang JS, Yeh RF, Xiao Y, Decker PA, et al. Variants in the CDKN2B and RTEL1 regions are associated with high grade glioma susceptibility. Nat Genet 2009; 41(8): 905–908. DOI: 10.1038/ng.408.

[26] Dueñas JM, Candanedo A, Santerre A, Orozco S, Sandoval H, Feria R, et al. Aromatase and estrogen receptor alpha mRNA expression as prognostic biomarkers in patients with astrocytomas. J Neurooncol 2014; 119(2): 275–284. DOI: 10.1007/s11060-014-1509-z.

[27] Batistatou A, Kyzas PA, Goussia A, Arkoumani E, Voulgaris S, Polyzoidis K, et al. Estrogen receptor beta (ER – β), protein expression correlates with BAG – 1, and prognosis in brain glial tumors. J Neurooncol 2006; 77(1): 17–23. DOI: 10.1007/s11060-005-9005-0

[28] Batistaou A, Stefanou D, Goussia A, Arkoumani E, Papavassiliou AG, Agnatis N. Estrogen receptor beta (ERβ) is expressed in brain astrocytic tumors and declines with

differentiation of the neoplasm. J Cancer Res Clin Oncol 2004; 130(7): 405–410. DOI: 10.1007/s00432-004-0548-9

[29] Sareddy GR, Nair BC, Gonugunta VK, Zhang QG, Brener A, Brann DW, et al. Therapeutic Significance of estrogen receptor β agonists in gliomas. Mol Cancer Ther 2012; 11(5): 1174–1182. DOI: 10.1158/1535-7163.MCT-11-0960

[30] Oñate SA, Tsai SY, Tsai MJ, O'Malley BW. Sequence and characterization of a coactivator for the steroid hormone receptor superfamily. Science 1995; 270(5240): 1354–1357. DOI: 10.1126/science.270.5240.1354

[31] Anzick SL, Kononen J, Walker RL, Azorsa DO, Tanner MM, Guan XY, et al. ALB1, a steroid receptor coactivator amplified in breast and ovarian cancer. Science. 1997; 277(5328): 965–968. DOI: 10.1126/science.277.5328.965

[32] Tetel MJ, Auger AP, Charlier TD. Who´s in charge? Nuclear receptor coactivator and corepressor function in brain and behavior. Front Neuroendocrinol 2009; 30(3): 328–342. DOI: 10.1016/j.yfrne.2009.04.008

[33] Molenda-Figueira HA, Murphy SD, Shea K, SIegal NK, Zhao Y, Chadwick JG. Steroid receptor coactivator – 1 from brain physically interacts differentially with steroid receptor subtypes. Endocrinology 2008; 149(10): 5272–5279. DOI: 10.1210/en.2008-0048

[34] Vienonen A, Miettinen S, Mannien T, Altuci L, Willhelm E, Ylikomi T. Regulation of nuclear receptor and cofactor expression in breast cancer cell lines. Eur J Endocrinol 2003; 148(4): 469–479. DOI: 10.1530/eje.0.1480469

[35] Weldon CB, Elliott S, Zhu Y, Clayton JL, Curiel TJ, Jaffe BM, Burow ME. Regulation of estrogen-mediated cell survival and proliferation by p160 coactivators. Surgery 2004;136(2): 346–354. DOI: 10.1016/j.surg.2004.05.010

[36] Apostolakis ED, Ramamurphy M, Zhou D, Oñate S, O´Malley BW. Acute disruption of select steroid receptor coactivators prevents reproductive behavior in rats and unmasks genetic adaptation in knockout mice. Mol Endocrinol 2002; 16(7): 1511–1523. DOI: 10.1210/mend.16.7.0877

[37] Nishihara E, Yoshida H, Chan C-S, Liao L, Davis RL, O'Malley BW, et al. SRC–1 null mice exhibit moderate motor dysfunction and delayed development of cerebellar Purkinje cells. J Neurosci 2003; 23(1): 213–222.

[38] Tognoni CM, Chadwick JG, Ackeifi CA, Tetel MJ. Nuclear receptor coactivators are coexpressed with steroid receptors and regulated by estradiol in mouse brain. Neuroendocrinology. 2011; 94: 49–57. DOI: 10.1159/000323780

[39] Lonard DM, Lanz RB, O´Malley BW. Nuclear receptor coregulators and human disease. Endocr Rev. 2007; 28(5): 575–587. DOI: 10.1210/er.2007-0012

[40] Sakaguchi H, Fujimoto J, Sun W-S, Tamaya T. Clinical implications of steroid receptor coactivator (SRC – 3) in uterine endometrial cancers. J Steroid Biochem Mol Biol 2007; 104(3–5): 237–240. DOI: 10.1016/j.jsbmb.2007.03.007

[41] Sakakura C, Hagiwara A, Yasuoka R, Fujita Y, Nakanishi M, Masuda K, et al. Amplification and over expression of the AIB1 nuclear receptor coactivator gene in primary gastric cancers. Int J Cancer 2000; 89(3): 217–223. DOI: 10.1002/1097-0215(20000520)89:3<2

[42] Hernández O, Rodríguez M, González A, Camacho I. Progesterone and estradiol effects on SRC–1 and SRC–3 expression in human astrocitoma cell lines. Endocrine 2010; 37(1): 194–200. DOI: 10.1007/s12020-009-9288-6

[43] González A, Hansberg V, Hernández O, González T, Henderson J, Lemus D, et al. Estradiol increases cell growth in human astrocitoma cell lines through ERα activation and its interaction with SCR–1, SCR–3, coactivators. Biochim Biophys Acta. 2002; 1823(2): 379–386. DOI: 10.1016/j.bbamcr.2011.11.004

[44] Giangrande P, McDonnel DP. The A and B isoforms of the human progesterone receptor: two functionally different transcription factors encoded by a single gene. Recent Prog Horm Res 1999; 54: 291–313.

[45] Tora L, Gronemeyer H, Turcotte B, Gaub MP, Chambon P. The N-terminal region of the chicken progesterone receptor specifies target gene activation. Nature 1988; 333(6169): 185–188. DOI: 10.1038/333185a0

[46] Vegeto E, Shahbaz MM, Wen DX, Goldman ME, O´Malley BW, McDonnell DP. Human Progesterone receptor A for is a cell – and promoter – specific repressor of human progesterone receptor B function. Mol Endocinol 2013; 7(10): 1244–1255. DOI: org/10.1210/mend.7.10.8264658#sthash.FjZjmlYb.dpuf

[47] Khalid H, Shibata S, Kishikawa M, Yasunaga A, Iseki M, Hiura T. Inmunohistochemical analysis of progesterone receptor and Ki – 67 labelling index in astrocytic tumors. Cancer. 1997; 80(11): 2133–2140. DOI: 10.1002/(SICI)1097-0142(19971201)80:11<2133::AID-CNCR13>3.

[48] Atif F, Patel N, Yosuf S, Stein D. The synergistic effect of combination progesterone and temozolamide on human glioblastoma cells. Plos One 2015; 10(6): e0131441. DOI: 10.1371/journal.pone.0131441

[49] Yong GC, Kim HK, Kap Lee H, Chan Lee K. Expression of androgen receptors in astrocytoma. J Korean Med Sci 1996; 11(6): 517–521. DOI: 10.3346/jkms.1996.11.6.517

[50] Yu X, Jiang Y, Wei W, Cong P, et al. Androgen receptor signalling regulates growth of glioblastoma multiforme in men. Tumor Biol 2015; 36(2): 967–972. DOI: 10.1007/s13277-014-2709-z

[51] Miller W, Larionov A. Aromatase 2004, Edinburgh, UK, 6–8 September 2004. Breast Cancer Res 2004; 7: E2. DOI: 10.1186/bcr964

[52] Simpson E, Clyne C, Rubin G, Boon W, Robertson K, Britt K, et al. Aromatase—a brief overview. Annu Rev Physiol 2002; 64: 93–127. DOI: 10.1146/annurev.physiol.64.081601.142703

[53] Kleihues P, Luois D, Scheithauer B, Rorke L, Reifenberger G, Burger P, et al. The WHO classification of tumors of the nervous system. J Neuropathol Exp Neurol. 2002; 61(3): 215–225. DOI: org/10.1093/jnen/61.3.215

[54] Stupp R, Weber D. The role of radio and chemotherapy in glioblastoma. Onkologie. 2005; 28(6–7): 315–317. DOI: 10.1159/000085575

[55] Gilbert M, Dignam J, Armstrong T, Wefel J, Blumenthal D, Vogelbaum M, et al. A randomized trial of bevacizumab for newly diagnosed glioblastoma. N Engl Med. 2014; 370(8): 699–708. DOI: 10.1056/NEJMoa1308573

[56] Chinot O, Reardon D. The future of antiangiogenic treatment in glioblastoma. Curr Opin Neurol 2014; 26(6): 675–682. DOI: 10.1097/WCO.0000000000000142.

[57] Stupp R, Picard M, Weller M. Does cilentigide deserve another chance? – Authors reply. Lancel Oncol 2014; 15(13): 585–586. DOI: 10.1016/S1470-2045(14)71121-0

[58] Westphal M, Heese O, Steinbach J, Schnell O, Schackert G, Mehdorn M, et al. A randomised, open label phase III trial with nimotuzumab, an anti epidermal growth factor receptor monoclonal antibody in the treatment of newly diagnosed adult glioblastoma. Eur J Cancer 2015; 51(4): 522–532. DOI: 10.1016/j.ejca.2014.12.019.

[59] Kim I, Park C, Heo D, Kim C, Rhee C, Nam D, et al. Radiotherapy followed by adjuvant temozolomide with or without neoadjuvant ACNU—CDDP chemotherapy in newly diagnosed glioblastomas: a prospective randomized controlled multicenter phase III trial. J Neurooncol 2011; 103(3): 595–602. DOI: 10.1007/s11060-010-0427

[60] Wick W, Steinbach J, Platten M, Hartmann C, Wenz F, von Deimiling, et al. Enzastaurin before and concomitant with radiation therapy, followed by enzastaurin maintenance therapy, in patients with newly diagnosed glioblastoma without MGMT promoter hypermethylation. Neuro Oncol 2013; 15(10): 1405–1412. DOI: 10.1093/neuonc/not100.

[61] Ducassou A, Uro-Coste E, Verelle P, Filleron T, Benouaich A, Lubrano V, et al. $\alpha v\beta 3$ integrin and Fibroblast growth factor receptor (FGFR1): pronostic factors in a phase I-II clinical trial associating continuous administration of tipifarnib with radiotherapy for patients with newly diagnosed glioblastoma. Eur J Cancer 2013; 49(9): 2161–2169. DOI: 10.1016/j.ejca.2013.02.033

[62] Hainswoth J, Shih K, Shepard G, Tillinghast G, Brinker B, Spigel D. Phase II study of concurrent radiation therapy, temozolamide, and bevacizumab followed by bevacizumab /everolimus as first line treatment for patients with glioblastoma. Cin Adv Hematol Oncol. 2012; 10(4): 240–246.

[63] Burtsein H, Prestud A, Seidenfeld J, Anderson H, Bucholz T, Davidson N, et al. American Society of Clinical Oncology Clinical Practice guideline: update on adjuvant

endocrine therapy for women with hormone receptor –positive breast cancer. J Clin Oncol. 2010; 34(7): 3784–3796.

[64] Geisler J, Haynes B, Anker G, Dowselt M, Lonning E. Influence of letrozole and anastrozole estrogen levels in postmenopausal breast cancer patients evaluated in a randomized, cross – over Study. J Clin Oncol. 2002; 3: 751–757.DOI:10.1038/bjc.2011.58

[65] Amaral C, Varela C, Borges M, Tavares da Silva E, Roleira F, Correia da Silva G, et al. Steroidal aromatase inhibitors inhibit growth of hormone–dependent breast cancer cells by inducing cell cycle arrest and apoptosis. Apoptosis 2013; 18(11): 1426–1436. DOI: 10.1007/s10495-013-0879-6

[66] Kovacs M, Kineman R, Schally A, Zarandi M, Groot K, Frohman L. Effects of antagonist of growth hormone—releasing hormone (GHRH) on GH and insulin—like growth factor 1 levels in transgenic mice overexpression the human GHRH, an animal model of acromegaly. Endocrinology 1997; 138(11): 4536–4542. DOI: org/10.1210/endo. 138.11.5498

[67] Kovacs M, Schally A, Lee E, Busto R, Armatis P, Groot K, Varga J. Inhibitory effects of antagonistic analogues of GHRH on GH3 pituitary cells overexpressing the human GHRH receptor. J Endocrinol. 2002; 175(2): 425–434. DOI: 10.1677/joe.0.1750425

[68] Jenkins PJ, Bustin SA Evidence for a link between IGF-I and cancer. Eur J Endocrinol. 2004; 151:S17–S22. DOI: 10.1530/eje.0.151S017

[69] Kahan Z, Gardi J, Nyari T, Foldesi I, Ormandi K, Lazar G, et al. Elevated levels of circulating insulin-like growth factor-I, IGF-binding globulin-3 and testosterone predict hormone-dependent breast cancer in postmenopausal women a case–control study. Int J Oncol 2006; 29(1):193–200. DOI: 10.3892/ijo.29.1.193

[70] Le Roith D. The insulin - like growth factor system. Experimental Diab Res. 2003; 4(4): 205–212. DOI: 10.1155/EDR.2003.205

[71] Kovacs M, Schally A, Varga J, Zaradi M. Endocrine and antineoplasic actions of growth actions of hormone – releasing hormone antagonists. Curr Med Chem 2008; 15(4): 314–321. DOI: 10.2174/092986708783497355

[72] Schally A, Varga J, Engel J. Antagonists of growth – hormone – releasing hormone: an emerging new therapy for cancer. Nat Clin Pract Endocrinol Metab. 2008; 4(1): 33–43. DOI:10.1038/ncpendmet0677

[73] Hohla F, Buchholz S, Schally A, Rick F, Szalontay L, Varga J, et al. GHRH antagonist causes DNA damage leading to pcell c21 mediated cell cycle arrest and apoptosis in human colon cancer cells. Cell Cycle 2009; 8(19): 3149–3156.

[74] Kanashiro C, Schally A, Zaradi M, Hammann B, Varga J. Alterations of EGFR/HER, angiogenesis and apoptosis pathways after therapy with antagonists of growth hormone releasing and bombesin in non – small cell lung cancer. Int J Oncol 2007; 30(4): 1019–1028. DOI: 10.3892/ijo.30.4.1019

[75] Havt A, Schally A, Halmos G, Varga J, Toller G, Hovarh J, et al. The expression of the pituitary growth hormone – releasing hormone receptor and its splice variants in normal and neoplastic human tissues. PNAS 2005; 102(48): 17424–17429. 18. DOI: 10.1073/pnas.

[76] Heinrih E, Schally A, Bulchholz S, Rock F, Halmos G, Mile M, et al. Dose dependent growth inhibition in vivo of PC – 3 prostate cancer with a reduction in tumoral growth factors after therapy with GHRH antagonist MZ – J – 7 – 138. Prostate 2008; 68(16): 1763–1772.

[77] Resaki Z, Czompoly T, Shally A, Halmos G. Isolation and sequencing of CDNA for splice variants of growth hormone—releasing hormone receptors from human cancers. PNAS 2000; 97(19): 10561–10566. DOI: 10.1073/pnas.

[78] Kovacs M, Schally A, Hohla F, Rick F, Pozsagai E, Szalontay L. A correlation of endocrine and anticancer effects of some antagonists of GHRH. Peptides 2010; 31(10): 1839–1846. DOI: 10.1016/j.peptides.2010.07.006

[79] Chiot O, Reardon D. The future of antiangiogenic treatment in glioblastoma. Curr Opin Neurol. 2014; 27(6): 675–682. DOI: 10.1097/WCO.

[80] Kim I, Park C, Heo D, Kim C, Rhee C, Nam D, et al. Radiotherapy followed by adjuvant temozolomide with or without neoadjuvant ACNU—CDDP chemotherapy in newly diagnosed glioblastomas: a prospective randomized controlled multicenter phase III trial. J Neurooncol 2011; 103(3): 595–602. DOI: 10.1007/s11060-010-0427.

2

Critical Molecular and Genetic Markers in Primary Brain Tumors with Their Clinical Importance

Ilhan Yaylim, Sumeyya Azam,
Ammad Ahmad Farooqi, Özlem Küçükhüseyin,
Muhammad Ismail and Ali Metin Kafadar

Abstract

Classification of primary brain tumors is based mainly on histopathological characteristics. Due to the peculiarity of the central nervous system (CNS), the location of the tumor is also used in the naming of the CNS tumors. These features, histopathology, and location determine the main prognostic factors in these tumors. Updated molecular and genetic findings in the last two decades accumulated vast amount of knowledge about the biological behavior, response to the treatment, and consequently the prognosis of CNS tumors. After the clinical use of these data, a recent classification is proposed by the International Society of Neuropathology named as "integrated diagnosis."

This classification considers the histopathological classification, World Health Organization (WHO) grade along with the molecular information. The emerging molecular-genetic data about the CNS tumors will allow the translational researchers to deliberately understand the oncogenic mechanisms involved in the evolution of these tumors and judge the optional treatment strategies.

Evaluating the check points of cell cycle and apoptosis provides valuable information about the tumor biology (tumorigenesis). These mechanisms (pathways) also play an exclusive role in CNS tumors. Knowledge concerning the gene repressors and gene activators or some epigenetic changes in proliferative and antiproliferative pathways that regarded gliomas may yield new individualized treatment options.

In this chapter, we will review the basic and translational research molecular-genetic data of gliomas with special interest on proliferative and antiproliferative pathways. Further emerging treatment options and treatment responses in gliomas will be critically evaluated with regard to their histopathology, anatomical location, and molecular-genetic fingerprints.

Keywords: gliomas, proliferation, apoptosis, cell cycle, gene

---

1. Introduction

Primary brain tumors are a distinct group of pathologies due to their location, low incidence compared to other human tumors, histopathologic diversities, and unexpected response to treatment methods mainly caused by their peculiar genetic and molecular characteristics. Evaluating new important biomarkers which affect the etiopathogenesis of brain tumors may also help clinicians in consulting patients about prognosis, potential clinical studies, and following response to the treatment strategies [1]. Nowadays, the value of early detection of various types of cancer before metastasis has become a very significant issue. This approach may increase life expectancy and the quality of life in these patients [2]. It is known that one of the best management strategies of cancer is to predict its prognosis and response to the updated therapeutic procedures. In order to achieve this, it is significant to consider the blood, serum, plasma, or tissue biomarkers. Although the value of liquid biopsy in different human tumors is established, there is a lack of data regarding primary brain tumors [3]. Confluence of information suggested that genetic, epigenetic, functional or compositional heterogeneity of diseased and healthy tissues presented a major challenge to strategies to improve clinical outcome. [4]. Many molecules found in various fluids, tissues, and cell lines are produced either by the tumor itself, other tissues, or tumor microenvironment, in response to the presence of cancer or other associated conditions including inflammation. The scientists study on cancer search for proper candidate tumor markers and for identifying patients who face different diagnosis or clinical stages of cancer. This type of biomarkers must have some characteristics which can be used to estimate tumor volume, determine response to treatment, and assess disease recurrence through monitoring. Recent advancements have shown that amplifications/translocations, genetic mutations and changes in microarray-generated profiles (genetic signatures) are contributory in cancer development, metastasis and development of resistance against different therapeutics. These genetic signatures are referred according to the type of tumor marker or profile and may be associated with clinical outcomes or good prognosis or enhanced quality of life [3,4]. An ideal tumor marker is described as easily measurable, reliable, and cost-effective by use of an assay with high analytical sensitivity and specificity. Although we have developed a deeper understanding of the underlying mechanisms, there are only a few markers which have been used in routine applications and only a limited number of them can be used to identify patients or monitor progression of cancer types and clinical staging.

Gene overexpression is described as increase in copy number of genes or chromosomes (i.e., gene amplification) through increased transcriptional activity. It is known that imbalance between the gene repressors and gene activators or some epigenetic changes as DNA methylation or chromosomal translocations can alter transcriptional activity of the gene [3,4].

2. Defined molecular markers which changed our clinical attitude

The use of biomarkers in glioblastoma (GBM) has been evaluated in a recent survey by neuro-oncologists [5]. Current evidences indicate that MGMT, EGFR, 1p/19q, EGFR, p53, phosphatase and tensin homolog (PTEN) mutation or deletion, EGFRvIII, IDH1/2, PDGFR, and PIK3CA are the most commonly used markers. But, use of these biomarkers claimed to be prognostic in GBM cases is still debated. There exist significantly varying clinical representations and cases of GBM, and the structure of the signaling molecules is highly complex, and therefore, use of these markers is not very common as of now. In addition, glioblastoma, still a heterogeneous disease, also possesses additional difficulties such as having limited biomarkers to diagnosis and monitoring and therapeutic options, having poorly understood pathogenesis, and requiring individualized treatments. On the other hand, the discovery of new biomarkers together with currently used markers can enable us to better stratify patients regarding treatment paradigms and clinical trials (**Figure 1**) [6,7].

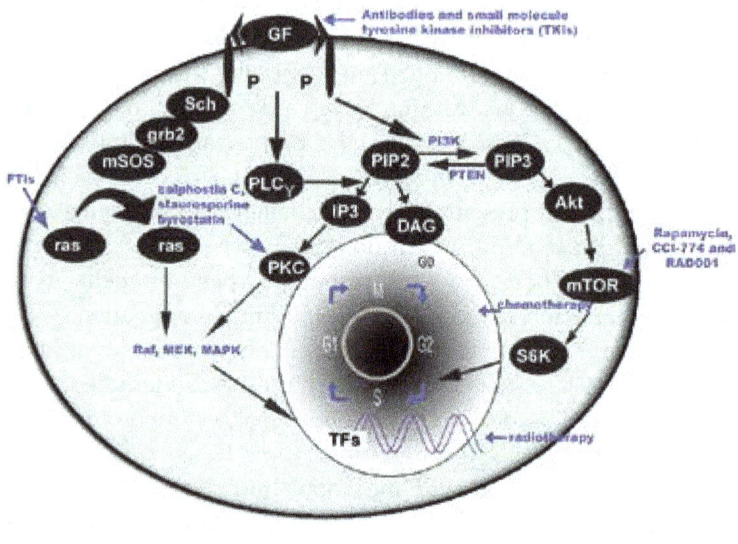

Figure 1. Some signaling pathways with therapeutic implications in gliomas [7]. Some abbreviations are shown below. EGF: epidermal growth factor; PIP2, phosphatidylinositol phosphate-2; PIP3, phosphatidylinositol phosphate-2; PKC, protein kinase C; Grb2, growth factor receptor-bound protein-2; VEGF, vascular endothelial growth factor; S6K, p70 S6 kinase; mTOR, mammalian target of rapamycin; TF, transcription factors; SOS, son of sevenless molecule.

3. Proliferative and antiproliferative pathways and their roles in gliomas

As more and more detailed studies into intracellular signaling cascades and modulators that regulate these pathways are published, intricacy of the fine-balance between celluar survival and death is revealed. A revolution in the signaling cascades has provided near complete resolution of how physiologically important signaling proteins interact with extracellular cues to trigger proliferation. More detailed understanding of the regulatory and activation processes of uncontrolled cellular proliferation is proving to be a key in identification of newer approaches to improve the efficacy of existing therapeutics. The homeostasis of mitogenic signaling is tactfully controlled by multiple mechanisms. The past several years have seen a dramatic leap in our understanding of how Receptor tyrosine kinase (RTK) mediated signaling is rewired during tumorigenesis to support the transformed phenotype. Activation of RTK results in receptor dimerization and autophosphorylation. More importantly, docking sites are created for different adaptor protein complexes such as Grb2/SOS. Mutant Ras is reportedly involved in 50% of all human tumors. There are direct pieces of evidence emphasizing on role of mutant Ras in gliomas. High Ras-GTP levels in advanced astrocytomas have been reported [8, 9].

Epidermal growth factor receptor (EGFR), coded as a cell-surface-bound receptor, is another important molecule involved in cell proliferation with potential effects on clinical prognosis of GBM. It is known that approximately <10% of secondary GBMs and 50% of primary GBMs have EGFR mutations [10]. The presence of EGFR variant III mutation (EGFRvIII) is known to upregulate mitogenic signaling pathways. There is a deletion of the regulator N-terminal domain (▪ 6–273) of EGFR in this pattern of EGFR. About 10–60% of the patients with GBM have EGFRvIII which can be detected in the peripheral blood of brain tumors. The detection of this mutation in brain cancer patients has great importance for anti-EGFRvIII therapies and patients can be monitored to track their response to these therapies [11,12]. Better and deeper knowledge of mechanistic insights that cause EGFR heterogeneity in GBM will prove to be helpful in identification of drugs with maximum efficacy. *EGFRvIII* mutation to identify patients for treatments such as erlotinib therapy for non-small cell lung cancer or RNA-directed treatments and vaccine therapies [13]. As of now, we still have a limited knowledge about downstream signaling pathways for EGFR and whether *EGFR* mutations affect these downstream signaling pathways, such as AKT, MAPK, and STAT3. On the other hand, it has been suggested that the clinical utility of this biomarker and its use for targeted treatment are complicated [1].

Platelet-derived growth factor receptor (PDGFR), a cell-surface tyrosine kinase, plays role in GBM proliferation and stem cell renewal. There are multiple isoforms of PDGFR, mutated in up to 30% of GBMs. One of them, the most significant one regarding GBM, is PDGFRA. The other isoform is also PDGFRAD (with a deletion of exons 8 and 9), seen in 40% of GBMs, and leads to constitutive activation [14,15]. According to the Cancer Genome Atlas, PDGFRA has a crucial role in the proneural subtype of GBM; however, no changes were observed in prognosis of the evaluated patients [16].

The phosphatidylinositol 3-kinase (PI3K)/AKT (PI3K/AKT) pathway is known as a crucial intracellular signaling pathway, taking role in regulating cell proliferation, migration, quiescence, proliferation, cancer, and longevity [17]. PI3K is an enzyme which phosphorylates phosphatidylinositol-4,5-bisphosphate (PIP2) to phosphatidylinositol-3,4,5-trisphosphate (PIP3) at the cell inner membrane. This activation process leads to recruit and upregulate various downstream pathways including AKT, a molecule localized in the plasma membrane [18].

Phosphatase and tensin homolog (PTEN) is known as a natural inhibitor of PI3K/AKT pathway. It has been shown to inhibit transduction of signals to downstream effectors via dephosphorylation of PIP_3 to PIP_2 [19]. It has been reported that an increased PI3K/Akt/mTOR signaling is seen in ~88% of all glioblastomas [20,21]. All of these biological pathways has been related to genetic alterations of key regulatory molecules involved in mitogenic signaling in RTKs and also in the PI3K-PTEN-Akt signaling axis.

Some regulatory and effector molecules play important role in classical cell death networks of both extrinsic (death receptor-mediated) and intrinsic (mitochondria-dependent) apoptosis signaling pathways [22]. Since the discovery of TNF (Tumor Necrosis Factor) family members, a new milestone in apoptosis-inducing cancer therapies has emerged. TRAIL (tumor necrosis factor-related apoptosis-inducing ligand) is a protein reportedly involved in selective killing of cancer cells while leaving normal cells intact. The major biological role of this 281-amino acid-type II transmembrane protein is apoptosis induction after interacting with its receptors to trigger extrinsically and intrinsically controlled pathways. Four different homologous human TRAIL receptors have been categorized into TRAIL-R1/DR4, TRAIL-R2/DR5 also known as Killer, TRAIL-R3 or DcR1, and TRAIL-R4 or DcR2. Substantial fraction of information has been added into the existing pool of knowledge related to TRAIL biology and known that different cancers are resistant to TRAIL-based therapeutics. Mechanistically it has been shown that downregulation of death receptors considerably impaired TRAIL-induced apoptosis in cancer cells. In the upcoming section, we briefly summarize advancements in our understanding related to the underlying mechanisms of resistance against TRAIL-induced apoptosis. We also discuss how TRAIL has shown as a potent anticancer agent in xenografted mice. Natural products have also added more options in the armory against brain tumor. Detailed mechanistic insights have provided a near complete resolution of protein network TRAIL-resistant glioblastoma and increasingly it is being realized that imbalance of stoichiometric ratios of proapoptotic and antiapoptotic proteins modulates response of cancer cells to TRAIL. Previously, it has been convincingly revealed that Znf domain of A20 E3 ligase ubiquitinated RIP1 through a K63-linked polyUB chain that structurally interacted with p18 domain of caspase-8 and blocked its dimerization and cleavage. Functionally inactive caspase-8 was unable to proteolytically process downstream effectors that resulted in impairment of TRAIL-induced apoptosis in glioblastoma [23]. Adeno-associated virus (AAV) vectors are being used to efficiently deliver secreted, soluble TRAIL in different preclinical studies. Additionally, these are also used in combination with TRAIL-sensitizing cardiac glycoside, lanatoside C (lan C). Tumor growth was considerably reduced in intracranial U87 tumor-bearing mice treated with AAV-sTRAIL and lanatoside C [24]. Mesenchymal stem cells (MSCs) have the ability to migrate toward intracranial glioma xenografts. Experimentally verified data indicated that MSCs expressing firefly luciferase (fluc) injected into the left hemisphere migrated rapidly toward right, tumor-bearing region of the brain. Results revealed that 11% of implanted MSCs were noted to be localized in right hemisphere within 2 hours after MSC inoculation. Coculture of GBM43 and U87 glioma cells with MSCs-TRAIL displayed notable rise in caspase-3 activity. Survival rate of tumor-bearing mice was enhanced intranasally delivered with MSCs-TRAIL [25]. Carbenoxolone (CBX), a derivative of 18-glycyrrhetinic acid, has been shown to effectively enhance killing activity of TRAIL-expressing MSCs. CBX considerably upregulated cell-surface expression of DR5 in CBX-treated ΔGli36 and U87MG cells. CBX also inhibited gap junction (GJ) communication via modulation of connexin (Cx43). CBX remarkably reduced expression levels of Cx43 in U87MG and ΔGli36 cells after 72 hours. Results revealed that TRAIL-induced apoptosis was markedly higher in cells transfected with Cx43-siRNA [26] .

Antibody-based anticancer therapies have attracted considerable attention and different structural variations are being tested for efficacies which involve smaller antibody fragments such as ScFvs, Fabs, and nanobodies. Single-chain Fv fragment (scFv) consists of a variable light-chain (VL) and variable heavy-chain (VH) domains, which contains whole antigen-binding site.

Multidrug resistance protein 3 (MRP3) is frequently overexpressed in glioblastoma multiforme cells. scFvM58-sTRAIL is an engineered protein formed by fusion of MRP3-specific scFv antibody M58 with N-terminus of soluble TRAIL. scFvM58-sTRAIL was effective against MRP3-positive GBM cells. Expectedly, scFvM58-sTRAIL did not show significant activity against MRP3-negative Jurkat cells. These results indicated that scFvM58-sTRAIL was effective against MRP3-positive cancer cells [27].

Various bivalent EGFR-targeting nanobodies (ENbs) have been designed and noted to be effective. Neural stem cells (NSC) are potent agents to deliver ENbs. Preclinical study revealed that tumor regression was significantly higher in xenografted mice treated with NSC-ENb2-TRAIL. Xenografted mice survived for 51 days upon treatment with control NSC-ENb2 and 80% of mice survived for 80 days after treatment with NSC-ENb2-TRAIL. These findings indicated that tumoritropic NSC-releasing ENb2 inhibited growth of glioblastoma and effectiveness of ENb2-based therapy was markedly improved by NSC-releasing ENb2-TRAIL [28].

Diethylamino-curcumin mimics with substituted triazolyl groups have previously been synthesized and reported to effectively sensitize resistant CRT-MG astroglioma cells to TRAIL [29].

Gingerol, a major bioactive component of ginger, has been shown to trigger expression of DR5 in a p53-dependent manner in U87 glioblastoma cells. Digitoxin (DT), a clinically approved cardiac glycoside, has been observed to overcome resistance against TRAIL in resistant U87MG glioblastoma cells. Digitoxin effectively enhanced DR5 expression on cell surface of resistant cancer cells [30].

4. Natural products mediated targeting of proliferative protein network in glioblastoma

Crude hydromethanolic extracts produced by maceration of *Spartium junceum* flowers and *Onopordum acanthium* leaves were tested for anticancer activity against glioblastoma U-373 cancer cells. *O. acanthium* was effective against glioblastoma cells and induced apoptosis [31] .

Aqueous extract of *Ruta graveolens* L. notably enhanced phosphorylated ERK1/2 and Akt levels in glioma cells. The results indicated that *Ruta graveolens* exerted inhibitory effects via activation of ERK1/2 and Akt-induced signaling pathways [32].

Triterpenoid saponins from *Albizia lebbeck* (L.) showed activity against TG1 and U-87 MG cancer cells with IC_{50} values of 2.10 and 2.24 μM for compound 2 and 3.46 and 1.36 μM for compound 1 [33].

Isocitrate Dehydrogenase 1 and 2 (IDH1/2) are two important enzymes involved in the Krebs cycle and oxidatively decarboxylate isocitrate to produce a-ketoglutarate and CO_2. IDH1 is a cytosolically located protein. IDH2 encodes a mitochondrial protein. Parsons et al. reported that IDH1/2 was mutated in approximately 60–80% of secondary gliomas and 5% of primary gliomas [34]. There are two common IDH mutation (IDH1R132H and IDH2172 mutations) types. It has been reported that these mutations are seen in GBM (>90% samples with IDH1/2 mutation). These mutations lead to increased production of the oncometabolite D-2-hydroxyglutarate. This metabolite has previously been noted to modify DNA methylation patterns in GBM and transcriptional activity of different target genes [35]. *IDH1* mutation may be correlated with several clinical factors such as younger patient age and frontal location. It has also been reported that additional survival benefit (median survival 9.75 years) was achieved from greater tumor resection (<5 cm^3 residual) in *IDH1* mutants, except for wild-type *IDH1*. It has also been suggested that the presence of *IDH1/2* mutation supports increased therapeutic efficacy with chemoradiotherapy and greater resection [1]. When IDH mutations occur, enzymatic activities of some important molecules can be altered. While alpha-ketoglutarate (α-KG) is decreased, produced 2-hydroxyglutarate (2-HG) can inhibit the activity of some enzymes. These enzymes play a significant role in regulating DNA and histone methylation (α-KG-dependent dioxygenase), including histone demethylases and the TET family of 5mC hydroxylases [36–38].

TET proteins are described as a new class of enzymes which can alter the methylation status of the DNA by converting 5-methylcytosine (5mC) to 5-hydroxymethylcytosine (5hmC). The biological function of 5hmC is not clear. It has been suggested that it is an intermediate in DNA demethylation process. 5hmC offers remarkable reduction in human gliomas as compared to normal brain. An inverse relationship has been reported between 5hmC levels and cell proliferation [39,40].

p53 is a very important protein involved in many physiological and pathological process in the regulation of cell viability in terms of cell cycle, apoptosis, cell differentiation, and other mechanisms of cell regulation during exposure to DNA-damaging agents (e.g., ultraviolet radiation, toxins, chemotherapeutic agents) [1]. It has been reported that P53 gene is mutated in 28% of primary GBMs [41]. There are three patterns regarding p53 dysfunction. One is called loss of function. This pattern may describe a lot of endogenous growth inhibitor effects of wild-type p53. The other is gain of function. This means that mutant p53 upregulates a distinct subset of genes from wild-type p53. The last one is dominant-negative effects of p53. It is associated with a tetramer pattern of mutant p53/wild-type p53 and leads to downregulate activity [42]. It is known that some other mechanisms of p53 inactivation include mutations of its modulators including MDM2 inhibitor or deletion of p14ARF [43,44]. Whether there is a correlation between p53 and GBM prognosis is still unclear due to the complexity of the p53 signaling pathway. P53 pathway includes many important regulators and the heterogeneity of p53 mutation types can also affect the p53 molecule. Because of those mentioned, therapies targeting P53 have been limited in this field [42].

The deletion of 1p and 19q, occurring early in tumorigenesis, is known as an important genetic signature. The deletion is seen in 50–70% of patients with low-grade oligodendrogliomas. This can be predictive for the tumor's chemosensitivity to some agents [46,47]. It has been reported that *P190RhoGAP,* localized on 19q13.3, can be one of the candidate genes as a tumor suppressor [48]. A large-scale genomic analysis by array CGH has reported two different patterns about 1p deletion for prognostic factors. One of them is the whole 1p (associated with the deletion of the whole 19q). This may be associated with a good prognosis for oligodendrogliomas. Another is 1p deletion (not associated with 19q loss). This deletion has a negative prognostic value and improves progression-free survival (PFS) and overall survival (OS). It is mostly associated with astrocytomas [49]. It is also related to the response to chemotherapy and radiation in oligodendroglioma. Data obtained from EORTC 26951 and RTOG 9402 trials showed an improvement in OS with the addition of radiation to procarbazine/lomustine/vincristine chemotherapy in anaplastic oligodendroglioma with 1p/19q mutation [50]. There are some studies correlated with these similar findings, In GBM, similar findings have been demonstrated in some studies [51,52], but not in others [53,54]. It has also been reported that codeletion of 1p and 19q is related with *IDH1* mutation and *MGMT* hypermethylation [47,55].

O-6-Methylguanine-DNA-methyltransferase (MGMT) is involved in removal of alkylation at the O6 position of guanine. Hypermethylation of *MGMT* transcriptionally down-regulated its expression. This situation results in impaired repair capability response to chemotherapeutic agents and radiation. Some clinical trials have confirmed the prognostic and predictive roles of *MGMTm* [56]. It has been suggested that patients with *MGMTm* are responsive to chemotherapy. However, *MGMT* status was not distinguished between patients with glioblastoma (GBM) and those with anaplastic astrocytoma (AA) and this restricts interpretation of the study. The European Organisation for Research and Treatment of Cancer (EORTC) 26981/22981 and National Cancer Institute of Canada (NCIC) trials also indicates increased responsiveness to temozolomide for patients with MGMTm [57]. It has been suggested that a standard marker both following prognosis and identifying patients for clinical trials, in which alkylation therapies and/or radiation therapy are applied, may be used for MGMTm [1].

5. Epigenetics in human gliomas with some details

Acetylation of lysine residues is a post-tranlational modification controlled by the opposing action of histone deacetylases (HDACs) and histone acetyl transferases (HATs) [58–60]. Histone methylation may generally occur on the side chains of lysines and arginines, which can alter the activity of effector proteins of the transcriptional machinery [58–60]. It has been reported that some mutations in some regulatory genes such as HDACs (HDAC2 and HDAC9), histone demethylases (JMJD1A and JMJD1B), and histone methyltransferases (SET7, SETD7, MLL, MLL3, and MLL4) have been detected to a large extent in genomic analysis of GBM samples [34]. However, it is still unclear whether histone modifications play significant roles in gliomas and their potential can serve as biomarkers and/or therapeutic targets. Noncoding RNAs are known to play an important role in the epigenetic regulation of gene expression [61,62].

One group of RNAs are described as microRNAs (miRNAs). miRNAs are important regulators for gene expression. miRNAs post-transcriptionally regulate expression of target genes. miRNAs are double-stranded RNA molecules of approximately 22 nucleotides (nt) in length. miRNA binds to specific recognition sequences within the 3′-untranslated region (3′-UTR) of target mRNAs [61–63]. miRNAs are characterized functionally into tumor suppressors and oncogenic miRNAs. Tumor suppressor miRNAs are frequently down-regulated in gliomas as compared to normal brain [64–67]. In contrast, some miRNAs are defined as oncogenes with enhanced expression in glioma such as miR-21, targeting regulators, miR-10b and miR-221, targeting cell cycle inhibitors, miR-30e, and targeting IjBa [68–71]. It has been suggested that there is a link between miRNAs and well-known stem cell-regulating proteins [72]. It has also been reported that miR-17-92 plays a critical role in regulation of glioma stem cell (GSC) differentiation, apoptosis, and proliferation [73]. miR-451 expression reduced notably in cancer cells kept in low glucose conditions. Results revealed that cancer cells kept in low glucose conditions had reduced cell proliferation but an enhanced rate of cell migration and survival in glioblastomas. Glucose sufficiency induced upregulation of miR-451 notably inhibited LKB1/AMPK pathway activation [74]. miR-128, downregulated in glioblastoma tissue, has a tumor-suppressive function. Both in vitro and in vivo, miR-128 expression significantly reduces glioma cell proliferation via downregulation of *Bmi-1 oncogene,* a component of the polycomb repressor complex (PRC). In addition, miR-128 inhibits GSC self-renewal [75]. The PRC has been shown to induce normal and cancer stem cell self-renewal and plays role in GSC regulation [76]. When miR-124 has overexpression, it can inhibit the CD133+ cell subpopulation of the neurosphere and downregulate stem cell markers, such as *BMI1, Nanog,* and *Nestin* [77]. Both miR-124 and miR-137 are up-regulated during adult neural stem cell differentiation and down-regulated in high-grade gliomas [78]. Although there are comprehensive studies about miRNa in gliomas, it should not be forgotten that one miRNA can affect the expression of various target genes. It must be reconsidered in terms of several important aspects before miRNAs may be used therapeutically [79].

LncRNAs which have more than 200 nucleotides and are up to 100 kb in length are described as an important RNA molecule that plays role in some biological cellular actions such as stemness, development, and cell survival [80–82]. Maternally expressed gene 3 (*MEG3*) is a maternally expressed imprinted gene that can also act as an lncRNA. Its expression in glioma tissues is lower than that in normal adjacent tissues [83]. The tumor-suppressive role of *MEG3* is confirmed by the fact that it can associate with p53. It is known that this association is needed for p53 activation [84].

6. Possible relationships between location and genetic signature in primary brain tumors

A unique finding is that the location of certain primary brain tumors determines their genetic characteristics. Cranial base meningiomas are less malignant compared to the non-cranial base meningiomas [85]. The frequencies of grade II and III cranial base and non-cranial base meningiomas are 3.5 and 12.1%, respectively. These findings origin from a clinical-pathological observation. The biological, molecular, and genetic basis of this fact requires further explanation. A simple answer would be the diverse embryological origins of the dura mater in various locations of human skull [86]. A recently published paper showed (utmost) intriguing data about meningioma biology, which is going to help our understanding of this tumor, of which 85–90% is classified as benign (grade I), but has in certain locations an aggressive course. Meningiomas regarding their genetic origin are divided as NF2 and non-NF2 meningiomas. The non-NF2 meningiomas behave clinically different and are generally always benign, with chromosomal stability, and originate from the medial skull base. In contrast to these findings, meningiomas with mutant NF2 and/or chromosome 22 loss are more likely to be atypical and demonstrate genomic instability and are localized to the cerebral and cerebellar hemispheres. This group concludes their study: "Collectively, these findings identify distinct meningioma subtypes, suggesting avenues for targeted therapeutics" [87]. There is a mutational profile of a meningioma, which can be predicted based on its anatomical location in human calvarium. This finding may provide a unique treatment strategy for midline tumors, which may have a response to medical treatment like hedgehog inhibitors. There are treatment-resistant meningiomas, which are surgically unresectable, recurrent, or invasive. In these patients one can reserve surgery or irradiation, bearing in mind that there is an independent risk factor for progression of these generally benign considered primary brain tumors. This location-based molecular and genetic data provides an updated information about prognosis and treatment response of meningiomas. This update research, which is collected over 300 meningiomas, is a valuable finding, regarding designing personalized management strategies for meningiomas.

Another fact about meningioma is that there is a subgroup of meningiomas, which are histopathologically classified as grade I meningioma, but recurs during follow-up in a short distance unexpectedly as grade II and later as grade III meningiomas. Although the malignant progression of gliomas is considerably well defined and researched entity, there is lack of scientific data about meningiomas, regarding which one is going to transform malignantly. Al-Mefty et al. explained this clinical observation with their FISH analysis of primary and recurring meningiomas with malignant progression in their series. They studied 175 recurrent meningiomas and found that 11 tumors showed histopathologically verified progression to a higher grade. In this study, the cytogenetic analysis with FISH showed deletions of 22, 1p, and 14q. The interesting finding was that in all but one case, these aberrations have been shown to be also present in the previous specimen despite their lower histopathological grades [88].

The conclusion of this translational paper from 2004 was defined: "Tumors that present with complex genetic alterations, even those with a benign histopathological grade are potentially aggressive and require closer follow-up." After 12 years this sentence is still valid for meningiomas and other primary brain tumors, which are genetically prone to upgrade. The designated malignant progression of primary brain tumors is an important issue for designing molecular-genetic-based therapeutic approaches in the near future. The finding that oligodendrogliomas show allelic deletions on 19q and 1p has been defined in 1994 by Reifenberger et al. [89]. Clinical relevance and its implication in changing management strategies followed this genetic finding. The chemotherapeutic response and survival in patients with anaplastic oligodendrogliomas were explained with the over-mentioned genetic background [90]. Its relationship with better prognosis and response to chemotherapy is today an established fact and will be considered in the update "integrated-layered" classification of central nervous system tumors after Haarlem consensus [91]. The location of oligodendrogliomas and its relationship with 1p19q deletion further changed our direction in a phylogenetic explanation of primary brain tumor development and coexisting molecular-genetic mechanisms. Frontal location of oligodendroglioma was suggested to be a favorable prognostic factor. The accumulated data clearly demonstrated that frontal location was strongly correlated with 1p19q deletion [92]. Prognostic variables in oligodendroglial tumors: a single-institution study of 95 cases. This translational information eased (helped) to predict the prognosis of these peculiar tumors. The embryological developmental basis of oligodendroglioma and its molecular-genetic relationship are other issues, which require further investigation.

Lucius Annaeus Seneca, known as Seneca the Younger (c. 4 BC–AD 65), stated: "No one can wear a mask for very long." We can further apply this wise quote to our update neuro-oncological approach, which requires redefinition in the coming decades: "No tumor can wear a mask for very long." The molecular-genetic data and determining its relationship with primary brain tumors will further relieve "the mask" of the primary brain tumors. The upcoming new WHO classification of central nervous system tumors will consider this issue.

Author details

Ilhan Yaylim[1], Sumeyya Azam[2], Ammad Ahmad Farooqi[3], Özlem Küçükhüseyin[1], Muhammad Ismail[3] and Ali Metin Kafadar[4*]

*Address all correspondence to: ctfkafadar@gmail.com

1 Institute of Experimental Medicine, Department of Molecular Medicine, Istanbul University, Istanbul, Turkey

2 First Affiliated Hospital of Xinjiang Medical University, Xinjiang, Urumqi, PR China

3 Institute of Biomedical and Genetic Engineering (IBGE), Islamabad, Pakistan

4 Department of Neurosurgery, Cerrahpaşa Medical Faculty, Istanbul University, Istanbul, Turkey

References

[1] Karsy M, Neil JA, Guan J, Mahan MA, Colman H, Jensen RL: A practical review of prognostic correlations of molecular biomarkers in glioblastoma. Neurosurg Focus. 2015;38(3):E4. doi: 10.3171/2015.1.FOCUS14755.

[2] Etzioni R, Urban N, Ramsey S, McIntosh M, Schwartz S, Reid B, Radich J, Anderson G, Hartwell L: The case for early detection. Nat Rev Cancer. 2003;3(4):243–252.

[3] Kulasingam V, Diamandis EP: Strategies for discovering novel cancer biomarkers through utilization of emerging technologies. Nat Clin Pract Oncol. 2008;5:588–599.

[4] Hayes DF, Bast RC, Desch CE, Fritsche H Jr, Kemeny NE, Jessup JM, Locker GY, Macdonald JS, Mennel RG, Norton L, Ravdin P, Taube S, Winn RJ: Tumor marker utility grading system: a framework to evaluate clinical utility of tumor markers. J Natl Cancer Inst. 1996;88(20):1456–1466.

[5] Holdhoff M, Ye X, Blakeley JO, Blair L, Burger PC, Grossman SA, et al: Use of personalized molecular biomarkers in the clinical care of adults with glioblastomas. J Neurooncol. 2012;110:279–285.

[6] Westhoff MA, Karpel-Massler G, Brühl O, Enzenmüller S, La Ferla-Brühl K, Siegelin MD, Nonnenmacher L Debatin KM: A critical evaluation of PI3K inhibition in glioblastoma and neuroblastoma therapy. Mol Cell Ther. 2014;2:32.

[7] Rao RD, James CD: Altered molecular pathways in gliomas: an overview of clinically relevant issues. Semin Oncol. 2004;31(5):595–604

[8] Guha A, Feldkamp MM, Lau N, Boss G, Pawson A: Proliferation of human malignant astrocytomas is dependent on Ras activation. Oncogene. 1997;15:2755–2765.

[9] Pandey V, Bhaskara VK, Babu PP: Implications of mitogen-activated protein kinase signaling in glioma. J Neurosci Res. 2016;94:114–127. doi: 10.1002/jnr.23687.

[10] Wong AJ, Ruppert JM, Bigner SH, Grzeschik CH, Humphrey PA, Bigner DS, et al: Structural alterations of the epidermal growth factor receptor gene in human gliomas. Proc Natl Acad Sci U S A. 1992;89:2965–2969.

[11] Frederick L, Wang XY, Eley G, James CD: Diversity and frequency of epidermal growth factor receptor mutations in human glioblastomas. Cancer Res. 2000;60:1383–1387.

[12] Salkeni MA, Zarzour A, Ansay TY, McPherson CM, Warnick RE, Rixe O, et al: Detection of EGFRvIII mutant DNA in the peripheral blood of brain tumor patients. J Neurooncol. 2013;115:27–35

[13] Taylor TE, Furnari FB, Cavenee WK: Targeting EGFR for treatment of glioblastoma: molecular basis to overcome resistance. Curr Cancer Drug Targets. 2012;12:197–209.

[14] Brennan C, Momota H, Hambardzumyan D, Ozawa T, Tandon A, Pedraza A, et al: Glioblastoma subclasses can be defined by activity among signal transduction pathways and associated genomic alterations. PLoS ONE. 2009;4:e7752.

[15] Ozawa T, Brennan CW, Wang L, Squatrito M, Sasayama T, Nakada M, et al: PDGFRA gene rearrangements are frequent genetic events in PDGFRA-amplified glioblastomas. Genes Dev. 2010;24:2205–2218.

[16] Verhaak RGW, Hoadley KA, Purdom E, Wang V, Qi Y, Wilkerson MD, et al: Integrated genomic analysis identifies clinically relevant subtypes of glioblastoma characterized by abnormalities in PDGFRA, IDH1, EGFR, and NF1. Cancer Cell. 2010;17:98–110.

[17] Sami A, Karsy M: Targeting the PI3K/AKT/mTOR signaling pathway in glioblastoma: novel therapeutic agents and advances in understanding. Tumour Biol. 2013;34:1991–2002.

[18] King D, Yeomanson D, Bryant HE: PI3King the lock: targeting the PI3K/Akt/mTOR pathway as a novel therapeutic strategy in neuroblastoma. J Pediatr Hematol Oncol. 2015;37:245–251.

[19] Rafalski VA, Brunet A: Energy metabolism in adult neural stem cell fate. Prog Neurobiol. 2011;93(2):182–203. doi: 10.1016/j.pneurobio.2010.10.007. PMID 21056618.

[20] Network CGAR: Comprehensive genomic characterization defines human glioblastoma genes and core pathways. Nature. 2008;455:1061–1068.

[21] Fan QW, Weiss WA: Targeting the RTK–PI3K–mTOR axis in malignant glioma: overcoming resistance. Curr Top Microbiol Immunol. 2010;347:279–296.

[22] Lavrik IN, Golks A, and Krammer PH: Caspases: pharmacological manipulation of cell death. J Clin Invest. 2005;115:2665–2672.

[23] Bellail AC, Olson JJ, Yang X, Chen ZJ, Hao C: A20 ubiquitin ligase-mediated polyubiquitination of RIP1 inhibits caspase-8 cleavage and TRAIL-induced apoptosis in glioblastoma. Cancer Discov. 2012;2(2):140–155.

[24] Crommentuijn MH, Maguire CA, Niers JM, Vandertop WP, Badr CE, Würdinger T, Tannous BA: Intracranial AAV–sTRAIL combined with lanatoside C prolongs survival in an orthotopic xenograft mouse model of invasive glioblastoma. Mol Oncol. 2015;11. pii: S1574-7891(15)00226-4.

[25] Balyasnikova IV, Prasol MS, Ferguson SD, Han Y, Ahmed AU, Gutova M, Tobias AL, Mustafi D, Rincón E, Zhang L, Aboody KS, Lesniak MS: Intranasal delivery of mesenchymal stem cells significantly extends survival of irradiated mice with experimental brain tumors. Mol Ther. 2014;22(1):140–148.

[26] Yulyana Y, Endaya BB, Ng WH, Guo CM, Hui KM, Lam PY, Ho IA: Carbenoxolone enhances TRAIL-induced apoptosis through the upregulation of death receptor 5 and

inhibition of gap junction intercellular communication in human glioma. Stem Cells Dev. 2013;22(13):1870–1882.

[27] Wang LH, Ni CW, Lin YZ, Yin L, Jiang CB, Lv CT, Le Y, Lang Y, Zhao CY, Yang K, Jiao BH, Yin J: Targeted induction of apoptosis in glioblastoma multiforme cells by an MRP3-specific TRAIL fusion protein in vitro. Tumour Biol. 2014;35(2):1157–1168.

[28] van de Water JA, Bagci-Onder T, Agarwal AS, Wakimoto H, Roovers RC, Zhu Y, Kasmieh R, Bhere D, Van Bergen en Henegouwen PM, Shah K: Therapeutic stem cells expressing variants of EGFR-specific nanobodies have antitumor effects. Proc Natl Acad Sci U S A. 2012;109(41):16642–16647

[29] Ahn Y, Oh S, Lee SJ, Park BG, Park YS, Shin WS, Jang HJ, Park JH, Kwon D, Lee S: Synthesis of diethylamino-curcumin mimics with substituted triazolyl groups and their sensitization effect of TRAIL against brain cancer cells. Bioorg Med Chem Lett. 2014;24(15):3346–3350.

[30] Lee DH, Lee CS, Kim DW, Ae JE, Lee TH: Digitoxin sensitizes glioma cells to TRAIL-mediated apoptosis by upregulation of death receptor 5 and downregulation of survivin. Anticancer Drugs. 2014;25(1):44–52.

[31] Abusamra YA, Scuruchi M, Habibatni S, Maammeri Z, Benayache S, D'Ascola A, Avenoso A, Campo GM, Spina E: Evaluation of putative cytotoxic activity of crude extracts from *Onopordum acanthium* leaves and Spartium junceum flowers against the U-373 glioblastoma cell line. Pak J Pharm Sci. 2015;28(4):1225–1232.

[32] Gentile MT, Ciniglia C, Reccia MG, Volpicelli F, Gatti M, Thellung S, Florio T, Melone MA, Colucci-D'Amato L: *Ruta graveolens* L. induces death of glioblastoma cells and neural progenitors, but not of neurons, via ERK 1/2 and AKT activation. PLoS One. 2015;10(3):e0118864.

[33] Noté OP, Jihu D, Antheaume C, Zeniou M, Pegnyemb DE, Guillaume D, Chneiwess H, Kilhoffer MC, Lobstein A: Triterpenoid saponins from *Albizia lebbeck* (L.) Benth and their inhibitory effect on the survival of high grade human brain tumor cells. Carbohydr Res. 2015;404:26–33.

[34] Parsons DW, Jones S, Zhang X, Lin JC, Leary RJ, Angenendt P, Mankoo P, Carter H, Siu IM, Gallia GL, Olivi A, McLendon R, Rasheed BA, Keir S, Nikolskaya T, Nikolsky Y, Busam DA, Tekleab H, Diaz LA Jr, Hartigan J, Smith DR, Strausberg RL, Marie SK, Shinjo SM, Yan H, Riggins GJ, Bigner DD, Karchin R,Papadopoulos N, Parmigiani G, Vogelstein B, Velculescu VE, Kinzler KW: An integrated genomic analysis of human glioblastoma multiforme. Science. 2008;321:1807–1812. doi: 10.1126/science.1164382.

[35] Noushmehr H, Weisenberger DJ, Diefes K, Phillips HS, Pujara K, Berman BP, et al: Identification of a CpG island methylator phenotype that defines a distinct subgroup of glioma. Cancer Cell. 2010;17:510–522.

[36] Lu C, Ward PS, Kapoor GS, Rohle D, Turcan S, Abdel-Wahab O, Edwards CR, Khanin R, Figueroa ME, Melnick A, Wellen KE, O'Rourke DM, Berger SL, Chan TA, Levine RL,

Mellinghoff IK, Thompson CB: IDH mutation impairs histone demethylation and results in a block to cell differentiation. Nature. 2012;483:474–478.

[37] Dang L, White DW, Gross S, Bennett BD, Bittinger MA, Driggers EM, Fantin VR, Jang HG, Jin S, Keenan MC, Marks KM, Prins RM, Ward PS, Yen KE, Liau LM, Rabinowitz JD, Cantley LC, Thompson CB, Vander Heiden MG, Su SM: Cancer-associated IDH1 mutations produce 2-hydroxyglutarate. Nature. 2010;465:966.

[38] Xu W, Yang H, Liu Y, Yang Y, Wang P, Kim SH, Ito S, Yang C, Wang P, Xiao MT, Liu LX, Jiang WQ, Liu J, Zhang JY, Wang B, Frye S, Zhang Y, Xu YH, Lei QY, Guan KL, Zhao SM, Xiong Y: Oncometabolite 2-hydroxyglutarate is a competitive inhibitor of alpha-ketoglutarate-dependent dioxygenases. Cancer Cell. 2011;19:17–30.

[39] Jin SG, Jiang Y, Qiu R, Rauch RA, Wang Y, Schackert G, Krex D, Lu Q, Pfeifer GP: 5-Hydroxymethylcytosine is strongly depleted in human cancers but its levels do not correlate with IDH1 mutations. Cancer Res. 2011;71:7360–7365.

[40] Kraus TF, Globisch D, Wagner M, Eigenbrod S, Widmann D, Munzel M, Muller M, Pfaffeneder T, Hackner B, Feiden W, Schuller U, Carell T, Kretzschmar HA: Low values of 5-hydroxymethylcytosine (5hmC), the "sixth base," are associated with anaplasia in human brain tumors. Int J Cancer. 2012, http://dx.doi.org/10.1002/ijc.27429.

[41] Ohgaki H, Kleihues P: Genetic profile of astrocytic and oligodendroglial gliomas. Brain Tumor Pathol. 2011;28:177–183.

[42] England B, Huang T, Karsy M: Current understanding of the role and targeting of tumor suppressor p53 in glioblastoma multiforme. Tumour Biol. 2013;34:2063–2074.

[43] Biernat W, Kleihues P, Yonekawa Y, Ohgaki H: Amplification and overexpression of MDM2 in primary (de novo) glioblastomas. J Neuropathol Exp Neurol. 1997;56:180–185.

[44] Nakamura M, Watanabe T, Klangby U, Asker C, Wiman K, Yonekawa Y, et al: p14ARF deletion and methylation in genetic pathways to glioblastomas. Brain Pathol. 2001;11:159–168.

[45] Blough MD, Beauchamp DC, Westgate MR, Kelly JJ, Cairncross JG: Effect of aberrant p53 function on temozolomide sensitivity of glioma cell lines and brain tumor initiating cells from glioblastoma. J Neurooncol. 2011;102:1–7.

[46] Ino Y, Betensky RA, Zlatescu MC, Sasaki H, Macdonald DR, Stemmer-Rachamimov AO, Ramsay DA, Cairncross JG, Louis DN: Molecular subtypes of anaplastic oligodendroglioma: implications for patient management at diagnosis. Clin Cancer Res. 2001;7:839–845.

[47] Jeuken JW, von Deimling A, Wesseling P: Molecular pathogenesis of oligodendroglial tumors. J Neurooncol. 2004;70:161–181.

[48] Wolf RM, Draghi N, Liang X, Dai C, Uhrbom L, Eklof C, Westermark B, Holland EC, Resh MD: p190RhoGAP can act to inhibit PDGF induced gliomas in mice: a putative

tumor suppressor encoded on human chromosome 19q13.3. Genes Dev. 2003;17:476–487.

[49] Idbaih A, Marie Y, Pierron G, Brennetot C, Hoang-Xuan K, Kujas M, Mokhtari K, Sanson M, Lejeune J, Aurias A, Delattre O, Delattre JY: Two types of chromosome 1p losses with opposite significance in gliomas. Ann Neurol. 2005;58:483– 487.

[50] Cairncross G, Wang M, Shaw E, Jenkins R, Brachman D, Buckner J, et al: Phase III trial of chemoradiotherapy for anaplastic oligodendroglioma: long-term results of RTOG 9402. J Clin Oncol. 2013;31:337–343.

[51] Boots-Sprenger SHE, Sijben A, Rijntjes J, Tops BBJ, Idema AJ, Rivera AL, et al: Significance of complete 1p/19q codeletion, IDH1 mutation and MGMT promoter methylation in gliomas: use with caution. Mod Pathol. 2013;26:922–929.

[52] Schmidt MC, Antweiler S, Urban N, Mueller W, Kuklik A, Meyer-Puttlitz B, et al: Impact of genotype and morphology on the prognosis of glioblastoma. J Neuropathol Exp Neurol. 2002;61:321–328.

[53] Hartmann C, Hentschel B, Simon M, Westphal M, Schackert G, Tonn JC, et al: Long-term survival in primary glioblastoma with versus without isocitrate dehydrogenase mutations. Clin Cancer Res. 2013;19:5146–5157.

[54] Laxton RC, Popov S, Doey L, Jury A, Bhangoo R, Gullan R, et al: Primary glioblastoma with oligodendroglial differentiation has better clinical outcome but no difference in common biological markers compared with other types of glioblastoma. Neuro Oncol. 2013;15:1635–1643.

[55] SongTao Q, Lei Y, Si G, YanQing D, HuiXia H, XueLin Z, et al: IDH mutations predict longer survival and response to temozolomide in secondary glioblastoma. Cancer Sci. 2012;103:269–273.

[56] Wick W, Hartmann C, Engel C, Stoffels M, Felsberg J, Stockhammer F, Sabel MC, Koeppen S, Ketter R, Meyermann R, Rapp M, Meisner C, Kortmann RD,Pietsch T, Wiestler OD, Ernemann U, Bamberg M, Reifenberger G, von Deimling A, Weller M: NOA-04 randomized phase III trial of sequential radiochemotherapy of anaplastic glioma with procarbazine, lomustine, and vincristine or temozolomide. J Clin Oncol. 2009;27(35):5874–5880. doi: 10.1200/JCO.2009.23.6497.

[57] Gorlia T, van den Bent MJ, Hegi ME, Mirimanoff RO, Weller M, Cairncross JG, Eisenhauer E, Belanger K, Brandes AA, Allgeier A, Lacombe D, Stupp R.: Nomograms for predicting survival of patients with newly diagnosed glioblastoma: prognostic factor analysis of EORTC and NCIC trial 26981-22981/CE.3. Lancet Oncol. 2008;9:29–38.

[58] Karlic R, Chung HR, Lasserre J, Vlahovicek K, Vingron M: Histone modification levels are predictive for gene expression. Proc Natl Acad Sci U S A. 2010;107:2926–2931.

[59] Bannister AJ, Kouzarides T: Regulation of chromatin by histone modifications. Cell Res. 2011;21:381–395.

[60] Santos-Rosa H, Schneider R, Bannister AJ, Sherriff J, Bernstein BE, Emre NC, Schreiber SL, Mellor J, Kouzarides T: Active genes are tri-methylated at K4 of histone H3. Nature. 2002;419:407–411.

[61] Costa FF: Non-coding RNAs, epigenetics and complexity. Gene. 2008;410:9–17.

[62] Esteller M: Non-coding RNAs in human disease. Nat Rev Genet. 2011;12:861–874.

[63] Mendell JT: MicroRNAs: critical regulators of development, cellular physiology and malignancy. Cell Cycle. 2005;4:1179–1184.

[64] Li Y, Guessous F, Zhang Y, diPierro C, Kefas B, Johnson E, Marcinkiewicz L, Jiang J, Yang Y, Schmittgen TD, Lopes B, Schiff D, Purow B, Abounader R: MicroRNA-34a inhibits glioblastoma growth by targeting multiple oncogenes. Cancer Res. 2009;69:7569–7576.

[65] Mei J, Bachoo R, Zhang CL: MicroRNA-146a inhibits glioma development by targeting Notch1. Mol Cell Biol. 2011;31:3584–3592.

[66] Kefas B, Godlewski J, Comeau L, Li Y, Abounader R, Hawkinson M, Lee J, Fine H, Chiocca EA, Lawler S, Purow B: MicroRNA-7 inhibits the epidermal growth factor receptor and the Akt pathway and is down-regulated in glioblastoma. Cancer Res. 2008;68:3566–3572.

[67] Zhang QQ, Xu H, Huang MB, Ma LM, Huang QJ, Yao Q, Zhou H, Qu LH: MicroRNA-195 plays a tumor-suppressor role in human glioblastoma cells by targeting signaling pathways involved in cellular proliferation and invasion. Neuro Oncol. 2012;14:278–287.

[68] Gabriely G, Yi M, Narayan RS, Niers JM, Wurdinger T, Imitola J, Ligon KL, Kesari S, Esau C, Stephens RM, Tannous BA, Krichevsky AM: Human glioma growth is controlled by microRNA-10b. Cancer Res. 2011;71;3563–3572.

[69] Gabriely G, Wurdinger T, Kesari S, Esau CC, Burchard J, Linsley PS, Krichevsky AM: MicroRNA 21 promotes glioma invasion by targeting matrix metalloproteinase regulators. Mol Cell Biol. 2008;28:5369–5380.

[70] Jiang L, Lin C, Song L, Wu J, Chen B, Ying Z, Fang L, Yan X, He M, Li J, Li M: MicroRNA-30e_ promotes human glioma cell invasiveness in an orthotopic xenotransplantation model by disrupting the NF-kappaB/IkappaBalpha negative feedback loop. J Clin Invest. 2012;122:33–47.

[71] Zhang CZ, Zhang JX, Zhang AL, Shi ZD, Han L, Jia ZF, Yang WD, Wang GX, Jiang T, You YP, Pu PY, Cheng JQ, Kang CS: MiR-221 and miR-222 target PUMA to induce cell survival in glioblastoma. Mol Cancer. 2010;9;229.

[72] Piccirillo SG, Reynolds BA, Zanetti N, Lamorte G, Binda E, Broggi G, et al: Bone morphogenetic proteins inhibit the tumorigenic potential of human brain tumour-initiating cells. Nature. 2006;444:761–765. doi: 10.1038/nature 05349.

[73] Ernst A, Campos B , Meier J, Devens F, Liesenberg F, Wolter M, et al: De-repression of CTGF via the miR-17-92 cluster upon differentiation of human glioblastoma spheroid cultures. Oncogene. 2010;29:3411–3422. doi: 10.1038/onc.2010.83.

[74] Godlewski J, Nowicki MO, Bronisz A,Nuovo G, Palatini J, DeLay M, et al: MicroRNA-451regulates LKB1/AMPKsignalingandallows adaptation to metabolic stress in glioma cells. Mol Cell. 2010;37:620–632. doi: 10.1016/j.molcel.2010.02.018.

[75] Godlewski J, Nowicki MO, Bronisz A, Williams S, Otsuki A, Nuovo G, et al: Targeting of the Bmi-1 oncogene/stemcell renewal factor by microRNA-128 inhibits glioma proliferation and self-renewal. Cancer Res. 2008;68:9125–9130. doi: 10.1158/0008-5472.CAN-08-2629.

[76] Natsume A, Ito M, Katsushima K,Ohka F, Hatanaka A,Shinjo K, et al: Chromatin regulator PRC2Is a key regulator of epigenetic plasticity in glioblastoma. Cancer Res. 2013;73:4559–4570.

[77] Xia H, Cheung WK, Ng SS, Jiang X, Jiang S, Sze J, et al: Loss of brain-enriched miR-124 microRNA enhances stem-like traits and invasiveness of glioma cells. J Biol Chem. 2012. 287:9962–9971. doi: 10.1074/jbc.M111.332627

[78] Silber J, Lim DA,Petritsch C, Persson AI, Maunakea AK, Yu M, et al: miR-124 and miR-137 inhibit proliferation of glioblastoma multiforme cells and induce differentiation of brain tumor stem cells. BMC Med. 2008;6:14. doi: 10.1186/1741-7015-6-14.

[79] Kreth S, Thon N, Kreth FW: Epigenetics in human gliomas. Cancer Lett. 2014;342:185–192

[80] Mercer TR, Dinger ME, Mattick JS: Long non-coding RNAs: insights into functions. Nat Rev Genet. 2009;10:155–159. doi: 10.1038/nrg2521

[81] Koziol MJ, Rinn JL: RNA traffic control of chromatin complexes. Curr Opin Genet Dev. 2010;20:142–148. doi: 10.1016/j.gde.2010.03.003.

[82] Zhang H, Chen Z, Wang X, Huang Z, He Z, Chen Y. Long non-coding RNA:a new player in cancer. J Hematol Oncol. 2013;6:37. doi: 10.1186/1756-8722-6-37.

[83] Wang P, Ren Z, Sun P: Overexpression of the long non-coding RNA MEG3 impairs in vitro glioma cell proliferation. J Cell Biochem. 2012;113:1868–1874. doi: 10.1002/jcb.24055

[84] Lu KH, Li W, Liu XH, Sun M, Zhang ML, Wu WQ, et al: Long non-coding RNA MEG3 inhibits NSCLC cells proliferation and induces apoptosis by affecting p53 expression. BMC Cancer. 2013;13:461. doi: 10.1186/1471-2407-13-461.

[85] Sade B, Chahlavi A, Krishnaney A, Nagel S, Choi E, Lee JH: World Health Organization grades II and III meningiomas are rare in the cranial base and spine. Neurosurgery. 2007;61:1194–1198.

[86] O'Rahilly R, Muller F: The meninges in human development. J Neuropathol Exp Neurol. 1986;45:588–608.

[87] Clark VE, Erson-Omay EZ, Serin A, Jun Yin J, Cotney J, Ozduman K, et al: Genomic analysis of non-NF2 meningiomas reveals mutations in TRAF7, KLF4, AKT1, and SMO. Science. 2013;339(6123)1077–1080.

[88] Al-Mefty O, Kadri P, Pravdenkova S, Sawyer JR, Stangeby C, Husain M: Malignant progression in meningioma: documentation of a series and analysis of cytogenetic findings. J Neurosurg. 2004;101:210–218.

[89] Reifenberger J, Reifenberger G, Liu L, James CD, Wechsler W, Collins VP: Molecular genetic analysis of oligodendroglial tumors shows preferential allelic deletions on 19q and 1p. Am J Pathol. 1994;145(5):1175–1190.

[90] Cairncross JG, Ueki K, Zlatescu MC, Lisle DK, Finkelstein DM, Hammond RR, Silver JS, Stark PC, Macdonald DR, Ino Y, Ramsay DA, Louis DN: Specific genetic predictors of chemotherapeutic response and survival in patients with anaplastic oligodendrogliomas. J Natl Cancer Inst. 1998;90:1473–1479.

[91] Louis DN, Perry A, Burger P, Ellison DW, Reifenberger G, von Deimling A, Aldape K, Brat D, Collins VP, Eberhart C et al.International society of neuropathology-haarlem consensus guidelines for nervous system tumor classification and grading. Brain Pathol. 2014;24:429–435.

[92] Scheie D, Meling TR, Cvancarova M, Skullerud K, Mørk S, Lote K, Eide TJ, Helseth E, Beiske K. Prognostic variables in oligodendroglial tumors: a single-institution study of 95 cases. Neuro Oncol. 2011;13:1225–1233.

3

Molecular Advances in Glioblastoma Neuropathology

Jens Schittenhelm and Marco Skardelly

Abstract

Glioblastoma is the most frequent and malignant brain tumor with a wide variety of morphological appearances. For a long time, the tumors were classified either as primary ("de novo") glioblastomas that develop rapidly in elderly patients or as secondary glioblastomas with clinical or histological progression from low-grade diffuse astrocytoma or anaplastic astrocytoma. Recent data from the comprehensive genetic characterization of these tumors identified a number of common and diverging alterations and pathways that allow future stratification of glioblastomas into several age-dependent biological subgroups. While the histological classification of diffuse gliomas based on the WHO grading scheme is still necessary, the use of additional meaningful immunohistochemical (and mutation-specific) markers, such as IDH R132H, ATRX, and H3F3A K27M, has improved routine diagnosis. In recent years, the spectrum of clinically relevant molecular markers has expanded. The utility of MGMT, ATRX, TERT, H3F3A and LOH 1p/19q in predicting prognosis and response to therapy in routine diagnostic settings is discussed.

Keywords: neuropathology, histopathology, immunohistochemistry, molecular classification, glioma

1. Introduction

Gliomas are diffusely growing neoplasms of the central nervous system that present high rates of morbidity and mortality. They are the most frequent CNS neoplasms, accounting for approximately 29% of all CNS neuroepithelial tumors [1]. In contrast to almost all other brain tumors, such diffuse gliomas are characterized by extensive, diffuse infiltration of tumor cells into the brain parenchyma—the neuropil. This infiltration is so extensive that even past attempts with radical resection of a hemisphere were not successful, as the tumors reemerged on the contralateral hemisphere [2]. Because of their similarity with non-neoplastic glial cells, these tumors are considered to be of astrocytic and/or oligodendroglial lineage and do not include the biologically different group of ependymomas [3]. The most common primary and malignant brain tumor among this group is glioblastoma, widely known by its acronym "GBM." The tumor was originally designated as "glioblastoma multiforme" because of the extensive variability of tumor histologies. However, some specific (and rare) entities have been isolated from this umbrella term, and individual glioblastomas can also appear quite monomorphic in histology. For this reason, the term "multiforme" is no longer in use following the WHO 2007 classification [4].

Glioblastomas are preferentially located in the subcortical or deep white matter of the cerebral hemispheres, but they may be observed in any other region of the brain, including the cerebellum and spinal cord [3]. Upon initial presentation, less than 2% of the tumors show multiple, clearly distant lesions [5]. In our institution, we prefer to use the term "multifocal" for such lesions without apparent MRI and histological continuum and the term "multicentric" for tumors with radiologically or macroscopically visible distinct tumor centers that have developed from a single lesion. Conventional radiological modalities tend to underestimate the extent of diffuse infiltrative glioma growth. Tumor cells are usually present even outside the peritumoral areas of low density in CT and hyperintensive regions on T2-weighted images in MRI [6]. Not surprisingly, the radiological distinction between multifocal and multicentric gliomas is slightly uncertain. The most extreme example of diffuse infiltrative glioma growth is represented by gliomatosis cerebri. This diagnosis requires the involvement of at least three cerebral lobes, usually bilaterally [3]. Because gliomatosis lacks molecular differences between more circumscribed tumors, this entity will most likely be removed in the next WHO revision. Unlike secondary/metastatic brain tumors, gliomas usually respect the blood-brain barrier, and extraneural metastasis, which is extremely rare, occurs due to ventriculo-peritoneal shunts [6]. In contrast, cerebrospinal fluid spread of glioblastoma cells is occasionally observed, but it is still far less common than in ependymomas or childhood primitive neuroectodermal tumors. Common routes of spread of glioblastoma include the fornix, corpus callosum, anterior commissure, and radiatio optica because of the high affinity of tumor cells to myelinated structures [7]. Symmetric tumors spread across the corpus callosum are called "butterfly gliomas." Tumors that reach the dura often show marked desmoplasia, leading to a firm texture that resembles gliosarcoma or meningioma [8].

2. Clinicopathological parameters of glioblastoma

Glioblastomas represent approximately 65% of all astrocytic or oligodendroglial neoplasms [1]. Incidence rates, estimated to be up to 4.6 per 100,000 people, tend to vary by region, with generally higher numbers in developed countries, increasing with patients' age and showing a slight predominance for males [9]. The vast majority of tumors are observed in adults, with a mean age at diagnosis of 61 years. However, GBM can be found in children, and due to their lower incidence, these tumors are often grouped together with anaplastic astrocytomas and intrinsic pontine gliomas as high-grade (i.e., WHO grade III and IV) tumors. As a matter of fact, comparing clinical and molecular data from such cohorts with adult tumors is difficult. Generally, a younger age of onset in non-pediatric GBM is one of the strongest predictive factors of prolonged survival [10]. Despite this fact, surprisingly, many publications do not include patients' age in multivariate analysis when analyzing biomarkers of patient survival. While almost all GBM occur sporadically, in individuals with Lynch syndrome, a constitutional mismatch repair defect results in an increase of brain tumors, including GBM, among families [11]. Glioblastomas have been reported in other inherited tumor syndromes, including neurofibromatosis type 1, Li-Fraumeni and Turcot-Syndrome and multiple enchondromatosis [3].

Because diffuse astrocytomas show a tendency to progress to a more malignant phenotype during disease progression, these tumors end up as the so-called secondary glioblastomas, (10–15% of all glioblastomas). However, the vast majority of glioblastomas (85–90%) develop without a precursor lesion—the so-called "de novo" or primary glioblastoma [12]. Based purely on histology, primary and secondary glioblastomas cannot be distinguished and it is expected will be rather separated in future WHO classification that glioblastomas will be separated by their molecular profile, than their clinical history (this will be discussed in more detail below). While there is no doubt that oligodendrogliomas undergo a similar malignant tumor progression as astrocytic neoplasms, there is still debate about how many of these truly develop into glioblastomas. As there is some overlap in preoperative imaging of GBM with solitary metastases or lymphomas, intraoperative cytology and frozen sectioning may help in the rapid diagnosis and decision making in neurosurgical procedures. In many cases, nuclear atypia, uneven cell distribution, and the presence of fibrillary processes should guide diagnosis. However, cellularity in frozen sections is often underestimated as a result of artifactual spaces (**Figure 1**).

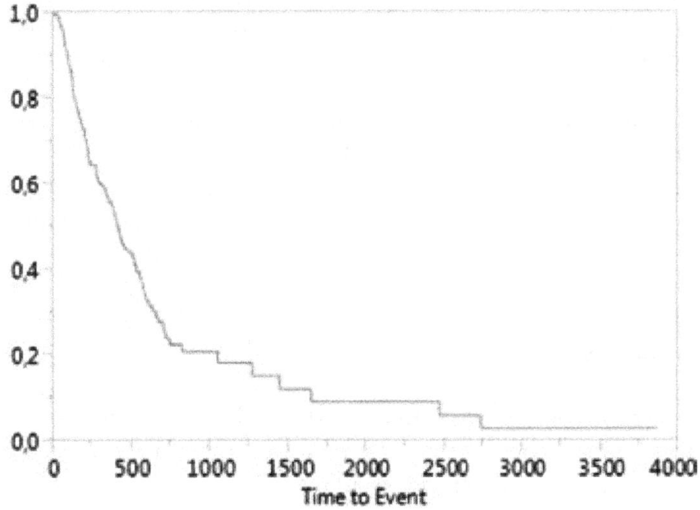

Figure 1. Glioblastomas have a poor prognosis. Kaplan–Meier overall survival Tübingen glioblastoma cohort (n = 205, median survival: 417 days, all cases IDH-wild-type, age <45 years, primary cases).

In newly diagnosed glioblastoma, current therapeutic strategies include surgery (from biopsy to gross total resection, depending on location, which itself is a prognostic marker [13]) followed by concomitant radiotherapy with temozolomide (TMZ) and up to 6 cycles of TMZ maintenance therapy in patients ≤65 years with a median overall survival (OS) of 14.6 months [14].

In addition to the well-established prognostic factors of survival in GBM patients, such as age, extent of resection (EOR), Karnofsky performance scale (KPS), and the treatment modality, molecular alterations (i.e., IDH mutation and MGMT gene promoter methylation, which we will discuss in more detail below) represent not only new significant prognostic factors of survival but also predictors of therapeutic responses in subgroups of GBM. MGMT gene promoter methylation status is a strong prognostic marker of survival in GBM with a median OS of 12.6 months in unmethylated and 23.4 months in methylated GBM treated by concomitant radio-chemotherapy with TMZ. Moreover, MGMT gene promoter methylation status also serves as a predictor of the response to TMZ therapy. In patients >65 years of age exclusive radiotherapy or chemotherapy is indicated according to the MGMT gene promoter methylation status. Patients with methylated GBM most benefit from monotherapy with TMZ, and patients with unmethylated GBM demonstrated the highest survival profit by exclusive radiotherapy [15, 16]. Recurring tumors with a methylated MGMT promoter (i.e., the silencing of the antagonistic effect of this repairing enzyme on alkylating chemotherapy) may thus benefit from a second round of treatment with TMZ [17]. Approximately 30–35% of glioblastoma samples contain a methylated MGMT promoter [18]. However, tumor treatment in diffuse gliomas lacks a persistent therapy response [19], which is why there is an increase of studies with direct ("personalized") targeting of driver mutations in glioblastomas. Alternative treatment approaches include the application of oncolytic parvoviruses to induce tumor cell cycle arrest and cell death [20], the application of low-energy alternating electric fields that affect dividing cells' viability [21], and the application of local hyperthermia induced by superparamagnetic iron oxide nanoparticles coated with hydrophilic polymers subjected to an alternating magnetic field [22].

One of the primary mechanisms related to treatment failure and tumor recurrence in GBM, even in targeted therapies, might be attributed to intratumoral molecular heterogeneity [23] and the presence of a subpopulation of cancer stem cells that contribute to tumor propagation and tumor maintenance through their ability to self-renew and differentiate [24].

2.1. Histologic tumor classification

Although serious advances in the neuroimaging of glioblastomas have been made in the past, histopathologic evaluation of neurosurgically removed tumor specimens is still required for definite classification and subsequent molecular stratification. In 1979, the World Health Organization (WHO) issued a publication for the classification of tumors of the central nervous system. This included a grading scheme based on the malignancy of tumor behavior. The grading of CNS tumors is performed with a four-tiered score, which ranges from grade II to grade IV in astrocytic/oligodendroglial tumors, to separate the histologic continuum of diffuse gliomas according to their expected clinical behavior. Grade IV has the worst prognosis and is reserved for glioblastoma [3].

On macroscopic view, the necrotic center of the tumor is often surrounded by a macroscopically visible gray rim and surrounded by yellowish-grayish texture blending into the surrounding white matter. Black hemorrhagic streaks and thrombosed veins are typically observed in glioblastomas [4]. Glioblastomas' tumor borders are usually diffuse, but rare cases (especially giant cell glioblastomas and gliosarcomas) can be very circumscribed, mimicking a carcinoma metastasis.

The astrocytic heritage of the glioblastoma is best appreciated in cases with prominent eosinophilic cytoplasm of pleomorphic tumor cells resting on a fibrillary background, but this is not the rule for all tumors [25]. As expected in a malignant tumor, marked nuclear atypia and elevated mitotic activity is common. The presence of microvascular proliferations, necrosis or both are required to determine the diagnosis of GBM [3, 4]. Intraoperative consultation with cryosection and smears can provide an initial histological diagnosis and the grade of malignancy. Therefore, intraoperative consultation is useful for neurosurgeons to a) confirm the region of interest in stereotaxic surgery, to b) decide the EOR in relation to the risk of developing new neurological deficits in patients with tumors in eloquent regions, and to c) distinguish between tumor infiltration and reactive astrocytosis.

In absence of these hallmarks, tumors must be classified as anaplastic astrocytomas, even when subsequent molecular data indicates that such tumors are underclassified glioblastomas [26]. On average, three pseudopalisading necroses are present in a glioblastoma specimen. Pseudopalisading cells are usually less proliferative and exhibit higher rates of apoptosis due to hypoxic conditions. More than half of the palisades show a central vascular lumen, and in approximately 20%, intravascular thrombosis is also observed [27]. The presence and extent of necrosis is an adverse prognostic factor [3]. Vascular proliferation in the form of glomeruloid bodies in glioblastomas is observed more frequently than in tumors from any other organ system [28]. Vascular proliferations tend to accumulate in the peripheral region of high cellularity corresponding to the contrast-enhancing ring observed in radiological images [3]. In addition to intrinsic tumor growth, the so-called secondary properties ("Scherer signs") indicate the presence of glioblastoma: perineuronal satellitosis, subpial growth along cortical surfaces and perivascular and intrafascicular growth along myelinated fibers in white matter tracts, mostly characterized by small undifferentiated cells [29]. In the spinal cord, tumor cells might extend into the subarachnoid space [4].

Tumor appearance can be so heterogeneous that diagnosis is often based on tissue patterns rather than individual tumor cell morphology. The 2007 WHO classification recognizes two distinct morphological variants, the giant cell glioblastoma and the gliosarcoma. The giant cell glioblastoma is often subcortically located, and the aptly named cells are regarded as a type of regressive change and harbor a high frequency of Tp53 mutations [3]. Diagnosis requires the presence of giant, often multinucleated cells in more than 50% of tumor cells that can be associated with reticulin deposits [30]. These tumors need to be distinguished from the more benign subependymal giant cell astrocytoma or pleomorphic xanthoastrocytoma. Gliosarcoma consists of often densely interwoven malignant glial and mesenchymal components and account for up to 2% of all glioblastoma samples. The alternating reticulin-free glial and reticulin-containing mesenchymal deposits can be additionally visualized through GFAP immunohistochemistry [3]. While the OS in giant cell glioblastoma is somewhat better, data from a large retrospective study (and others) did not show significant differences for gliosarcomas [31]. Currently considered as a pattern, not a morphological variant, gliomas can show focal areas of epithelial differentiation that range from the positive immunoreactivity of epithelial antigens to adenoid or squamous formations, leading to the misdiagnosis of carcinoma [32]. Among this group, the epithelioid GBM stands out with a younger age of onset and a high percentage of therapeutically relevant BRAF V600E hotspot mutations, and it is very likely that this tumor will become a third glioblastoma variant in the upcoming 2016 WHO classification [32]. These closely packed tumors have variably lipidized, small- to medium-sized cells with rounded cytoplasmic profiles, eosinophilic cytoplasm without stellate processes, and the absence of interspersed neuropils [33].

Small cells with little cytoplasm can appear so monomorphous that small cell glioblastomas mimic anaplastic oligodendrogliomas. Such tumor cells intermingled with gemistocytes are more likely observed in glioblastomas developing from a previous lower-grade gemistocytic astrocytoma. However, the tumors show the same aggressive course as primary GBM [34]. In some tumors, the nucleus-to-cytoplasm ratio is so high that sharply demarcated hypercellular tumor nodules with evidence of neuronal differentiation are present. These clonally expanded, often myc-amplified, so-called PNET components have a high risk of cerebrospinal fluid dissemination [35]. Some tumors may show prominent perivascular rosettes resembling anaplastic ependymomas but usually lack the more uniform roundness of ependymal tumor cells. Tumor cells can be elongated and arranged in fascicles so that upon first viewing them, a sarcoma comes to mind. In up to 15% of the tumors, perinuclear halos around nuclei in glioblastomas may resemble oligodendrogliomas on first viewing; however, the tumor nuclei usually lack the monotonous roundness of true oligodendrogliomas. Such tumors are often called glioblastoma with oligodendroglial component because initial studies suggested that these tumors might have a better prognosis than standard glioblastoma. Comprehensive reviews, including molecular analysis, indicated a pathogenetically heterogeneous group (including misdiagnosed oligodendrogliomas) without a prognostic role [36]. Another occasionally encountered pattern is the presence of adipocyte-like tumor cells that are clearly of astrocytic origin. These tumors are not genetically distinct from conventional glioblastoma [37]. In some cases, the xanthomatous/lipomatous changes are so prominent that the glial nature of these tumors is obscured [38]. Other morphologic variants include granular cell astrocytoma, which is characterized by large, PAS-positive cells with a degenerative granular lysosomal content. These look similar to the benign granular cell tumor of the pituitary stalk [39]. Metaplastic transformation can be so strong that chondroid and osseous formations in gliomas are possible [40]. Rare cases may show melanotic differentiation [41] or a rhabdoid phenotype with focal loss of INI-1 as observed in atypical teratoid/rhabdoid tumors (**Figure 2**) [42].

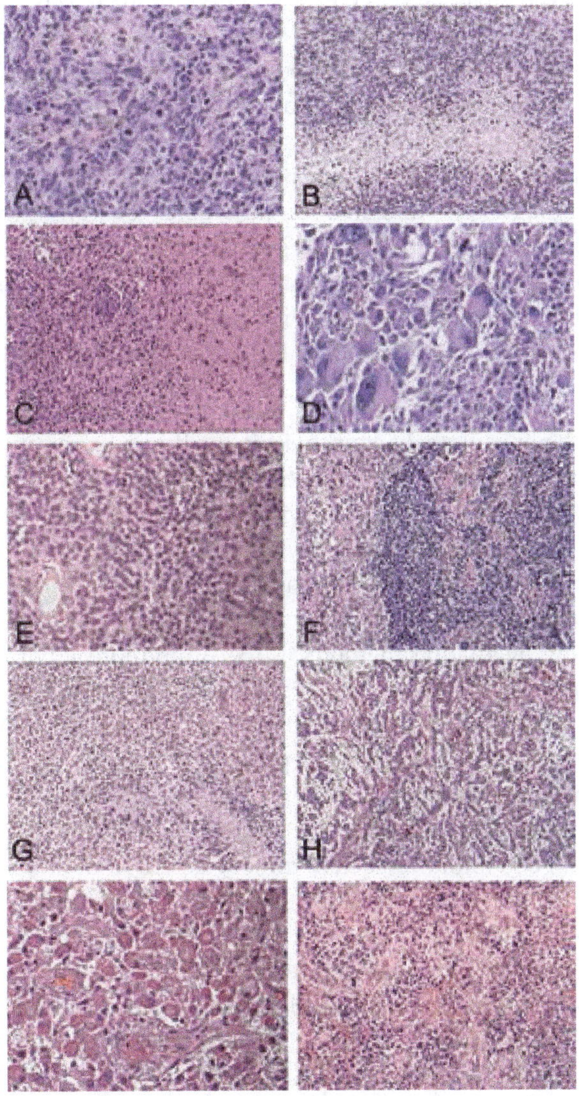

Figure 2. Glioblastoma histology consists of an anaplastic glial tumor with increased cellularity and mitotic activity (A), areas of pseudopalisading necrosis (B). The tumor diffusely invades the brain and has proliferating vessels (C). Morphological variants include giant cell glioblastoma (D), small cell glioblastoma (E), glioblastoma with PNET component (F), with oligodendroglial component (G), with adenoid features on a myxoid background (H), granular cell glioblastoma (I), and epithelioid glioblastoma (K).

2.2. Immunohistochemistry

In many instances, the diagnosis of GBM is straightforward in histology. However, confirmation of the diagnosis with a routine immunohistochemistry panel is mandatory for laboratory quality and improves diagnostic accuracy. Furthermore, some stains have not only diagnostic but also a prognostic role, and their results should be communicated back to clinicians.

The immunoprofile of the glial markers GFAP and EAAT1 in GBM is similar to astrocytomas [43]. In the vast majority of glioblastomas, these antigens are strongly expressed in the cytoplasm of the tumor cells, but they may be occasionally lacking (especially in small cell glioblastomas). The alternatives S-100, WT1, and MAP2 are less specific. Strong MAP2 and WT1 immunoreactivity in cytoplasmatic cell processes is observed in 90% of glioblastomas and is helpful in discriminating GBM from oligodendrogliomas [44, 45]. Vimentin is very unspecific and has no diagnostic value in brain tumors. Cytokeratin expression in glioblastomas (especially in giant cell glioblastomas and glioblastomas with epithelial differentiation) is an important diagnostic pitfall and should not lead to the erroneous diagnosis of carcinoma metastasis [32]. Dot-like EMA immunoreactivity is less frequently observed in GBM than in ependymomas, where usually more than 5 EMA-positive dots per high-power field are observed [46].

Identifying axons with neurofilament stains within the tumor can support the diffuse growth of GBM. In gliosarcomas, GFAP is lacking in reticulin-rich, sarcomatous areas. Usually 15–25% of the nuclei are MIB-1 positive, but the tumor proliferation rate varies greatly between individual GBM. We have observed gemistocytic tumors with less than 5% positive cells and small cell glioblastomas with 90% proliferating cells [25]. Recurrent tumors with history of previous radiation may show little proliferating activity. Because of inconsistent laboratory techniques and varying evaluation methods, MIB-1 immunoreactivity has little prognostic relevance. Nuclear Tp53 immunoreactivity in primary GBM is less present than in astrocytomas and their GBM recurrences, but it may be considerably high in giant cell glioblastomas. Tp53 expression alone is not an independent prognostic marker, but in combination with a methylated MGMT promoter, p53 nuclear staining in more than 50% of tumor cells indicates a less favorable course, similar to GBM with an unmethylated MGMT promoter [47]. It is noteworthy, that not all p53 immunoreactive tumors contain mutations in the Tp53 gene [48] and molecular determination of p53 mutation status in GBM does not correlate with patients' outcome [49]. Several studies have attempted to obtain the MGMT status by immunohistochemistry for MGMT protein expression, but results are hampered by diverging cut-off values and poor correlations with clinical outcome. MGMT immunohistochemistry therefore should be avoided unless there is a consensus with clinical data [50]. Microglial markers, such as CD68- and CD163-positive cells, are regularly found in GBM and can be very widespread, especially in tumors with granular cell components, and must be distinguished from demyelinating lesions.

The NADP-dependent enzymes IDH1 and IDH2 catalyze the conversion from isocitrate to alpha-ketoglutarate. Mutations of the catalytic center in brain tumors result in the accumulation of the oncogenic metabolite D-2-hydroxyglutarate [51]. Because IDH1 mutations are associated with a significantly more favorable outcome in GBM, confirmed in several independent studies, IDH analysis has become the major biomarker in neuropathology practice [52, 53]. The prognostic role of IDH1/2 mutations becomes obvious in WHO grade IV IDH-positive glioblastomas because they show a better prognosis than WHO grade III IDH-negative anaplastic astrocytomas [54]. The upcoming 2016 WHO tumor classification therefore separates glioblastomas according their IDH status. The vast majority of IDH1 hotspot mutations lead to a distinct amino acid substitution on codon 132 (Arg132His), for which a mutation-specific antibody is available [55]. This antibody, however, does not recognize other non-canonical IDH1 and IDH2 mutations, and negative staining results do not imply an IDH wild-type status. IDH1 R132H antibody expression is found in 4% of primary and in 71% of glioblastomas with a lower-grade precursor [55]. In elderly GBM patients above 65 years, the incidence of IDH mutations is rare—one study reported only 2 positive cases out of 167 samples, accounting for the unfavorable prognosis of this age class [56]. Another important clinical aspect is the association of epileptic seizures in IDH1 mutant tumors (**Figure 3**) [57].

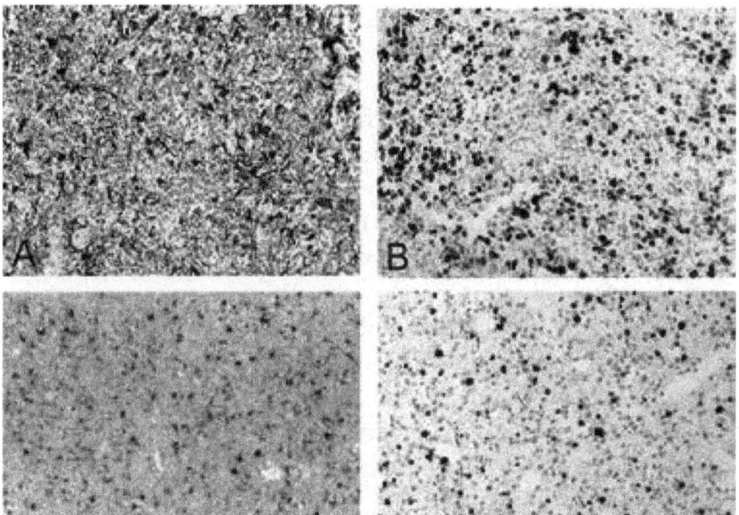

Figure 3. Immunohistochemistry: (A) Limited GFAP expression in a glioblastoma with an oligodendroglial component. The absence of an IDH mutation and partial 19q deletion excluded pure oligodendroglioma in this case. (B) Elevated proliferative activity (MIB-1 index) in the same case. (C) Prognostically relevant IDH1 R132H expression in a glioblastoma arising from a grade II astrocytoma seven years ago. The same case shows nuclear ATRX loss in tumor cells (D).

Some studies aimed to identify antigens to detect the tumor subpopulation with stem cell-like properties, i.e., the cells that have a marked capacity for proliferation, self-renewal, and differentiation. In glioblastoma, the most widely propagated marker for cancer stem cell ability is CD133 along with SOX2 and nestin [58]. However, recent studies indicate that CD133-negative tumor cells may also have stem cell abilities and that different subtypes associated with divergent molecular glioblastoma profiles, discussed below, may exist [59].

2.3. The genetic landscape

Like other tumors, GBM shows an accumulation of several epigenetic and genetic alterations in neoplastic cells within the brain. Recent data from the comprehensive multiplatform genomic characterization of GBM samples identified a number of common and diverging alterations and indicate that glioblastoma consists of biologically heterogeneous subgroups with similar histological appearances. The pilot project of The Cancer Genome Atlas Consortium in 2008 analyzed more than 20000 genes in 90 primary glioblastomas and identified the most common somatic genetic alterations/mutations: Tp53 (42% of the tumors mutated), PTEN (33%), NF1 (21%), EGFR (18%), RB1 (11%), and PI3K-pathway genes (7–10%) [60]. Interestingly, Tp53 mutations are found in almost all GBM with a giant cell component [61]. In addition, pediatric glioblastomas also show a high frequency of Tp53 mutations, as in up to 60% of tumors examined [62].

The most surprising finding was the discovery of isocitrate dehydrogenase (IDH) mutations that occurred in younger patients; these mutations are always heterozygous and are associated with an increase in OS [63, 64]. So far, several hotspot mutations were identified in the catalytic active centers in IDH1 R132, IDH2 R140, and R172 codons, and the most common, R132H, comprises over 80% of all mutations observed to date. The IDH1/2 mutations are present in 50–88% of the so-called secondary glioblastomas (the same point mutation is always present in lower grade precursor tumors, and in cases of a IDH1 R132C mutation, strongly associated with an astrocytoma phenotype). In contrast, IDH1 mutations are observed in only 3–7% of primary glioblastomas and gliosarcomas [54, 65]. In these tumors, IDH2 mutations are virtually absent, except for a single reported case. There is ongoing discussion of whether anaplastic astrocytomas that are IDH1/2 wild-type should be considered glioblastomas without vascular proliferation and/or necrosis because they show the same clinical course and also contain similar genomic alterations as primary GBM. Because IDH1 R132H also represents a tumor-specific antigen, immunotherapy trials currently aim at vaccination to induce antitumor immunoreactions [66].

The activation of receptor tyrosine kinases (RTKs) and the associated RAS/PI3K signaling pathway are common events in GBM. Approximately 45–50% of all primary GBM show high-level genomic amplification of epidermal growth factor receptor (EGFR). Among 30–50% of these amplified cases, intragenic rearrangements with the deletion of exons 2–7, the EGFRvIII variant is detected as a late event. The resulting overexpression leads to the constitutive activity of the receptor in the absence of its ligand and trigger the downstream pathways, resulting in increased cellular proliferation and radiation resistance of the tumor [67]. GBM with small cell morphology are often EGFRvIII-positive tumors [34]. Another important fact is that EGFR mutations in GBM significantly differ from those mutations found in other cancer types, such as non-small-cell lung cancer, where mutations are often located in the intracellular domain [26].

Like EGFR, other RTKs, such as PDGFR and MET, are often amplified in GBM. Platelet-derived growth factor receptor α amplification is significantly enriched for pontine tumors and the pediatric GBM cohort. These tumors are often grouped by the German Cancer Research Center (DKFZ) tumor methylation profiles as RTK class I tumors, while EGFR amplified tumors are classified as RTK-II tumors [68]. Approximately 40% of all PDGFR amplified tumors contain an intragenic deletion of exons 8 and 9 in PDGFRA, which induces an aggressive growth phenotype. Detailed cellular analysis in GBM samples showed that independent focal amplification of PDGFR α and EGFR could coexist in the same tumor [69].

Other common oncogenic alterations in GBM involve the extended PI3K-AKT-mTor and RAS-MAPK pathways. Mutations of the important primary negative regulator PTEN are found in up to 30% of GBM, and the RAS antagonist neurofibromin 1 (NF1) is mutated in 15% of all primary tumors. NF1 germline mutations result in neurofibromatosis type 1, and although rare in comparison to the prevalence of pilocytic astrocytoma, the occurrence of GBM in NF1 syndrome has been reported in a handful of cases [70]. The loss of NF1 is usually associated with concomitant Tp53 mutations, and the additional deletion of PTEN results in the progression of astrocytoma to GBM [48]. Interestingly, PTEN loss and subsequent PI3K-AKT pathway activation results in increased expression of the programmed death ligand-1 (PD-L1), which in turn contributes to GBM immunoresistance and immune escape [71]. Consequently, studies with immune-checkpoint inhibitor treatment in GBM are currently ongoing, although there are conflicting data on the prognostic role and predictive role of PD-L1 gene and protein expression in glioblastoma [72].

Up to 78% of GBMs show alterations of the retinoblastoma (Rb)/CDKN2A-p16^{ink4a} pathway [73]. This pathway plays a central role in proliferation and cell cycle regulation, and alterations include deletions and point mutations in several involved genes. Interestingly, the Rb promoter is far less methylated in primary GBM than in secondary GBM, consistent with the observation that the CDKN2A-p16^{ink4a} gene is affected by the commonly observed chromosomal 9q loss in primary GBM [74]. Although CDKN2A deletion is associated with tumor progression of astrocytomas to GBM and is one of the key molecular marker used to determine a "classical GBM," its prognostic role remains to be elucidated.

Mutations in the promoter region of the telomerase reverse transcriptase (TERT), the catalytic subunit of the telomerase complex, are found in 70–80% of GBM. Similar high frequencies in brain tumors are only observed in oligodendrogliomas [75]. The presence of a TERT mutation in IDH1/2 wild-type tumors is associated with poor outcome and indicates underdiagnosed glioblastoma in a small specimen with otherwise low-grade glioma [76]. TERT itself may also contribute to glioma genesis, as there is evidence that the TERT SNP genetic rs2736100 may influence glioma risk, although it is not a prognostic marker itself [77]. Glioblastomas that do not carry a TERT mutation were recently designated as "triple negative" tumors, i.e., lacking, IDH mutation, 1p/19q codeletion and TERT mutation, again highlighting the importance of these three markers for tumor stratification. TERT mutations are rare in pediatric glioblastomas, where whole exome sequencing recently identified H3F3A mutations, often combined with Tp53 and ATRX/DAXX alterations [78]. The H3F3A mutations are concentrated on two hotspots, K27M and G34V/R, which are mutually exclusive. Both show distinct clinicopathological tumor profiles. H3F3A K27M mutations alter the di- and tri-methylation state of endogenous histone H3 at the Lys27 position and are mainly found in pontine and thalamic tumors [79]. In contrast, the mainly supratentorially located H3F4A G34 mutant tumors presented as a histopathologically heterogeneous group of neoplasms, overlapping classical GBM with central nervous system primitive neuroectodermal tumors (CNS-PNET) [80]. There is growing evidence that G34 mutations may have an alternative mechanism to drive MCYN overexpression for tumor growth [68]. While K27M mutant tumors show a very unfavorable course, the three-year survival rate without this mutation in the pediatric cohort is approximately 70% [81]. Alpha-thalassemia C-linked mental retardation (ATRX) mutations are found in approximately 30% of pediatric GBM and in 6% of adult glioblastoma. Interestingly, in pediatric GBM, ATRX mutations occur around a hotspot near the carboxy-terminal helicase, while they are widely distributed across the gene in adult GBM [82].

ATRX and its binding partner DAXX (death-associated protein) belong to a complex with a role in regulating chromatin remodeling, nucleosome assembly and telomere maintenance. ATRX mutant tumors are associated with alternative lengthening of telomeres, the so-called ALT phenotype [78]. Because nuclear ATRX is diminished in tumors with the ALT phenotype, ATRX immunohistochemistry has become useful in identifying potential IDH mutants, H3F3A alterations or secondary GBM (usually showing ATRX loss and being mutually exclusive of LOH 1p/19q) [83]. Furthermore, retrospective analysis of ATRX in samples from the NOA-04 clinical trial showed a survival benefit of ATRX mutant tumors [84].

2.4. Epigenetics and molecular profiling

The DNA repair enzyme O-methylguanine-DNA methyltransferase (MGMT) removes alkyl groups from the O^6 position. Methylation of the MGMT promoter region results in decreased MGMT activity, which in turn results in decreased tumor resistance to alkylating agent therapy with TMZ, and is therefore a predictive molecular marker [36]. Usually, MGMT is determined in formalin-fixated paraffin-embedded specimens, and approximately 40% of all primary GBM carry a methylated promoter [18]. Less than 15% of gliosarcomas have a methylated phenotype [65]. In pediatric glioblastomas, approximately half of the tumors are methylated, mainly due to the association between H3F3A mutations and the methylated MGMT profile, but the prognostic and predictive role of MGMT methylation in children remains a matter of controversy [62, 68]. MGMT analysis is essential for almost all clinical studies and one of the most requested molecular analyses in routine neuropathology practice.

Unsupervised hierarchical clustering of GBM identified four tumor subclasses called proneural (characterized by mostly IDH/Tp53 mutations, PDGFRα amplifications, PI3K pathway dysregulation), classic (large-scale EGFR amplification, PTEN, and CDKN2A loss), mesenchymal (NF1, Tp53, and CDKN2A alterations), and neuronal (currently no specific genetic alterations). As expected from the IDH mutation data, the patients with a proneural tumor profile were younger and showed the best outcome [60]. The proneural group exhibited a robust hypermethylated glioma-CpG island methylator phenotype (G-CIMP) that is also present in most secondary GBM indicating a common gliomagenesis for IDH-mutated GBMs [85]. Glioma stratification according the IDH status therefore has widely replaced the previous clinic-based separation of primary and secondary GBM. Computational modeling to predict the temporal sequence of driver events during tumorigenesis indicates that most non-GCIMP mesenchymal GBMs arise from a PDGFA-driven proneural-like precursor though additional NF1 loss [86]. However, assignment with established glioblastoma subtype classifiers becomes difficult in cases with substantial tumor heterogeneity and may change further during patient treatment [73].

Glioblastoma intratumoral heterogeneity contributes to therapy resistance. This is exemplified in a whole genome sequencing report that showed not only extensive mutational and copy-number heterogeneity within the primary tumor but also uncovered the recurrence of a double-minute chromosome converging on the KIT/PDGFRA/PI3K/mTOR axis, superseding the IDH1 mutation in dominance in a mutually exclusive manner [87]. Despite targeted therapy with imatinib, the patient succumbed to progressive disease. Another good example is the recent discovery that EGFRvIII mutant cells are expressed only in a fraction of GBM cells of EGFR amplified tumors and enhance the proliferative activity of their neighboring EGFR wild-type tumor cells though cytokine secretion [88]. Because the majority of GBMs exhibit the activation of three or more RTKs, this highlights the need for the combined approach of several specific inhibitors for successful treatment.

Although there is increasing knowledge of divergent molecular alterations in histologically similarly appearing glioblastoma specimens, clinical decision-making on molecular alterations of glioblastoma subtypes is still limited. Notable exceptions include the determination of chromosomal allelic losses in 1p/19q in younger GBM patients, as such tumors respond far better to a combined Procarbazine-CCNU-Vincristine (PCV) therapy regimen [89]. The 1p/19q co-deletion is strongly associated with oligodendroglial tumor morphology and will become a diagnostic marker to be reassigned in future glioblastoma with this signature into the anaplastic oligodendroglioma group [26]. Up to 75% of co-deleted tumors also show either additional IDH1 or IDH2 mutations [90]. This combined molecular signature is so robust and remains visible in tumor recurrences, even in cases with increased intratumoral heterogeneity, and overlaps with "proneural" expression profile of the TCGA genomic landscape [91].

2.5. Conclusion

Glioblastomas have an extensive variety of histological appearances and divergent immunohistochemical and molecular profiles, making diagnosis somewhat difficult for those who are not familiar in working with brain tumors. The histological classification of diffuse gliomas based on the latest WHO grading scheme is a prerequisite to optimal decision-making regarding patient treatment. In addition to core features (microvascular proliferations, necrosis, and secondary structures of Scherer), the clinically relevant pattern and variants (gliosarcoma, giant cell glioblastoma, epithelioid, small cell GBM, and GBM with PNET component) should be clearly depicted in neuropathology reports. Immunohistochemistry and molecular biology have contributed to an improved classification and were shown in some cases to be of prognostic value. A panel of different antibodies is very helpful in securing the diagnosis and avoids potential differential diagnostic pitfalls. The advantages and limitations of the most commonly used antibodies, such as GFAP, WT1, MAP2, MIB-1, P53, IDH1R132H, and ATRX, in GBM have been outlined. The GBM subtype, patient's age, tumor location, and staining results subsequently guide a staged approach to therapeutically relevant molecular analysis, such as the 1p19q codeletion, MGMT promoter methylation, H3F3A screening, TERT promoter and IDH hotspot mutations. The classic concept of primary and secondary glioblastomas has been challenged by the discovery of clinically divergent molecular GBM cohorts, providing a good example of "convergent evolution showing a similar phenotype of genotypically different tumor cells" [92]. The implementation of these additional molecular markers into routine diagnoses has already started, including the routine determination of

MGMT gene promoter methylation status to guide therapy and the re-classification of tumors for appropriate treatment according to LOH1p/19q analysis, and it is expected to further evolve. The heterogenous landscape within and across GBMs underscores the difficulty in developing multimodal targeted therapies and is also a challenge to stratify patients for clinical trials. However, the recent identification of recurring driver mutations as illustrated here provides a rationale to identify tumor-specific peptides and antibody targets that may improve glioblastoma treatment.

Acknowledgements

The authors thank their colleagues at the Department of Neuropathology and Neurooncology for valuable feedback in discussion rounds.

Author details

Jens Schittenhelm[1,2*] and Marco Skardelly[1,2]

*Address all correspondence to: jens.schittenhelm@med.uni-tuebingen.de

1 Department of Neuropathology, Institute of Pathology and Neuropathology, Germany

2 Department of Neurosurgery, University Medical Clinic, University of Tübingen, Germany

References

[1] Ostrom QT, Gittleman H, Fulop J, Liu M, Blanda R, Kromer C, Wolinsky Y, Kruchko C, Barnholtz-Sloan JS. CBTRUS Statistical report: primary brain and central nervous system tumors diagnosed in the United States in 2008–2012. Neuro Oncol. 2015;17(Suppl. 4):iv1–iv62. DOI: 10.1093/neuonc/nov189

[2] Dandy W. Removal of right cerebral hemisphere for certain tumors with hemiplegia. JAMA 1928;90:823–825.

[3] Louis DN, Ohgaki H, Wiestler OD, Cavenee WK, editors. WHO Classification of Tumours of the Central Nervous system, 4th ed. Lyon: IARC Press; 2007.

[4] Burger PC, Scheithauer BW, editors. Tumors of the Central Nervous System. AFIP Atlas of Tumor Pathology Series 4. Washington, DC: ARP Press; 1994.

[5] Barnard RO, Geddes JF. The incidence of multifocal cerebral gliomas. A histologic study of large hemisphere sections. Cancer 1987;60:1519–1531. DOI: 10.1002/1097–0142(19871001)60:7<1519::AID-CNCR2820600719>3.0.CO;2-1

[6] Elena A, Melina C, Raffaele N, Carlo B, Vittoria N, Francesco A, Gaetano F, Marica E. Extraneural metastases in glioblastoma patients: two cases with YKL-40-positive glioblastomas and a meta-analysis of the literature. Neurosurg Rev. 2016;39:37–46. DOI: 10.1007/s10143-015-0656-9

[7] Ganslandt O, Stadlbauer A, Fahlbusch R, Kamada K, Buslei R, Blumcke I, Moser E, Nimsky C. Proton magnetic resonance spectroscopic imaging integrated into image-guided surgery: correlation to standard magnetic resonance imaging and tumor cell density. Neurosurgery 2005;56:291–298. DOI: 10.1227/01.NEU.0000156782.14538.78

[8] Burger PC, Dubois PJ, Schold SC, Smith KR, Odom GL, Crafts DC, Giangaspero F. Computerized tomographic and pathologic studies of the untreated, quiescent, and recurrent glioblastoma multiforme. J Neurosurg. 1983;58:159–169.

[9] Ohgaki H, Kleihues P. Population-based studies on incidence, survival rates, and genetic alterations in astrocytic and oligodendroglial gliomas. J Neuropathol Exp Neurol. 2005;64:479–489. DOI: 10.1093/jnen/64.6.479

[10] Kita D, Ciernik IF, Vaccarella S, Franceschi S, Kleihues P, Lütolf UM, Ohgaki H. Age as a predictive factor in glioblastomas: population-based study. Neuroepidemiology 2009;33:17–22. DOI: 10.1159/000210017

[11] Therkildsen C, Ladelund S, Rambech E, Persson A, Petersen A, Nilbert M. Glioblastomas, astrocytomas and oligodendrogliomas linked to Lynch syndrome. Eur J Neurol. 1995;22:717–724. DOI: 10.1111/ene.12647

[12] Ohgaki H, Kleihues P. Genetic pathways to primary and secondary glioblastoma. Am J Pathol. 2007;170:1445–1453. DOI: 10.2353/ajpath.2007.070011

[13] Marko NF, Weil RJ, Schroeder JL, Lang FF, Suki D, Sawaya RE. Extent of resection of glioblastoma revisited: personalized survival modeling facilitates more accurate survival prediction and supports a maximum-safe-resection approach to surgery. J Clin Oncol. 2014;32:774–782. DOI: 10.1200/JCO.2013.51.8886

[14] Hegi ME, Diserens AC, Gorlia T, Hamou MF, de Tribolet N, Weller M, Kros JM, Hainfellner JA, Mason W, Mariani L, Bromberg JE, Hau P, Mirimanoff RO, Cairncross JG, Janzer RC, Stupp R. MGMT gene silencing and benefit from temozolomide in glioblastoma. N Engl J Med. 2005;352:997-1003. DOI: 10.1056/NEJMoa043331

[15] Malmström A, Grønberg BH, Marosi C, Stupp R, Frappaz D, Schultz H, Abacioglu U, Tavelin B, Lhermitte B, Hegi ME, Rosell J, Henriksson R, Nordic Clinical Brain Tumour Study Group (NCBTSG). Temozolomide versus standard 6-week radiotherapy versus hypofractionated radiotherapy in patients older than 60 years with glioblastoma: the

Nordic randomised, phase 3 trial. Lancet Oncol. 2012;13:916–926. DOI: 10.1016/S1470-2045(12)70265-6

[16] Wick W, Platten M, Meisner C, Felsberg J, Tabatabai G, Simon M, Nikkhah G, Papsdorf K, Steinbach JP, Sabel M, Combs SE, Vesper J, Braun C, Meixensberger J, Ketter R, Mayer-Steinacker R, Reifenberger G, Weller M, NOA-08 Study Group of Neuro-oncology Working Group (NOA) of German Cancer Society. Temozolomide chemotherapy alone versus radiotherapy alone for malignant astrocytoma in the elderly: the NOA-08 randomised, phase 3 trial. Lancet Oncol. 2012;13:707–715. DOI: 10.1016/S1470-2045(12)70164-X

[17] Weller M, Tabatabai G, Kästner B, Felsberg J, Steinbach JP, Wick A, Schnell O, Hau P, Herrlinger U, Sabel MC, Wirsching HG, Ketter R, Bähr O, Platten M, Tonn JC, Schlegel U, Marosi C, Goldbrunner R, Stupp R, Homicsko K, Pichler J, Nikkhah G, Meixensberger J, Vajkoczy P, Kollias S, Hüsing J, Reifenberger G, Wick W, DIRECTOR Study Group. MGMT promoter methylation is a strong prognostic biomarker for benefit from dose-intensified temozolomide rechallenge in progressive glioblastoma: the DIRECTOR trial. Clin Cancer Res. 2015;21:2057–2064. DOI: 10.1158/1078-0432.CCR-14-2737

[18] Tabatabai G, Stupp R, van den Bent MJ, Hegi ME, Tonn JC, Wick W, Weller M. Molecular diagnostics of gliomas: the clinical perspective. Acta Neuropathol. 2010;120:585–592. DOI: 10.1007/s00401-010-0750-6

[19] Stupp R, Hegi ME, Mason WP, van den Bent MJ, Taphoorn MJ, Janzer RC, Ludwin SK, Allgeier A, Fisher B, Belanger K, Hau P, Brandes AA, Gijtenbeek J, Marosi C, Vecht CJ, Mokhtari K, Wesseling P, Villa S, Eisenhauer E, Gorlia T, Weller M, Lacombe D, Cairncross JG, Mirimanoff RO, European Organisation for Research and Treatment of Cancer Brain Tumour and Radiation Oncology Groups; National Cancer Institute of Canada Clinical Trials Group. Effects of radiotherapy with concomitant and adjuvant temozolomide versus radiotherapy alone on survival in glioblastoma in a randomised phase III study: 5-year analysis of the EORTC-NCIC trial. Lancet Oncol. 2009;10:459–466. DOI: 10.1016/S1470–2045(09)70025-7

[20] Marchini A, Bonifati S, Scott EM, Angelova AL, Rommelaere J. Oncolytic parvoviruses: from basic virology to clinical applications. Virol J. 2015;12:6. DOI: 10.1186/s12985-014-0223-y

[21] Swanson KD, Lok E, Wong ET. An overview of alternating electric fields therapy (NovoTTF Therapy) for the treatment of malignant glioma. Curr Neurol Neurosci Rep. 2016;16:8. DOI: 10.1007/s11910-015-0606-5

[22] Legendre C, Garcion E. Iron metabolism: a double-edged sword in the resistance of glioblastoma to therapies. Trends Endocrinol Metab. 2015;26:322–331. DOI: 10.1016/j.tem.2015.03.008

[23] Ellis HP, Greenslade M, Powell B, Spiteri I, Sottoriva A, Kurian KM. Current challenges in glioblastoma: intratumour heterogeneity, residual disease, and models to predict disease recurrence. Front Oncol. 2015;5:251. DOI: 10.3389/fonc.2015.00251

[24] Sundar SJ, Hsieh JK, Manjila S, Lathia JD, Sloan A. The role of cancer stem cells in glioblastoma. Neurosurg Focus 2014;37:E6. DOI: 10.3171/2014.9.FOCUS14494

[25] Schittenhelm J. Diagnostic Evaluation of Diffuse Gliomas, Advances in the Biology, Imaging and Therapies for Glioblastoma, Prof. Clark Chen (Ed.). Rijeka: InTech; 2011. DOI: 10.5772/24225

[26] Aldape K, Zadeh G, Mansouri S, Reifenberger G, von Deimling A. Glioblastoma: pathology, molecular mechanisms and markers. Acta Neuropathol. 2015;129:829–848. DOI: 10.1007/s00401-015-1432-1

[27] Brat DJ, Castellano-Sanchez AA, Hunter SB, Pecot M, Cohen C, Hammond EH, Devi SN, Kaur B, Van Meir EG. Pseudopalisades in glioblastoma are hypoxic, express extracellular matrix proteases, and are formed by an actively migrating cell population. Cancer Res. 2004;64:920–927.

[28] Plate KH. Mechanisms of angiogenesis in the brain. J Neuropathol Exp Neurol. 1999;58:313–320. DOI: 10.1097/00005072-199904000-00001

[29] Scherer HJ. Structural development in gliomas. Am J Cancer 1938;34:333–351.

[30] Palma L, Celli P, Maleci A, Di Lorenzo N, Cantore G. Malignant monstrocellular brain tumours. A study of 42 surgically treated cases. Acta Neurochir (Wien) 1989;97:17–25.

[31] Ortega A, Nuño M, Walia S, Mukherjee D, Black KL, Patil CG. Treatment and survival of patients harboring histological variants of glioblastoma. J Clin Neurosci. 2014;21:1709–1713. DOI: 10.1016/j.jocn.2014.05.003

[32] Rodriguez FJ, Scheithauer BW, Giannini C, Bryant SC, Jenkins RB. Epithelial and pseudoepithelial differentiation in glioblastoma and gliosarcoma: a comparative morphologic and molecular genetic study. Cancer 2008;113:2779–2789. DOI: 10.1002/cncr.23899

[33] Fuller GN, Goodman JC, Vogel H, Ghorbani R. Epithelioid glioblastoma: a distinct clinicopathologic entity. J Neuropathol Exp Neurol. 1998;57:501. DOI: 10.1097/00005072-199805000-00145

[34] Perry A, Aldape KD, George DH, Burger PC. Small cell astrocytoma: an aggressive variant that is clinicopathologically and genetically distinct from anaplastic oligodendroglioma. Cancer 2004;101:2318–2326. DOI: 10.1002/cncr.20625

[35] Perry A, Miller CR, Gujrati M, Scheithauer BW, Zambrano SC, Jost SC, Raghavan R, Qian J, Cochran EJ, Huse JT, Holland EC, Burger PC, Rosenblum MK. Malignant gliomas with primitive neuroectodermal tumor-like components: a clinicopathologic

and genetic study of 53 cases. Brain Pathol. 2009;19:81–90. DOI: 10.1111/j.1750-3639.2008.00167.x

[36] Hegi ME, Janzer RC, Lambiv WL, Gorlia T, Kouwenhoven MC, Hartmann C, von Deimling A, Martinet D, Besuchet Schmutz N, Diserens AC, Hamou MF, Bady P, Weller M, van den Bent MJ, Mason WP, Mirimanoff RO, Stupp R, Mokhtari K, Wesseling P, European Organisation for Research and Treatment of Cancer Brain Tumour and Radiation Oncology Groups; National Cancer Institute of Canada Clinical Trials Group. Presence of an oligodendroglioma-like component in newly diagnosed glioblastoma identifies a pathogenetically heterogeneous subgroup and lacks prognostic value: central pathology review of the EORTC_26981/NCIC_CE.3 trial. Acta Neuropathol. 2012;123:841–852. DOI: 10.1007/s00401-011-0938-4

[37] Rickert CH, Riemenschneider MJ, Schachenmayr W, Richter HP, Bockhorn J, Reifenberger G, Paulus W. Glioblastoma with adipocyte-like tumor cell differentiation--histological and molecular features of a rare differentiation pattern. Brain Pathol. 2009;19:431–438. DOI: 10.1111/j.1750-3639.2008.00199.x

[38] Kepes JJ, Rubinstein LJ. Malignant gliomas with heavily lipidized (foamy) tumor cells: a report of three cases with immunoperoxidase study. Cancer 1981;47:2451–2459.

[39] Schittenhelm J, Psaras T. Glioblastoma with granular cell astrocytoma features: a case report and literature review. Clin Neuropathol. 2010;29:323–329.

[40] Schittenhelm J, Erdmann T, Maennlin S, Will BE, Beschorner R, Bornemann A, Meyermann R, Mittelbronn M. Gliosarcoma with chondroid and osseous differentiation. Neuropathology 2007;27:90–94. DOI: 10.1111/j.1440-1789.2006.00747.x

[41] Jaiswal S, Agrawal V, Vij M, Sahu RN, Jaiswal AK, Behari S. Glioblastoma with melanotic differentiation. Clin Neuropathol. 2010;29:330–333. DOI: 10.1002/1097-0142(19810515)47:10<2451::AID-CNCR2820471024>3.0.CO;2–5

[42] Kleinschmidt-De Masters BK, Alassiri AH, Birks DK, Newell KL, Moore W, Lillehei KO. Epithelioid versus rhabdoid glioblastomas are distinguished by monosomy 22 and immunohistochemical expression of INI-1 but not claudin 6. Am J Surg Pathol. 2010;34:341–354. DOI: 10.1097/PAS.0b013e3181ce107b

[43] Waidelich J, Schittenhelm J, Allmendinger O, Meyermann R, Beschorner R. Glutamate transporters in diagnostic neurooncology. Brain Pathology 2010;20(Suppl. 1):1–99.

[44] Blümcke I, Müller S, Buslei R, Riederer BM, Wiestler OD. Microtubule-associated protein-2 immunoreactivity: a useful tool in the differential diagnosis of low-grade neuroepithelial tumors. Acta Neuropathol. 2004;108:89–96. DOI: 10.1007/s00401-004-0873-8

[45] Schittenhelm J, Beschorner R, Simon P, Tabatabai G, Herrmann C, Schlaszus H, Capper D, Weller M, Meyermann R, Mittelbronn M. Diagnostic value of WT1 in neuroepithelial

tumours. Neuropathol Appl Neurobiol. 2009;35:69–81. DOI: 10.1111/j.1365-2990.2008.00957.x

[46] Hasselblatt M, Paulus W. Sensitivity and specificity of epithelial membrane antigen staining patterns in ependymomas. Acta Neuropathol. 2003;106:385–388. DOI: 10.1007/s00401-003-0752-8

[47] Ogura R, Tsukamoto Y, Natsumeda M, Isogawa M, Aoki H, Kobayashi T, Yoshida S, Okamoto K, Takahashi H, Fujii Y, Kakita A. Immunohistochemical profiles of IDH1, MGMT and P53: practical significance for prognostication of patients with diffuse gliomas. Neuropathology 2015;35:324–335. DOI: 10.1111/neup.12196

[48] Kwon CH, Zhao D, Chen J, Alcantara S, Li Y, Burns DK, Mason RP, Lee EY, Wu H, Parada LF. Pten haploinsufficiency accelerates formation of high-grade astrocytomas. Cancer Res. 2008;68:3286–3294. DOI: 10.1158/0008-5472.CAN-07-6867

[49] Weller M, Felsberg J, Hartmann C, Berger H, Steinbach JP, Schramm J, Westphal M, Schackert G, Simon M, Tonn JC, Heese O, Krex D, Nikkhah G, Pietsch T, Wiestler O, Reifenberger G, von Deimling A, Loeffler M. Molecular predictors of progression-free and overall survival in patients with newly diagnosed glioblastoma: a prospective translational study of the German Glioma Network. J Clin Oncol. 2009;27:5743–5750. DOI: 10.1200/JCO.2009.23.0805

[50] Preusser M, Charles Janzer R, Felsberg J, Reifenberger G, Hamou MF, Diserens AC, Stupp R, Gorlia T, Marosi C, Heinzl H, Hainfellner JA, Hegi M. Anti-O6-methylguanine-methyltransferase (MGMT) immunohistochemistry in glioblastoma multiforme: observer variability and lack of association with patient survival impede its use as clinical biomarker. Brain Pathol. 2008;18:520–532. DOI: 10.1111/j.1750-3639.2008.00153.x

[51] Dang L, White DW, Gross S, Bennett BD, Bittinger MA, Driggers EM, Fantin VR, Jang HG, Jin S, Keenan MC, Marks KM, Prins RM, Ward PS, Yen KE, Liau LM, Rabinowitz JD, Cantley LC, Thompson CB, Van der Heiden MG, Su SM. Cancer-associated IDH1 mutations produce 2-hydroxyglutarate. Nature 2010;462(7273):739–744.

[52] Nobusawa S, Watanabe T, Kleihues P, Ohgaki H. IDH1 mutations as molecular signature and predictive factor of secondary glioblastomas. Clin Cancer Res. 2009;15:6002–6007. DOI: 10.1158/1078–0432.CCR-09-0715

[53] Sanson M, Marie Y, Paris S, Idbaih A, Laffaire J, Ducray F, El Hallani S, Boisselier B, Mokhtari K, Hoang-Xuan K, Delattre JY. Isocitrate dehydrogenase 1 codon 132 mutation is an important prognostic biomarker in gliomas. J Clin Oncol. 2009;27:4150–4154. DOI: 10.1200/JCO.2009.21.9832

[54] Hartmann C, Hentschel B, Wick W, Capper D, Felsberg J, Simon M, Westphal M, Schackert G, Meyermann R, Pietsch T, Reifenberger G, Weller M, Loeffler M, von Deimling A. Patients with IDH1 wild type anaplastic astrocytomas exhibit worse prognosis than IDH1-mutated glioblastomas, and IDH1 mutation status accounts for

the unfavorable prognostic effect of higher age: implications for classification of gliomas. Acta Neuropathol. 2010;120:707–718. DOI: 10.1007/s00401-010-0781-z

[55] Capper D, Weissert S, Balss J, Habel A, Meyer J, Jäger D, Ackermann U, Tessmer C, Korshunov A, Zentgraf H, Hartmann C, von Deimling A. Characterization of R132H mutation-specific IDH1 antibody binding in brain tumors. Brain Pathol. 2010;20:245–254. DOI: 10.1111/j.1750-3639.2009.00352.x

[56] Wiestler B, Claus R, Hartlieb SA, Schliesser MG, Weiss EK, Hielscher T, Platten M, Dittmann LM, Meisner C, Felsberg J, Happold C, Simon M, Nikkhah G, Papsdorf K, Steinbach JP, Sabel M, Grimm C, Weichenhan D, Tews B, Reifenberger G, Capper D, Müller W, Plass C, Weller M, Wick W, Neuro-oncology Working Group (NOA) of the German Cancer Society. Malignant astrocytomas of elderly patients lack favorable molecular markers: an analysis of the NOA-08 study collective. Neuro Oncol. 2013;15:1017–1026. DOI: 10.1093/neuonc/not043

[57] Skardelly M, Brendle E, Noell S, Behling F, Wuttke TV, Schittenhelm J, Bisdas S, Meisner C, Rona S, Tatagiba MS, Tabatabai G. Predictors of preoperative and early postoperative seizures in patients with intra-axial primary and metastatic brain tumors: a retrospective observational single center study. Ann Neurol. 2015;78:917–928. DOI: 10.1002/ana.24522

[58] Singh SK, Clarke ID, Terasaki M, Bonn VE, Hawkins C, Squire J, Dirks PB. Identification of a cancer stem cell in human brain tumors. Cancer Res. 2003;63:5821–5828.

[59] Stopschinski BE, Beier CP, Beier D. Glioblastoma cancer stem cells—from concept to clinical application. Cancer Lett. 2013;338:32–40. DOI: 10.1016/j.canlet.2012.05.033

[60] Verhaak RG, Hoadley KA, Purdom E, Wang V, Qi Y, Wilkerson MD, Miller CR, Ding L, Golub T, Mesirov JP, Alexe G, Lawrence M, O'Kelly M, Tamayo P, Weir BA, Gabriel S, Winckler W, Gupta S, Jakkula L, Feiler HS, Hodgson JG, James CD, Sarkaria JN, Brennan C, Kahn A, Spellman PT, Wilson RK, Speed TP, Gray JW, Meyerson M, Getz G, Perou CM, Hayes DN, Cancer Genome Atlas Research Network. Integrated genomic analysis identifies clinically relevant subtypes of glioblastoma characterized by abnormalities in PDGFRA, IDH1, EGFR, and NF1. Cancer Cell 2010;17:98–111. DOI: 10.1016/j.ccr.2009

[61] Srivastava A, Jain A, Jha P, Suri V, Sharma MC, Mallick S, Puri T, Gupta DK, Gupta A, Sarkar C. MGMT gene promoter methylation in pediatric glioblastomas. Childs Nerv Syst. 2010;26:1613–1618. DOI: 10.1007/s00381-010-1214-y

[62] Meyer-Puttlitz B, Hayashi Y, Waha A, Rollbrocker B, Boström J, Wiestler OD, Louis DN, Reifenberger G, von Deimling A. Molecular genetic analysis of giant cell glioblastomas. Am J Pathol. 1997;151:853–857.

[63] Parsons DW, Jones S, Zhang X, Lin JC, Leary RJ, Angenendt P, Mankoo P, Carter H, Siu IM, Gallia GL, Olivi A, Mc Lendon R, Rasheed BA, Keir S, Nikolskaya T, Nikolsky Y, Busam DA, Tekleab H, Diaz LAJr, Hartigan J, Smith DR, Strausberg RL, Marie SK,

Shinjo SM, Yan H, Riggins GJ, Bigner DD, Karchin R, Papadopoulos N, Parmigiani G, Vogelstein B, Velculescu VE, Kinzler KW. An integrated genomic analysis of human glioblastoma multiforme. Science 2008;321:1807–1812. DOI: 10.1126/science.1164382

[64] Yan H, Parsons DW, Jin G, Mc Lendon R, Rasheed BA, Yuan W, Kos I, Batinic-Haberle I, Jones S, Riggins GJ, Friedman H, Friedman A, Reardon D, Herndon J, Kinzler KW, Velculescu VE, Vogelstein B, Bigner DD. IDH1 and IDH2 mutations in gliomas. N Engl J Med. 2009;360:765–773. DOI: 10.1056/NEJMoa0808710

[65] Lee D, Kang SY, Suh YL, Jeong JY, Lee JI, Nam DH. Clinicopathologic and genomic features of gliosarcomas. J Neurooncol. 2012;107:643–650.

[66] Schumacher T, Bunse L, Pusch S, Sahm F, Wiestler B, Quandt J, Menn O, Osswald M, Oezen I, Ott M, Keil M, BalßJ, Rauschenbach K, Grabowska AK, Vogler I, Diekmann J, Trautwein N, Eichmüller SB, Okun J, StevanovićS, Riemer AB, Sahin U, Friese MA, Beckhove P, von Deimling A, Wick W, Platten M. A vaccine targeting mutant IDH1 induces antitumour immunity. Nature 2014;512:324–327. DOI: 10.1038/nature13387

[67] Hatanpaa KJ, Burma S, Zhao D, Habib AA. Epidermal growth factor receptor in glioma: signal transduction, neuropathology, imaging, and radioresistance. Neoplasia 2010;12:675–684.

[68] Sturm D, Bender S, Jones DT, Lichter P, Grill J, Becher O, Hawkins C, Majewski J, Jones C, Costello JF, Iavarone A, Aldape K, Brennan CW, Jabado N, Pfister SM. Paediatric and adult glioblastoma: multiform (epi)genomic culprits emerge. Nat Rev Cancer 2014;14:92–107. DOI: 10.1038/nrc3655

[69] Szerlip NJ, Pedraza A, Chakravarty D, Azim M, Mc Guire J, Fang Y, Ozawa T, Holland EC, Huse JT, Jhanwar S, Leversha MA, Mikkelsen T, Brennan CW. Intratumoral heterogeneity of receptor tyrosine kinases EGFR and PDGFRA amplification in glioblastoma defines subpopulations with distinct growth factor response. Proc Natl Acad Sci U S A 2012;109:3041–3046. DOI: 10.1073/pnas.1114033109

[70] Jeong TS, Yee GT. Glioblastoma in a patient with neurofibromatosis type 1: a case report and review of the literature. Brain Tumor Res Treat. 2014;2:36–38. DOI: 10.14791/btrt.2014.2.1.36

[71] Parsa AT, Waldron JS, Panner A, Crane CA, Parney IF, Barry JJ, Cachola KE, Murray JC, Tihan T, Jensen MC, Mischel PS, Stokoe D, Pieper RO. Loss of tumor suppressor PTEN function increases B7-H1 expression and immunoresistance in glioma. Nat Med. 2007;13:84–88. DOI: 10.1038/nm1517

[72] Preusser M, Berghoff AS, Wick W, Weller M. Clinical Neuropathology mini-review 6-2015: PD-L1: emerging biomarker in glioblastoma? Clin Neuropathol. 2015;34:313–321.

[73] Patel AP, Tirosh I, Trombetta JJ, Shalek AK, Gillespie SM, Wakimoto H, Cahill DP, Nahed BV, Curry WT, Martuza RL, Louis DN, Rozenblatt-Rosen O, SuvàML, Regev A,

Bernstein BE. Single-cell RNA-seq highlights intratumoral heterogeneity in primary glioblastoma. Science 2014;344:1396–1401. DOI: 10.1126/science.1254257

[74] Appin CL, Brat DJ. Molecular genetics of gliomas. Cancer J. 2014;20:66–72. DOI: 10.1097/PPO.0000000000000020

[75] Koelsche C, Sahm F, Capper D, Reuss D, Sturm D, Jones DT, Kool M, Northcott PA, Wiestler B, Böhmer K, Meyer J, Mawrin C, Hartmann C, Mittelbronn M, Platten M, Brokinkel B, Seiz M, Herold-Mende C, Unterberg A, Schittenhelm J, Weller M, Pfister S, Wick W, Korshunov A, von Deimling A. Distribution of TERT promoter mutations in pediatric and adult tumors of the nervous system. Acta Neuropathol. 2013;126:907–915. DOI: 10.1007/s00401-013-1195-5

[76] Labussière M, Boisselier B, Mokhtari K, Di Stefano AL, Rahimian A, Rossetto M, Ciccarino P, Saulnier O, Paterra R, Marie Y, Finocchiaro G, Sanson M. Combined analysis of TERT, EGFR, and IDH status defines distinct prognostic glioblastoma classes. Neurology 2014;83:1200–1206. DOI: 10.1212/WNL

[77] Mosrati MA, Malmström A, Lysiak M, Krysztofiak A, Hallbeck M, Milos P, Hallbeck AL, Bratthäll C, Strandéus M, Stenmark-Askmalm M, Söderkvist P. TERT promoter mutations and polymorphisms as prognostic factors in primary glioblastoma. Oncotarget 2015;6:16663–166673. DOI: 10.18632/oncotarget.4389

[78] Schwartzentruber J, Korshunov A, Liu XY, Jones DT, Pfaff E, Jacob K, Sturm D, Fontebasso AM, Quang DA, Tönjes M, Hovestadt V, Albrecht S, Kool M, Nantel A, Konermann C, Lindroth A, Jäger N, Rausch T, Ryzhova M, Korbel JO, Hielscher T, Hauser P, Garami M, Klekner A, Bognar L, Ebinger M, Schuhmann MU, Scheurlen W, Pekrun A, Frühwald MC, Roggendorf W, Kramm C, Dürken M, Atkinson J, Lepage P, Montpetit A, Zakrzewska M, Zakrzewski K, Liberski PP, Dong Z, Siegel P, Kulozik AE, Zapatka M, Guha A, Malkin D, Felsberg J, Reifenberger G, von Deimling A, Ichimura K, Collins VP, Witt H, Milde T, Witt O, Zhang C, Castelo-Branco P, Lichter P, Faury D, Tabori U, Plass C, Majewski J, Pfister SM, Jabado N. Driver mutations in histone H3.3 and chromatin remodelling genes in paediatric glioblastoma. Nature 2012;482:226–231. DOI: 10.1038/nature10833

[79] Chan KM, Han J, Fang D, Gan H, Zhang Z. A lesson learned from the H3.3K27M mutation found in pediatric glioma: a new approach to the study of the function of histone modifications in vivo? Cell Cycle 2013;12:2546–2552. DOI: 10.4161/cc.25625

[80] Korshunov A, Capper D, Reuss D, Schrimpf D, Ryzhova M, Hovestadt V, Sturm D, Meyer J, Jones C, Zheludkova O, Kumirova E, Golanov A, Kool M, Schüller U, Mittelbronn M, Hasselblatt M, Schittenhelm J, Reifenberger G, Herold-Mende C, Lichter P, von Deimling A, Pfister SM, Jones DT. Histologically distinct neuroepithelial tumors with histone 3 G34 mutation are molecularly similar and comprise a single nosologic entity. Acta Neuropathol. 2016; 131: 137-146. DOI: 10.1007/s00401-015-1493-1

[81] Korshunov A, Ryzhova M, Hovestadt V, Bender S, Sturm D, Capper D, Meyer J, Schrimpf D, Kool M, Northcott PA, Zheludkova O, Milde T, Witt O, Kulozik AE,

Reifenberger G, Jabado N, Perry A, Lichter P, von Deimling A, Pfister SM, Jones DT. Integrated analysis of pediatric glioblastoma reveals a subset of biologically favorable tumors with associated molecular prognostic markers. Acta Neuropathol. 2015;129:669–678. DOI: 10.1007/s00401-015-1405-4

[82] Jiao Y, Killela PJ, Reitman ZJ, Rasheed AB, Heaphy CM, de Wilde RF, Rodriguez FJ, Rosemberg S, Oba-Shinjo SM, Nagahashi Marie SK, Bettegowda C, Agrawal N, Lipp E, Pirozzi C, Lopez G, He Y, Friedman H, Friedman AH, Riggins GJ, Holdhoff M, Burger P, Mc Lendon R, Bigner DD, Vogelstein B, Meeker AK, Kinzler KW, Papadopoulos N, Diaz LA, Yan H. Frequent ATRX, CIC, FUBP1 and IDH1 mutations refine the classification of malignant gliomas. Oncotarget 2012;3:709–722. DOI: 10.18632/oncotarget.588

[83] Reuss DE, Sahm F, Schrimpf D, Wiestler B, Capper D, Koelsche C, Schweizer L, Korshunov A, Jones DT, Hovestadt V, Mittelbronn M, Schittenhelm J, Herold-Mende C, Unterberg A, Platten M, Weller M, Wick W, Pfister SM, von Deimling A. ATRX and IDH1-R132H immunohistochemistry with subsequent copy number analysis and IDH sequencing as a basis for an "integrated" diagnostic approach for adult astrocytoma, oligodendroglioma and glioblastoma. Acta Neuropathol. 2015;129:133–146. DOI: 10.1007/s00401-014-1370-3

[84] Wiestler B, Capper D, Holland-Letz T, Korshunov A, von Deimling A, Pfister SM, Platten M, Weller M, Wick W. ATRX loss refines the classification of anaplastic gliomas and identifies a subgroup of IDH mutant astrocytic tumors with better prognosis. Acta Neuropathol. 2013;126:443–451. DOI: 10.1007/s00401-013-1156-z

[85] Noushmehr H, Weisenberger DJ, Diefes K, Phillips HS, Pujara K, Berman BP, Pan F, Pelloski CE, Sulman EP, Bhat KP, Verhaak RG, Hoadley KA, Hayes DN, Perou CM, Schmidt HK, Ding L, Wilson RK, Van Den Berg D, Shen H, Bengtsson H, Neuvial P, Cope LM, Buckley J, Herman JG, Baylin SB, Laird PW, Aldape K, Network Cancer Genome Atlas Research. Identification of a CpG island methylator phenotype that defines a distinct subgroup of glioma. Cancer Cell 2010;17:510–522. DOI: 10.1016/j.ccr.2010.03.017

[86] Ozawa T, Riester M, Cheng YK, Huse JT, Squatrito M, Helmy K, Charles N, Michor F, Holland EC. Most human non-GCIMP glioblastoma subtypes evolve from a common proneural-like precursor glioma. Cancer Cell 2014;26:288–300. DOI: 10.1016/j.ccr.2014.06.005

[87] Favero F, Mc Granahan N, Salm M, Birkbak NJ, Sanborn JZ, Benz SC, Becq J, Peden JF, Kingsbury Z, Grocok RJ, Humphray S, Bentley D, Spencer-Dene B, Gutteridge A, Brada M, Roger S, Dietrich PY, Forshew T, Gerlinger M, Rowan A, Stamp G, Eklund AC, Szallasi Z, Swanton C. Glioblastoma adaptation traced through decline of an IDH1 clonal driver and macro-evolution of a double-minute chromosome. Ann Oncol. 2015;26:880–887. DOI: 10.1093/annonc/mdv127

[88] Inda MM, Bonavia R, Mukasa A, Narita Y, Sah DW, Van den berg S, Brennan C, Johns TG, Bachoo R, Hadwiger P, Tan P, Depinho RA, Cavenee W, Furnari F. Tumor

heterogeneity is an active process maintained by a mutant EGFR-induced cytokine circuit in glioblastoma. Genes Dev. 2010;24:1731–1745. DOI: 10.1101/gad.1890510

[89] Cairncross G, Wang M, Shaw E, Jenkins R, Brachman D, Buckner J, Fink K, Souhami L, Laperriere N, Curran W, Mehta M. Phase III trial of chemoradiotherapy for anaplastic oligodendroglioma: long-term results of RTOG 9402. J Clin Oncol. 2013;31:337–343. DOI: 10.1200/JCO.2012.43.2674

[90] Kim YH, Nobusawa S, Mittelbronn M, Paulus W, Brokinkel B, Keyvani K, Sure U, Wrede K, Nakazato Y, Tanaka Y, Vital A, Mariani L, Stawski R, Watanabe T, De Girolami U, Kleihues P, Ohgaki H. Molecular classification of low-grade diffuse gliomas. Am J Pathol. 2010;177:2708–2714. DOI: 10.2353/ajpath.2010.100680

[91] Riemenschneider MJ, Jeuken JW, Wesseling P, Reifenberger G. Molecular diagnostics of gliomas: state of the art. Acta Neuropathol. 2010;120:567–584. DOI: 10.1007/s00401-010-0736-4

[92] Basanta D, Scott JG, Rockne R, Swanson KR, Anderson AR. The role of IDH1 mutated tumour cells in secondary glioblastomas: an evolutionary game theoretical view. Phys Biol. 2011;8:015016. DOI 10.1088/1478-3975/8/1/015016

4

Molecular Imaging of Brain Tumors

W. Phillip Law

Abstract

This chapter is a review of the most common radiotracers currently used in clinical brain tumour imaging, and an update of future potentially useful radiotracers for imaging brain tumours with positron emission tomography (PET). It will focus mainly on glioma —the most common type of primary brain tumour—and intracranial metastases, as the cause of the majority of morbidity and mortality in neurooncology. Emerging data support the use of somatostatin analogue PET in the treatment planning and surveillance of meningiomas. There is currently a limited role of PET in other non-glial brain neoplasms including neuronal tumours, pineal and pituitary tumours, germ cell tumours and embryonal tumours (PNET, neuroblastoma). Finally, the newest hybrid imaging modality of PET/MRI and the promise it holds for obtaining state-of-the-art structural and functional imaging data simultaneously, are concisely reviewed.

Keywords: PET, molecular imaging, brain tumour, neurooncology, radiotracer

1. Introduction

Structural imaging using contrast-enhanced computed tomography (CT) and magnetic resonance imaging (MRI) is crucial for the initial detection and diagnosis of brain tumours. However, it has limitations in post-treatment surveillance where tumour- and therapy-related changes can appear similarly. Molecular imaging with positron emission tomography (PET) provides additional information that can better delineate tumour extent and burden, for example fluorodeoxyglucose (FDG) depicts the metabolic activity and fluroethyltyrosine (FET) and fluorodihydroxyphenylalanine (FDOPA) depict the amino acid turnover of otherwise nonspecific soft tissue changes on CT and MRI. This could ultimately improve clinical decision-making and anatomical targeting of tumour for biopsy, radiotherapy or surgery.

2. Brain tumour types

Brain tumours affect approximately 5–10 persons per 100,000 populations. In adults, about half of all brain neoplasms are primary tumours and the other half are metastatic. In childhood, brain neoplasms account for up to 20% of all cancers. Seventy percentage of childhood brain tumours arise from the posterior cranial fossa, whereas in adults, a similar proportion arises above the tentorium [1].

Intracranial tumours may spread directly to adjacent structures, along white matter tracts, or through the cerebrospinal fluid (CSF) spaces. It is rare for brain malignancy to metastasise to other parts of the body.

The most widely accepted system for classifying brain tumours is the World Health Organisation (WHO) classification of tumours of the central nervous system (CNS), which is based on the histological characteristics of the tumour. The latest revision was published in 2007 [2].

2.1. Gliomas

Gliomas are tumours of glial cells and include astrocytomas, oligodendrogliomas and ependymomas. Unlike most neurons, glial cells retain the ability to undergo cell division in the adult CNS. Since carcinogenesis is related to the sequential accumulation of genetic aberrations through cell division, it is not surprising that gliomas are the most common primary brain malignancy and account for about half of all adult brain tumours. The WHO classification of CNS tumours additionally classifies gliomas into Grade I to IV depending on the degree of tumour histological differentiation (**Table 1**).

	I	II	III	IV		I	II	III	IV
Astrocytic tumours									
Subependymal giant cell astrocytoma	•				Central neurocytoma		•		
Pilocytic astrocytoma	•				Extraventricular neurocytoma		•		
Pilomyxoid astrocytoma		•			Cerebellar liponeurocytoma		•		
Diffuse astrocytoma		•			Paraganglioma of the spinal cord	•			
Pleomorphic xanthoastrocytoma		•			Papillary glioneuronal tumour	•			
Anaplastic astrocytoma			•		Rosette-forming glioneuronal tumour of the fourth ventricle	•			
Glioblastoma				•					
Giant cell glioblastoma				•					
Gliosarcoma				•	**Pineal tumours**				
					Pineocytoma	•			
Oligodendroglial tumours					Pineal parenchymal tumour of intermediate differentiation		•	•	
Oligodendroglioma		•			Pineoblastoma				•
Anaplastic oligodendroglioma			•		Papillary tumour of the pineal region		•	•	
Oligoastrocytic tumours									
Oligoastrocytoma		•			**Embryonal tumours**				
Anaplastic oligoastrocytoma			•		Medulloblastoma				•
					CNS primitive neuroectodermal tumour (PNET)				•
Ependymal tumours					Atypical teratoid / rhabdoid tumour				•
Subependymoma	•								
Myxopapillary ependymoma	•				**Tumours of the cranial and paraspinal nerves**				
Ependymoma		•			Schwannoma	•			

	I	II	III	IV		I	II	III	IV
Anaplastic ependymoma			•		Neurofibroma	•			
					Perineurioma	•	•	•	
Choroid plexus tumours					Malignant peripheral nerve sheath tumour (MPNST)		•	•	•
Choroid plexus papilloma	•								
Atypical choroid plexus papilloma		•			**Meningeal tumours**				
Choroid plexus carcinoma			•		Meningioma	•			
					Atypical meningioma		•		
Other neuroepithelial tumours					Anaplastic/malignant meningioma			•	
Angiocentric glioma	•				Haemangiopericytoma		•		
Chordoid glioma of the third ventricle		•			Anaplastic haemangiopericytoma			•	
					Haemangioblastoma	•			
Neuronal and mixed neuronal-glial tumours									
Gangliocytoma	•				**Tumours of the sellar region**				
Ganglioglioma	•				Craniopharyngioma	•			
Anaplastic ganglioglioma			•		Granular cell tumour of the neurohypophysis	•			
Desmoplastic infantile astrocytoma and ganglioglioma	•				Pituicytoma	•			
Dysembryoplastic neuroepithelial tumour	•				Spindle cell oncocytoma of the adenohypophysis	•			

Table 1. WHO grading of tumours of the CNS.

2.2. Brain metastases

The most common primary malignancies that metastasise to the brain are carcinomas of the lung, breast and melanoma [3]. The meninges are also a frequent site of metastatic disease involvement.

The following sections on molecular imaging with PET radiotracers will focus on gliomas and intracranial metastases as the cause of the majority of morbidity and mortality in neurooncology.

3. Fluorodeoxyglucose

3.1. Tumour detection

F-18 FDG is an analogue of glucose (**Figure 1**). Its active transport into the cell is mediated by a group of structurally related glucose transport proteins (GLUT) and once intracellular, FDG

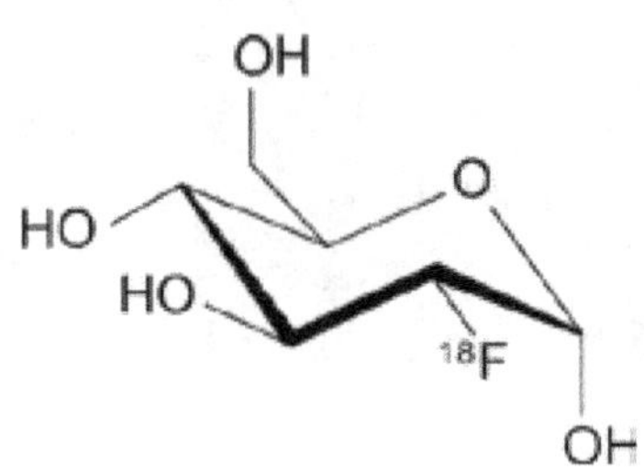

Figure 1. Chemical structure of F-18 fluorodeoxyglucose.

is phosphorylated by the enzyme hexokinase as the first step towards glycolysis. However, unlike glucose, once phosphorylated FDG-6-phosphate cannot continue along the glycolytic pathway and effectively becomes trapped intracellularly. FDG uptake in PET is thus an indication of the metabolic activity of the structure in which it is being taken up. Most malignant cells are metabolically active and demonstrate an increased expression of glucose transport proteins, particularly GLUT-1 and GLUT-3, as well as higher levels of hexokinase.

FDG is the single most important, widely used and explored radiotracer in PET; however, its current role in brain tumour imaging is limited due to the presence of intense physiological FDG uptake in the normal brain resulting in poor tumour-to-background contrast. Thus, an underlying brain tumour, even if FDG-avid, can escape detection on FDG PET (**Figure 2**). In some studies, increased FDG uptake in gliomas was only reported in 21–47% of high-grade tumours and as few as 3–6% of low-grade tumours [4, 5]. Delayed imaging (e.g. 6 h) following FDG administration instead of the usual imaging performed 60–90 min post-radiotracer can improve discrimination between tumour and physiological background uptake as FDG is retained in tumour longer than in normal brain parenchyma [6].

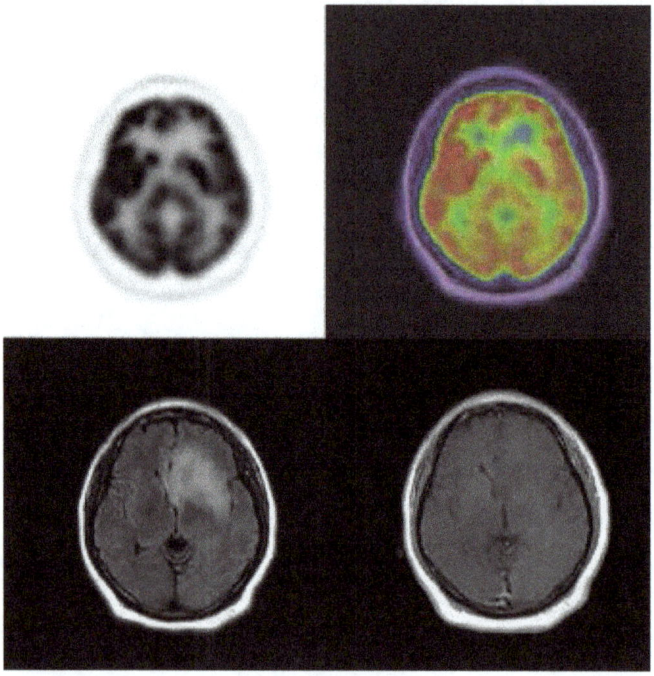

Figure 2. FDG uptake in a left frontal cerebral glioma on PET/CT. *Top row:* The tumour is not readily discernible from intense physiological FDG activity in the adjacent cerebral parenchyma. *Bottom row:* The tumour is much better depicted on MRI FLAIR imaging (*bottom left panel*) and shows no contrast enhancement due to its low grade (*bottom right panel*).

3.2. Tumour grading and prognosis

The uptake of FDG in a neoplasm is a consequence of the increased expression and activity of glucose transporter proteins and of hexokinase, a glucose phosphorylating enzyme. FDG uptake generally correlates with tumour grade [7–9], with low-grade tumours showing similar FDG uptake as white matter, and high-grade tumours similar uptake as grey matter. Tumours can be heterogeneous and contain areas of low- and high-grade dedifferentiation.

FDG uptake in gliomas has also been shown to correlate with survival [10, 11]. Median survival for intracranial metastases is typically less than 1 year, with these metastases generally showing a high-grade pattern of FDG uptake.

3.3. Localisation for biopsy

FDG PET can be useful in selection of a biopsy site where uptake is highest in the tumour, thereby ensuring sampling of the most malignant tissue [12–16].

3.4. Radiotherapy planning

MRI is the current technique of choice for radiotherapy planning. Due to its relatively low tumour-to-background contrast, FDG PET has limited utility for conventional treatment planning. More recently, the addition of PET imaging of some radiotracers—in particular the amino acid analogues—in radiotherapy planning has been shown to be promising in the identification of microscopic residual tumour post-surgery and differentiation of tumour from brain tissue, thereby improving local control and reducing radiation to healthy brain parenchyma (see Section 4).

3.5. Assessment of treatment response

The differentiation of tumour recurrence from radiation necrosis following treatment is one of the most common and important clinical indications for MRI and PET. Both viable tumour and post-radiotherapy necrosis demonstrate contrast enhancement on MRI. Similarly, increased FDG uptake cannot reliably differentiate residual/recurrent tumour from radiation necrosis. Furthermore, false-negative MRI and FDG PET can result from decreased enhancement (due to antiangiogenic therapy) and poor tumour-to-background contrast, respectively.

Whilst the criteria for Response Assessment in Neuro-Oncology have been updated to mitigate these potentially confounding factors in MRI [17–19], advancements in response assessment in PET have focused on other (non-metabolic) radiotracers.

4. Amino acid radiotracers

Amino acids are the building blocks of proteins and critical to nearly every biological process in the human body. They serve as components in metabolic cycles which are upregulated in cancer cells with increased proliferative activity. Because the brain uses glucose almost exclusively for fuel (except during prolonged starvation), PET imaging of brain tumours with amino acid and amino acid analogue radiotracers has a significant advantage of high tumour-to-background contrast (**Figure 3**).

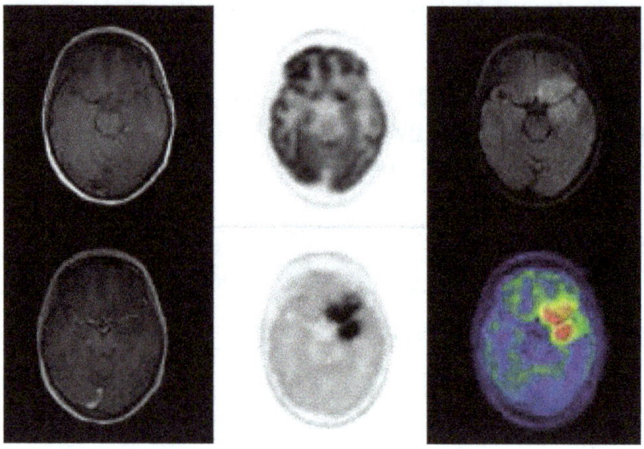

Figure 3. F-18 FDG PET/CT (*top row*) and F-18 FDOPA PET/CT (*bottom row*) of a left frontotemporal low-grade non-enhancing cerebral glioma showing the high tumour-to-background contrast of amino acid imaging compared with metabolic imaging.

4.1. Methionine

Methionine (MET) is a sulphur-containing naturally occurring amino acid (**Figure 4**) whose transport into malignant glioma cells and the supporting vasculature of these tumours is strongly upregulated [20–22].

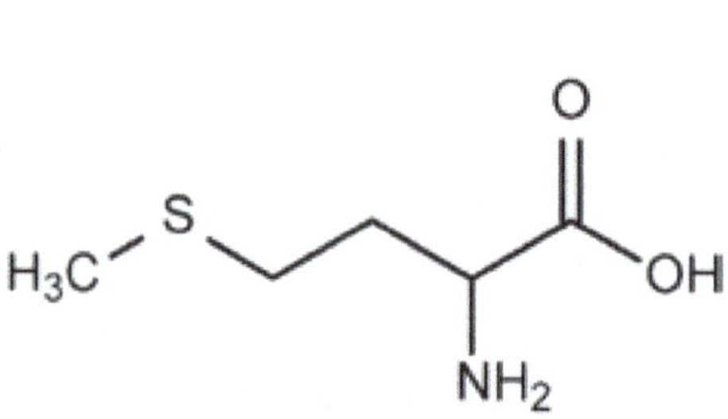

Figure 4. Chemical structure of methionine.

C-11 MET is one of the most widely used amino acid radiotracers for PET imaging in neuro-oncology, mainly due to its relative ease of production that can be performed rapidly with high yield and without the need for complicated purification steps.

The overall sensitivity of MET PET for malignant gliomas ranges from 76 to 95%, with higher rates of detection for higher grade tumours [23]. Increased uptake of MET is also seen in low-grade gliomas—with reported sensitivities of 65–85% [23, 24]—in which there is typically little or absent contrast enhancement on MRI and low uptake on FDG PET [24, 25].

MET is also generally regarded as the reference in prognostication of disease, image-guided biopsy and radiotherapy planning, and the detection of tumour recurrence [26–34], making it the most important radiotracer in the amino acid category.

The main limitation of C-11 MET is its short half-life (20 min), confining its use to centres with a cyclotron on-site or very nearby. It has also been shown to accumulate in brain abscesses and inflammation (cerebritis) [35], important false positives to exclude in the diagnosis of brain tumour.

F-18 has a much longer half-life (110 min) than C-11 and opens up the possibility of radiotracer transport to another centre for diagnostic imaging. F-18 labelled amino acids include F-18-labelled fluoroethyltyrosine (FET) and dihydroxyfluorophenylalanine (FDOPA).

4.2. Fluoroethyltyrosine

FET is an artificial amino acid (**Figure 5**) taken up by upregulated tumour cells but not incorporated into proteins (unlike naturally occurring amino acids such as methionine). As such, its use in the characterisation of brain lesions and the grading of gliomas requires dynamic analysis of activity over time [36]. Its overall accuracy in the diagnosis of gliomas is comparable to MET [37, 38]. It is an excellent tool for differentiating tumour from non-tumour causes in the initial evaluation of newly diagnosed brain lesions [39] (**Figure 6**). FET PET can also distinguish active tumour from radiation necrosis following treatment [40, 41].

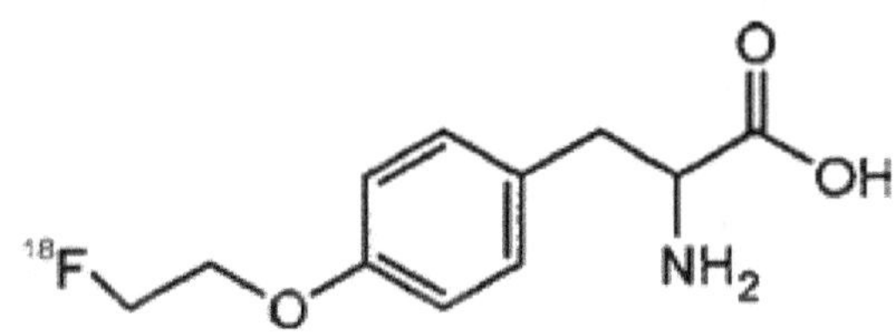

Figure 5. Chemical structure of F-18 fluoroethyltyrosine.

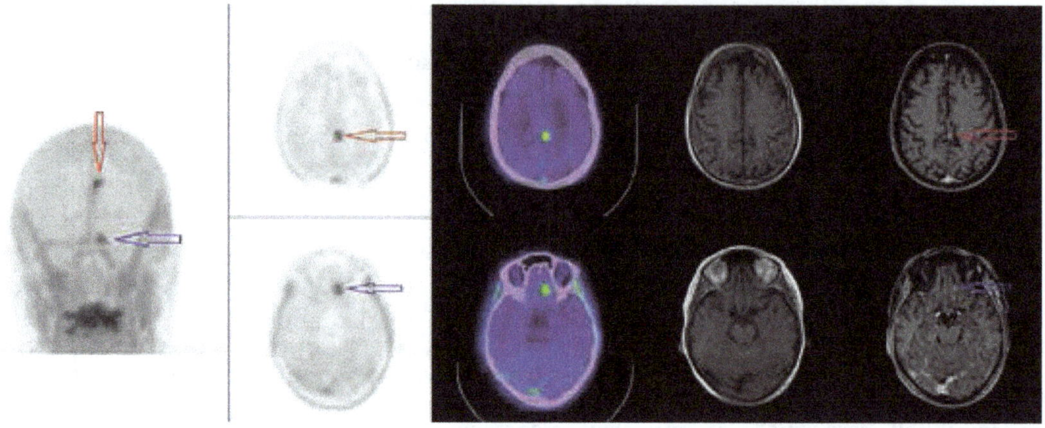

Figure 6. FET PET/CT (*left-sided panels*) and pre/post intravenous gadolinium MRI (*right-sided panels*) in a patient with two small cerebral melanoma metastases (*red and blue arrows*).

4.3. Fluorodihydroxyphenylalanine

FDOPA was originally developed for imaging the DOPA-decarboxylase pathway in Parkinson's disease and other neurodegenerative diseases. It is a fluorinated form of L-DOPA (**Figure 7**) which is used to increased dopamine concentrations in the treatment of Parkinson's disease. FDOPA has since been shown to be a marker of amino acid transport in brain tumours and metastases.

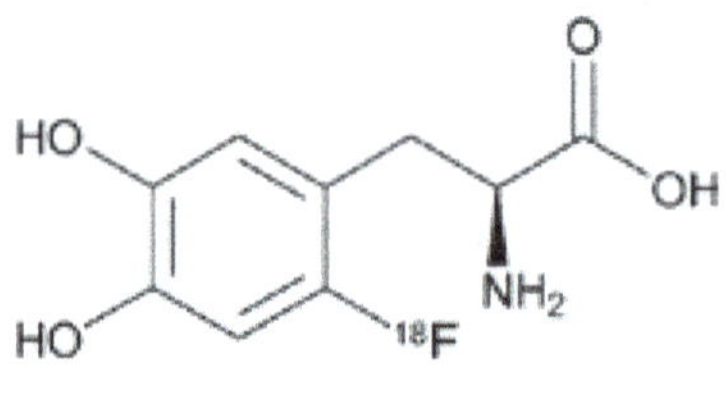

Figure 7. Chemical structure of F-18 fluorodihydroxyphenylalanine.

FDOPA uptake has been shown to correlate with tumour proliferation and grade [42], and more accurate than FDG for evaluating low-grade tumours and distinguishing tumour recurrence from radiation necrosis [43].

It also accumulates in neuroendocrine tumours (NETs) such as phaeochromocytomas and paragangliomas.

5. Fluorothymidine

Thymidine (T) is the pyrimidine deoxynucleoside in DNA that pairs with deoxyadenosine (A). F-18 fluorothymidine (FLT) is a thymidine analogue (**Figure 8**) and a substrate for thymidine kinase 1 (responsible for synchronising cells in G1/early S phase), but unlike thymidine, FLT is a poor substrate for mitochondrial thymidine kinase 2 and its uptake is therefore specific to the cell cycle and a marker of cellular proliferation.

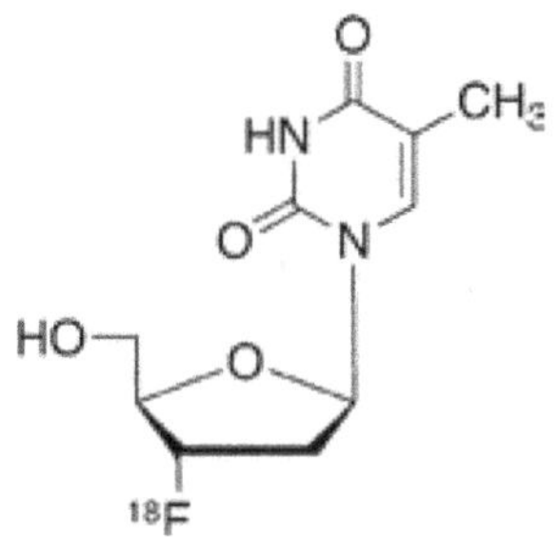

Figure 8. Chemical structure of F-18 fluorothymidine.

FLT uptake in normal brain cells is limited by the blood–brain barrier, thus FLT PET provides higher tumour-to-background contrast than FDG PET. FLT is more sensitive than FDG PET for the detection of recurrent high-grade glioma and also correlates better with tumour progression and survival [44].

However, its use as a quantitative marker of the activity of DNA synthesis in gliomas remains a subject of debate, particularly whether FLT can discriminate moderately proliferative tumours driven by thymidine salvage pathway utilisation from highly proliferative tumours primarily driven by de novo synthesis of thymidine. Quantitative FLT PET with kinetic modelling may also be useful for distinguishing glioma recurrence from radiation necrosis [45].

6. Choline

Choline is a water-soluble B-complex vitamin (**Figure 9**), normally found in blood, which is phosphorylated and subsequently integrated into lecithin, a component of cell membrane phospholipids. Malignant tumour cells demonstrate increased proliferation which results in increased cell membrane turnover and a greater demand for cell membrane components such as choline.

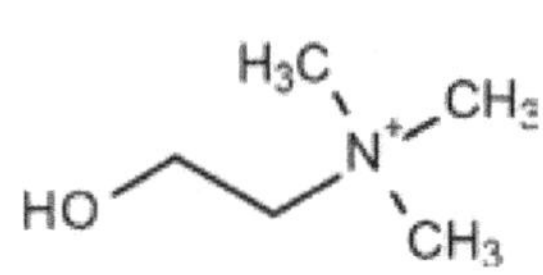

Figure 9. Chemical structure of choline.

Like the amino acid radiotracers, PET imaging with choline offers excellent delineation of tumour from brain with a 10:1 contrast ratio achievable within 5 min of radiotracer injection

[46]. Higher choline uptake generally corresponds with more malignant tumours, and choline PET also appears promising for radiotherapy planning because of more precise delineation of biological target volume [47]. It also has higher accuracy than FDG PET and MRI for the differentiating radiation necrosis and tumour recurrence [47].

Choline can be radiolabelled with C-11 or F-18, permitting its use in centres without an on-site cyclotron.

It has also been investigated extensively for imaging in prostate cancer, with some studies also suggesting a potential role in oesophageal and lung cancer [46, 48–50].

7. Hypoxia radiotracers

Hypoxia is an important factor in the malignant progression of tumour and its resistance to therapy. The majority of hypoxia PET radiotracers belong to a group of compounds known as nitroimidazoles that freely cross the blood–brain barrier, enter cells by diffusion and are subsequently reduced by nitroreductases at a rate inversely proportional to oxygen tension. Thus, in an oxygen-rich environment, they are able to diffuse back out of the cell again, whereas under hypoxic conditions, they are reduced and become irreversibly trapped in the cell. Another favourable property of the nitroimidazoles is their rapid equilibration within the brain parenchyma independently of perfusion.

7.1. Fluoromisonidazole

F-18 fluoromisonidazole (FMISO) was the first of the nitroimidazole radiotracers (**Figure 10**) to be developed for imaging with PET and has been widely used in preclinical and clinical studies.

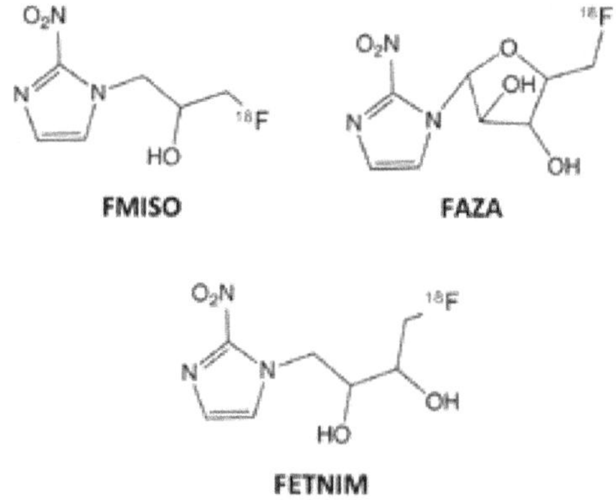

Figure 10. Nitroimidazoles are the most commonly used hypoxia PET radiotracers. FMISO: fluoromisonidazole; FAZA: fluoroazomycin; FETNIM: fluoroerythronitroimidazole.

Hypoxia can be quantified by analysing FMISO PET images using a simple tissue-to-blood ratio of radiotracer activity, with a ratio of 1.2 or greater useful for discriminating and quantifying hypoxic tissue. Hypoxic tumour volume and maximal tumour-to-blood ratio calculated in this way has been shown to predict worse prognosis independent of other factors [51]. FMISO can also differentiate lower from higher grade gliomas better than FDG [52].

More recently, an image-derived region to assess blood activity on FMISO PET has been shown to be an accurate surrogate for serial blood sampling in the quantification of hypoxia [53] and this may obviate the need for routine venous sampling in patients undergoing FMISO PET in the future.

7.2. Fluoroazomycin

F-18 fluoroazomycin (FAZA) is a second-generation nitroimidazole derivative (Figure 10) with more favourable pharmacokinetics than FMISO. FAZA demonstrates faster clearance of unbound radiotracer from non-hypoxic areas (thereby resulting in shorter waiting time for imaging) and improved biodistribution (does not cross the intact blood–brain barrier due to its increased hydrophilicity). Consequently, there is improved hypoxia-to-normoxia contrast, and FAZA shows considerable promise and is expected to overcome the disadvantages of FMISO for imaging hypoxia in brain tumours.

8. Meningiomas

Meningiomas are predominantly benign tumours in adults arising from the meningothelium of the arachnoid mater. Consequently, they occur at the brain surface—over the cerebral convexity, parafalcine region or along the skull base. Rarely, they can occur in intraventricular or intraosseous locations. Meningiomas account for 20–25% of all intracranial neoplasms, with women affected more commonly than men. They are commonly associated with loss of heterozygosity of the long arm of chromosome 22.

On CT and MRI, meningiomas typically appear as rounded or ovoid avidly enhancing masses with dural tails at the tumour margins, variable compressive effect on adjacent brain parenchyma (mainly depending on tumour size) and occasional hyperostosis of the adjacent skull.

Molecular imaging of meningiomas can be accurately performed using somatostatin analogue radiotracers [54] (**Figure 11**).

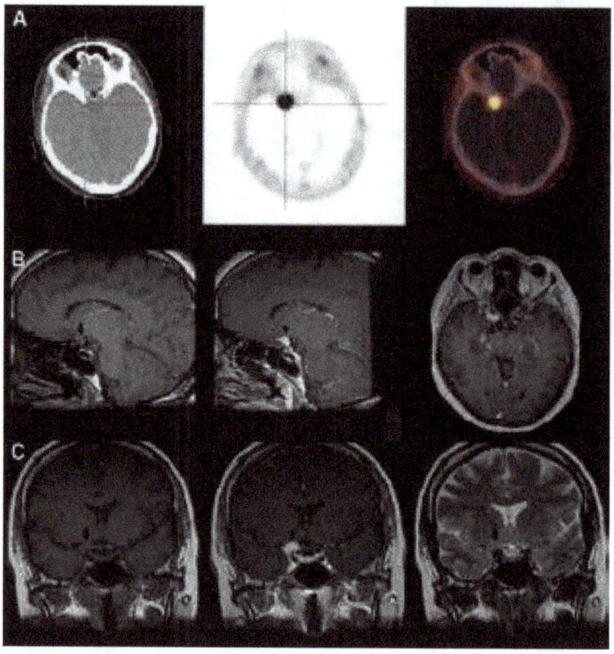

Figure 11. *Row A*: Fusion PET/CT shows a Ga-68 DOTATATE-avid focus directly adjacent to the right anterior clinoid process of the sphenoid bone. *Rows B and C*: Multiplanar MRI sequences show characteristic features of an intracranial meningioma on non-enhanced (*arrows*) and gadolinium-enhanced (*arrowheads*) imaging.

8.1. Somatostatin analogue radiotracers

Currently, the primary indication for using gallium-68 (Ga-68)-labelled somatostatin analogue radiotracers is for PET imaging of carcinoid and other NETs which usually express a high density of somatostatin receptors to which these peptides bind with high affinity [55]. Some non-NETs are also known to express somatostatin receptors, including meningiomas [56–58] which express all of the five somatostatin receptor (SSTR) subtypes but predominantly SSTR1 and SSTR2.

Traditional scintigraphic imaging of meningiomas utilised indium-111-labelled octreotide and single-photon emission computed tomography (SPECT). However, PET imaging with Ga-68-labelled somatostatin analogue radiotracers such as 1,4,7,10-tetraazacyclododecane-1,4,7,10-tetraacetic acid (DOTA)-Tyr^3-octreotate (TATE), DOTA-1-Nal^3-octreotide (NOC) and DOTA-Phe^1-Tyr^3-octreotide (TOC) offers superior count statistics and spatial resolution compared with SPECT. It also provides much higher target-to-background ratio of radiotracer uptake and more detailed tumour characterisation and has largely replaced octreotide SPECT imaging. This detailed spatial characterisation of meningiomas, when coupled with anatomical imaging by CT and MRI (in particular), allows for more accurate radiotherapy planning in patients with large, non-resectable tumours.

The demonstration of DOTATATE avidity in an intracranial lesion with only some features of meningioma on CT or MRI could permit differentiation of a meningioma from other tumours such as metastasis or craniopharyngioma, which can have a significant impact on clinical management.

There are also emerging data that DOTATATE uptake on PET improves diagnostic accuracy by delineating meningioma from tumour-free tissue [58] that can potentially enhance on CT and MRI especially in the setting of previous therapy.

FET PET in the late phase may be useful for the non-invasive grading of meningiomas [59].

9. Lymphoma

Almost all patients with primary CNS lymphoma have brain parenchymal lesions which have a predilection for the periventricular and superficial regions. Contrast-enhanced MRI remains the technique of choice when CNS lymphoma is suspected, although it is usually not possible to conclusively differentiate CNS lymphoma from other malignant brain lesions on MRI.

FDG remains the most widely explored radiotracer for PET imaging in CNS lymphoma, though its utility is limited compared with FDG PET in extracranial lymphoma, due to the poor tumour-to-background contrast in the brain. FDG uptake is typically intense in lymphoma—metabolic imaging with PET may help to differentiate lymphoma in the brain from low-grade gliomas and meningiomas [60–62] and may also be suitable for early evaluation of post-treatment response [60]. Infectious pathologies in the brain of immunocompromised subjects can be discerned from lymphoma by their usually hypometabolic nature on FDG PET [63], and high uptake ratio on thallium-201 (Tl-201) imaging [64]. Steroid treatment can cause false-negative results by reducing FDG uptake in CNS lymphoma [62].

MET PET typically shows intense uptake in CNS lymphomas which often involves a larger area than the corresponding enhancing abnormality on CT and MRI and may more accurately delineate the actual tumour margins [65]. It may also be more accurate for the detection of residual or recurrent lymphoma after treatment [65].

10. Other non-glial neoplasms

There is currently a limited role of PET in other non-glial brain neoplasms including neuronal tumours, pineal and pituitary tumours, germ cell tumours and embryonal tumours (PNET, neuroblastoma), although anecdotal evidence, case reports and series exist for some of these tumours.

PET imaging with MET, for example, detected all but one CNS germinoma in a case series of 10 patients [66], and choline uptake correlated with residual intracranial non-seminomatous germ cell tumour in a series of four patients [67].

Pituitary adenomas can appear as hypermetabolic lesions on FDG PET [68, 69], with higher uptake seen in macroadenomas than in microadenomas [69]. Increased DOTATATE uptake has been reported in intracranial metastases of pituitary carcinoma and may be useful in the decision to treat with peptide receptor radionuclide therapy [70, 71]. MET successfully detected all cases of craniopharyngioma in 10 patients [72].

11. PET/MRI

PET/MRI is a relatively novel hybrid diagnostic imaging device that can simultaneously acquire PET and MR images of the brain and other body regions. PET images show the distribution of an intravenously injected radiotracer, whilst MRI depicts the local responses of atomic nuclei to high-frequency radio waves when placed in a strong magnetic field. PET/MRI represents an advance on hybrid PET/CT imaging systems that are currently used in routine clinical practice for the assessment of patients with cancer and other diseases.

The integration of PET with MRI rather than CT has several advantages:

a. ***Reduced radiation exposure for patients.*** The use of MRI to correct PET images for the attenuation of emitted radiation by overlying tissue avoids the ionising radiation of CT. Because the acquisition time for MRI often exceeds that for PET, there are also opportunities to reduce the amount of radiotracer administered, by increasing PET acquisition time.

b. ***More accurate anatomical localisation of areas of radiotracer uptake.*** The simultaneous acquisition of MR and PET images reduces the likelihood of patient movement causing misregistration of the two image sets.

c. ***Compensation for some limitations of PET.*** The ability of PET to identify tumour sites is constrained by background physiological tracer uptake in some organs. For the most commonly used clinical PET radiotracer, FDG, these organs include the brain (as well as the liver and bone marrow) which are frequent sites of tumour recurrence after initial treatment. PET interpretation is also complicated by processes other than tumour infiltration that can cause radiotracer uptake, the most notably inflammation which can be particularly problematic when assessing cancer status after treatment, especially surgery or radiotherapy.

Many of these advantages are particularly relevant to brain tumour imaging, and indeed, the first exploration of feasibility of hybrid PET/MRI in clinical oncology was in brain tumours [73].

PET/MRI could theoretically harness the advantages of PET imaging with various radiotracers to accurately distinguish tumours from surrounding normal brain tissues—and the ability of advanced MRI techniques such as fMRI and diffusion tensor imaging to map the spatial relationship between tumours and adjacent functional brain tissues and white matter tracts—at the same time.

To date, studies in PET/MRI have shown that it can diagnose, grade and evaluate treatment response in glioma patients [74, 75]. Other studies have also shown that PET/MRI can identify areas of greater cellular proliferation and vascularity in brain tumours using a combination of advanced MRI techniques and PET radiotracers for treatment targeting [76–78]. FMISO PET/MRI can quantify hypoxia in recurrent glioma for risk stratification prior to commencement of angiogenesis inhibitor therapy (such as bevacizumab) and assess response to treatment [79, 80].

PET/MRI may gradually replace PET/CT in paediatric oncology due to the radiation dose saving achieved with performing MRI in place of CT, and more specifically in the field of neurooncology, the superior characterisation of brain tumours afforded by MRI over CT. In this arena, PET/MRI with choline and FDOPA have shown promise in the imaging of paediatric astrocytomas [81, 82].

The major disadvantages of PET/MRI currently relate to its high cost and consequent lack of access in many centres, need for optimisation of workflow and image acquisition parameters, and a greater body of evidence to evaluate its perceived superiority over existing techniques in neurooncology such as PET/CT, MRI or indeed PET/CT and MRI with software fusion of PET and MRI data. This would presumably require the results of large randomised controlled trials that should be a focus of future research efforts.

12. Conclusion

Whilst MRI remains the gold standard for imaging of brain tumours, future applications integrating PET—with its enlarging gamut of radiotracers—and MRI are likely forthcoming. This chapter briefly summarised the current status of the most commonly used radiotracers for the molecular imaging of brain tumours (**Table 2**). It will hopefully also serve as a useful guide that the reader can refer back to and build upon with future reading.

Radiotracer	Mechanism	Advantages	Disadvantages
FDG	Glucose analogue, active transport into cell mediated by GLUT transport proteins; phosphorylated by hexokinase and trapped intracellularly	Most widely used and explored radiotracer in PET	Poor tumour-to-background contrast due to intense physiological uptake in normal brain
MET	Essential amino acid transported into malignant glioma cells by LAT1 transporter and incorporated into proteins	Generally regarded as reference in glioma diagnosis, grading, prognosis, imaged-guided biopsy and	Short half-life (20 min) due to C-11 radiolabelling limits use to centres with cyclotron on-site or very nearby

Radiotracer	Mechanism	Advantages	Disadvantages
		radiotherapy planning, and detection of tumour recurrence in PET	
FET	Artificial amino acid transported into upregulated glioma cells but not incorporated into proteins	Overall accuracy for diagnosis of glioma comparable to MET; can distinguish active tumour from radiation necrosis; late phase FET PET may be useful for grading meningiomas	Use in grading of gliomas requires dynamic analysis of activity over time since not incorporated into proteins
FDOPA	Fluorinated form of L-DOPA, the precursor of dopamine that is transported physiologically into brain and abnormally (increased) into glioma	Uptake correlates with tumour proliferation and grade; more accurate than FDG for evaluating low-grade tumours and distinguishing tumour recurrence from radiation necrosis	Limited data outside of use for initial diagnosis of glioma
FLT	Thymidine analogue and substrate for cellular thymidine kinase 1 but poor substrate for mitochondrial thymidine kinase 2	More sensitive than FDG for detection of recurrent high-grade glioma; correlates better with tumour progression and survival	May accumulate in benign brain lesions with disrupted blood–brain barrier
Choline	Water-soluble B-complex vitamin phosphorylated and subsequently integrated into lecithin, a component of cell membrane phospholipids	Can be radiolabelled with C-11 and F-18; higher uptake generally corresponds with higher grade; more accurate than FDG for distinguishing tumour recurrence from radiation necrosis	May accumulate in benign inflammatory lesions
FMISO	First-generation nitroimidazole; enters cells by diffusion and subsequently reduced at a rate inversely proportional to oxygen tension	Permits quantification of hypoxia which has been shown to predict worse prognosis; can differentiate low from high grade gliomas	Requires venous blood sampling for quantification of hypoxia
FAZA	Second-generation nitroimidazole	Better hypoxia-to-normoxia contrast than FMISO	Requires venous blood sampling for quantification of hypoxia
Somatostatin analogues	Bind with high affinity to somatostatin receptors expressed richly by neuroendocrine tumours and some non-neuroendocrine tumours including meningiomas	Excellent tumour-to-background contrast for neuroendocrine tumours; appears promising for tumour delineation in radiotherapy planning	Limited data for use in radiotherapy planning

Table 2. Summary of radiotracers most commonly used in PET imaging of brain tumours.

Acknowledgements

W.P.L is supported by a Princess Alexandra Hospital Research Foundation grant.

Author details

W. Phillip Law*

Address all correspondence to: phil.law.au@gmail.com

Medical Imaging Department, Princess Alexandra Hospital, School of Medicine, University of Queensland, Brisbane, QLD, Australia

References

[1] Kumar V, Abbas AK, Aster JC. Robbins & cotran pathologic basis of disease. 9th ed. Philadelphia: Saunders; 2015.

[2] Louis DN, Ohgaki H, Wiestler OD, Cavenee WK (eds). WHO classification of tumours of the central nervous system. Lyon: IARC; 2007

[3] Cavaliere R, Schiff D. Cerebral metastases: a therapeutic update. Nat Clin Pract Neurol. 2006;2:426–436.

[4] Kato T, Shinoda J, Nakayama N, et al. Metabolic assessment of gliomas using 11C-methionine, [18F] fluorodeoxyglucose, and 11C-choline positron-emission tomography. AJNR Am J Neuroradiol. 2008;29:1176–1182.

[5] Pauleit D, Stoffels G, Bachofner A, et al. Comparison of (18)F-FET and (18)F-FDG PET in brain tumors. Nucl Med Biol. 2009;36:779–787.

[6] Spence AM, Muzi M, Mankoff DA, et al. ^{18}F-FDG PET of gliomas at delayed intervals: improved distinction between tumor and normal gray matter. J Nucl Med. 2004;45:1653–1659.

[7] Di Chiro G, Oldfield E, Bairamian D, et al. In vivo glucose utilization of tumors of the brain stem and spinal cord. In: Greitz T, Ingvar DH, Widen L, eds. The Metabolism of the Human Brain Studied with Positron Emission Tomography. New York: Raven Press;1985:351–361.

[8] Di Chiro G. Positron emission tomography using [18F] fluorodeoxyglucose in brain tumors: a powerful diagnostic and prognostic tool. Investig Radiol. 1987;22:360–371.

[9] Di Chiro G, DeLaPaz RL, Brooks RA, et al. Glucose utilization of cerebral gliomas measured by [18F] fluorodeoxyglucose and positron emission tomography. Neurology. 1982;32:1323–1329.

[10] Padma MV, Said S, Jacobs M, et al. Prediction of pathology and survival by FDG PET in gliomas. J Neurooncol. 2003;64:227–237.

[11] De Witte O, Levivier M, Violon P, et al. Prognostic value of positron emission tomography with [^{18}F]fluoro-2-D-glucose in the low-grade glioma. J Neurosurg. 1996;39:470–477.

[12] Goldman S, Levivier M, Pirotte B, et al. Regional glucose metabolism and histopathology of gliomas: a study based on positron emission tomography-guided stereotactic biopsy. Cancer. 1996;78:1098–1106.

[13] Hanson MW, Glantz MJ, Hoffman JM, et al. FDG PET in the selection of brain lesions for biopsy. J Comput Assist Tomogr. 1991;15:796–801.

[14] Herholz K, Pietryzk U, Voges J, et al. Correlation of glucose consumption and tumor cell density in astrocytomas: a stereotactic PET study. J Neurosurg. 1993;79:853–858.

[15] Pirotte B, Goldman S, David P, et al. Stereotactic brain biopsy guided by positron emission tomography (PET) with [F-18]fluorodeoxyglucose and [C-11]methionine. Acta Neurochir Suppl. 1997;68:133–138.

[16] Spence AM, Mankoff DA, Muzi M. Positron emission tomography imaging of brain tumors. Neuroimaging Clin N Am. 2003;13:717–739.

[17] Wen PY, Macdonald DR, Reardon DA, et al. Updated response assessment criteria for high-grade gliomas: response assessment in neuro-oncology working group. J Clin Oncol. 2010;28:1963–1972.

[18] Macdonald DR, Cascino TL, Schold SC Jr, Cairncross JG. Response criteria for phase II studies of supratentorial malignant glioma. J Clin Oncol. 1990;8:1277–1280.

[19] van den Bent MJ, Wefel JS, Schiff D, et al. Response assessment in neuro-oncology (a report of the RANO group): assessment of outcome in trials of diffuse low-grade gliomas. Lancet Oncol. 2011;12:583–593.

[20] Kim DK, Kim IJ, Hwang S, et al. System L-amino acid transporters are differently expressed in rat astrocyte and C6 glioma cells. Neurosci Res. 2004;50:437–446.

[21] Isselbacher KJ. Sugar and amino acid transport by cells in culture—differences between normal and malignant cells. N Engl J Med. 1972;286:929–933.

[22] Jager PL, Vaalburg W, Pruim J, de Vries EG, Langen KJ, Piers DA. Radiolabeled amino acids: basic aspects and clinical applications in oncology. J Nucl Med. 2001;42:432–445.

[23] Ogawa T, Shishido F, Kanno I, et al. Cerebral glioma: evaluation with methionine PET. Radiology. 1993;186:45–53.

[24] Herholz K, Holzer T, Bauer B, et al. ^{11}C-methionine PET for differential diagnosis of low-grade gliomas. Neurology. 1998;50:1316–1322.

[25] Chung JK, Kim YK, Kim SK, et al. Usefulness of ^{11}C-methionine PET in the evaluation of brain lesions that are hypo- or isometabolic on ^{18}F-FDG PET. Eur J Nucl Med Mol Imaging. 2002;29:176–182.

[26] De Witte O, Goldberg I, Wikler D, et al. Positron emission tomography with injection of methionine as a prognostic factor in glioma. J Neurosurg. 2001;95:746–750.

[27] Braun V, Dempf S, Weller R, Reske SN, Schachenmayr W, Rihter HP. Cranial neuronavigation with direct integration of 11C methionine positron emission tomography (PET) data—results of a pilot study in 32 surgical cases. Acta Neurochir (Wien). 2002;144:777–782.

[28] Kracht LW, Miletic H, Busch S, et al. Delineation of brain tumor extent with [11C]L-methionine positron emission tomography: local comparison with stereotactic histopathology. Clin Cancer Res. 2004;10:7163–7170.

[29] Pirotte B, Goldman S, Massager N, et al. Combined use of 18F-fluorodeoxyglucose and 11C-methionine in 45 positron emission tomography-guided stereotactic brain biopsies. J Neurosurg. 2004;101:476–483.

[30] Matsuo M, Miwa K, Shinoda J, et al. Target definition by C11-methionine-PET for the radiotherapy of brain metastases. Int J Radiat Oncol Biol Phys. 2009;74:714–722.

[31] Grosu A, Weber WA. PET for radiation treatment planning of brain tumours. Radiother Oncol. 2010;96:325–327.

[32] Terakawa Y, Tsuyuguchi N, Iwai Y, et al. Diagnostic accuracy of 11C-methionine PET for differentiation of recurrent brain tumors from radiation necrosis after radiotherapy. J Nucl Med. 2008;49:694–699.

[33] Tsuyuguchi N, Takami T, Sunada I, et al. Methionine positron emission tomography for differentiation of recurrent brain tumor and radiation necrosis after stereotactic radiosurgery—in malignant glioma. Ann Nucl Med. 2004;18:291–296.

[34] Tsuyuguchi N, Sunada I, Iwai Y, et al. Methionine positron emission tomography of recurrent metastatic brain tumor and radiation necrosis after stereotactic radiosurgery: is a differential diagnosis possible? J Neurosurg. 2003;98:1056–1064.

[35] van Waarde A, Elsinga PH. Proliferation markers for the differential diagnosis of tumor and inflammation. Curr Pharm Des. 2008;14:3326–3339.

[36] Popperl G, Kreth FW, Mehrkens JH, et al. FET PET for the evaluation of untreated gliomas: correlation of FET uptake and uptake kinetics with tumour grading. Eur J Nucl Med Mol Imaging. 2007;34:1933–1942.

[37] Weber WA, Wester HJ, Grosu AL, et al. O-2(18F)Fluorethyl-L-tyrosine and L-(methyl-11C)-methionine uptake in brain tumors: initial results of a comparative study. Eur J Nucl Med. 2000;27:542–549.

[38] Kunz M, Thon N, Eigenbrod S, et al. Hot spots in dynamic 18FET-PET delineate malignant tumor parts within suspected WHO grade II gliomas. Neuro-Oncology. 2011;13:307–316.

[39] Dunet V, Rossier C, Buck A, Stupp R, Prior JO. Performance of ^{18}F-fluoro-ethyl-tyrosine (^{18}F-FET) PET for the differential diagnosis of primary brain tumor: a systematic review and metaanalysis. J Nucl Med. 2012;53:207–214.

[40] Galldiks N, Rapp M, Stoffels G, et al. Response assessment of bevacizumab in patients with recurrent malignant glioma using [18F] fluoroethyl-L-tyrosine PET in comparison to MRI. Eur J Nucl Med Mol Imaging. 2013;40:22–33.

[41] Popperl G, Gotz, C, Rachinger W, Gildehaus FJ, Tonn JC, Tatsch K. Value of O-(2-[18F]fluoroethyl)-L-tyrosine PET for the diagnosis of recurrent glioma. Eur J Nucl Med Mol Imaging. 2004;31:1464–1470.

[42] Fueger BJ, Czernin J, Cloughesy T, et al. Correlation of 6-18F-fluoro-L-dopa PET uptake with proliferation and tumor grade in newly diagnosed and recurrent gliomas. J Nucl Med. 2010;51:1532–1538.

[43] Chen W, Silverman DH, Delaloye S, et al. ^{18}F-FDOPA PET imaging of brain tumors: comparison study with ^{18}F-FDG PET and evaluation of diagnostic accuracy. J Nucl Med. 2006;47:904–911.

[44] Chen W, Cloughesy T, Kamdar N, et al. Imaging proliferation in brain tumors with ^{18}F-FLT PET: comparison with ^{18}F-FDG. J Nucl Med. 2005;46:945–952.

[45] Spence AM, Muzi M, Link JM, et al. NCI-sponsored trial for the evaluation of safety and preliminary efficacy of 3′-deoxy-3′-[^{18}F]fluorothymidine (FLT) as a marker of proliferation in patients with recurrent gliomas: preliminary efficacy studies. Mol Imaging Biol. 2009;11:343–355.

[46] DeGrado TR, Baldwin SW, Wang S, et al. Synthesis and evaluation of ^{18}F-labeled choline analogs as oncologic PET tracers. J Nucl Med. 2001;42:1805–1814.

[47] Giovannini E, Lazzeri P, Milano A, Gaeta MC, Ciarmiello A. Clinical applications of choline PET/CT in brain tumors. Curr Pharm Des. 2015;21:121–127.

[48] Vallabhajosula S. ^{18}F-labeled positron emission tomographic radiopharmaceuticals in oncology: an overview of radiochemistry and mechanisms of tumor localization. Semin Nucl Med. 2007;37:400–419.

[49] Hara T. 18F-fluorocholine: a new oncologic PET tracer. J Nucl Med. 2001;42:1815–1817.

[50] Reske SN. [11C]Choline uptake with PET/CT for the initial diagnosis of prostate cancer: relation to PSA levels, tumour stage and anti-androgenic therapy. Eur J Nucl Med Mol Imaging. 2008;35:1740–1741.

[51] Spence AM, Muzi M, Swanson KR, et al. Regional hypoxia in glioblastoma multiforme quantified with [^{18}F]fluoromisonidazole positron emission tomography before radiotherapy: correlation with time to progression and survival. Clin Cancer Res. 2008;14:2623–2630.

[52] Hirata K, Terasaka S, Shiga T, et al. ^{18}F-fluoromisonidazole positron emission tomography may differentiate glioblastoma multiforme from less malignant gliomas. Eur J Nucl Med Mol Imaging. 2012;39:760–770.

[53] Muzi M, Peterson LM, O'Sullivan JN, et al. ^{18}F-Fluoromisonidazole quantification of hypoxia in human cancer patients using image-derived blood surrogate tissue reference regions. J Nucl Med. 2015;56:1223–1228.

[54] Law WP, Fiumara F, Fong W, Macfarlane DJ. The 'double pituitary hot spot' sign of skull base meningioma on gallium-68-labelled somatostatin analogue PET. J Med Imaging Radiat Oncol. 2013;57:680–683.

[55] Khan MU, Khan S, El-Refaie S, et al. Clinical indications for Gallium-68 positron emission tomography imaging. Eur J Surg Oncol. 2009;35:561–567.

[56] Klutmann S, Bohuslavizki KH, Brenner W, et al. Somatostatin receptor scintigraphy in postsurgical follow-up examinations of meningioma. J Nucl Med. 1998;39:1913–1917.

[57] Arena S, Barbieri F, Thellung S, et al., Expression of somatostatin receptor mRNA in human meningiomas and their implication in in vitro antiproliferative activity. J Neurooncol. 2004;66:155–166.

[58] Rachinger W, Stoecklein VM, Terpolilli NA, et al. Increased 68Ga-DOTATATE uptake in PET imaging discriminates meningioma and tumor-free tissue. J Nucl Med. 2015;56:347–353.

[59] Cornelius JF, Stoffels G, Filb C, et al. Uptake and tracer kinetics of O-(2-(18)F-fluoroethyl)-L-tyrosine in meningiomas: preliminary results. Eur J Nucl Med Mol Imaging. 2015;42:459–467.

[60] Go JL, Lee SC, Kim PE. Imaging of primary central nervous system lymphoma. Neurosurg Focus. 2006;21:E4.

[61] Palmedo H, Urbach H, Bender H, et al. FDG-PET in immunocompromised patients with primary central nervous system lymphoma: correlation with MRI and clinical follow-up. Eur J Nucl Med Mol Imaging. 2006;33:164–168.

[62] Rosenfeld SS, Hoffman JM, Coleman RE, et al. Studies of primary central nervous system lymphoma with fluorine-18-fluorodeoxyglucose positron emission tomography. J Nucl Med. 1992;33:532–536.

[63] Kasamon YL, Ambinder RF. AIDS-related primary central nervous system lymphoma. Hematol Oncol Clin N Am. 2005;19:665–687.

[64] Ruiz A, Ganz WI, Post MJ, et al. Use of thallium-201 brain SPECT to differentiate cerebral lymphoma from toxoplasma encephalitis in AIDS patients. AJNR Am J Neuroradiol. 1994;15:1885–1894.

[65] Ogawa T, Kanno I, Hatazawa J, et al. Methionine PET for follow-up of radiation therapy of primary lymphoma of the brain. Radiographics. 1994;14:101–110.

[66] Okochi Y, Nihashi T, Fujii M, et al. Clinical use of (11)C-methionine and (18)F-FDG-PET for germinoma in central nervous system. Ann Nucl Med. 2014;28:94–102.

[67] Tsouana E, Stoneham S, Fersht N, et al. Evaluation of treatment response using integrated 18F-labeled choline positron emission tomography/magnetic resonance imaging in adolescents with intracranial non-germinomatous germ cell tumours. Pediatr Blood Cancer. 2015;62:1661–1663.

[68] Ryu SI, Tafti BA, Skirboll SL. Pituitary adenomas can appear as hypermetabolic lesions in (^{18}F) F-FDG PET imaging. J Neuroimaging. 2010;20:393–396.

[69] Jeong SY, Lee S-W, Lee HJ, et al. Incidental pituitary uptake on whole-body 18F-FDG PET/CT: a multicentre study. Eur J Nucl Med Mol Imaging. 2010;37:2334–2343.

[70] Xiao J, Zhu Z, Zhong D, Ma W, Wang R. Improvement in diagnosis of metastatic pituitary carcinoma by 68Ga DOTATATE PET/CT. Clin Nucl Med. 2015;40:e129–131.

[71] Maclean J, Aldridge M, Bomanji J, Short S, Fersht N. Peptide receptor radionuclide therapy for aggressive atypical pituitary adenoma/carcinoma: variable clinical response in preliminary evaluation. Pituitary. 2014;17:530–538.

[72] Laser BS, Merchant TE, Indelicato DJ, Hua CH, Shulkin BL, Synder SE. Evaluation of children with craniopharyngioma using carbon-11 methionine PET prior to proton therapy. Neuro-oncology. 2013;15:506–510.

[73] Boss A, Bisdas S, Kolb A, et al. Hybrid PET/MRI of intracranial masses: initial experiences and comparison to PET/CT. J Nucl Med. 2010;51:1198–1205.

[74] Yoon JH, Kim JH, Kang WJ, et al. Grading of cerebral glioma with multiparametric MR imaging and 18F-FDG-PET: concordance and accuracy. Eur Radiol. 2014;24:380–389.

[75] Dunet V, Maeder P, Nicod-Lalonde M, et al. Combination of MRI and dynamic FET PET for initial glioma grading. Nuclearmedizin. 2014;53:155–161.

[76] Weber MA, Henze M, Tuttenberg J, et al. Biopsy targeting gliomas: do functional imaging techniques identify similar target areas? Investig Radiol. 2010;45:755–768.

[77] Widhalm G, Krssak M, Minchev G, et al. Value of 1H-magnetic resonance spectroscopy chemical shift imaging for detection of anaplastic foci in diffusely infiltrating

gliomas with non-significant contrast-enhancement. J Neurol Neurosurg Psychiatry. 2011;82:512–520.

[78] Bisdas S, Ritz R, Bender B, et al. Metabolic mapping of gliomas using hybrid MR-PET imaging: feasibility of the method and spatial distribution of metabolic changes. Investig Radiol. 2013;48:295–301.

[79] Barajas RF Jr, Pampaloni MH, Clarke JL, et al. Assessing biological response to bevacizumab using 18F-fluoromisonidazole PET/MR imaging in a patient with recurrent anaplastic astrocytoma. Case Rep Radiol. 2015;73:1361.

[80] Kickingereder P, Radbruch A, Burth S, et al. MR perfusion-derived hemodynamic parametric response mapping of bevacizumab efficacy in recurrent glioblastoma. Radiology. 2015. doi:10.1148/radiol.2015151172

[81] Fraioli F, Shankar A, Hargrave D, et al. 18F-fluoroethylcholine (18F-Cho) PET/MRI functional parameters in pediatric astrocytic brain tumors. Clin Nucl Med. 2015;40:e40–e45.

[82] Morana G, Piccardo A, Milanaccio C, et al. Value of 18F-3,4-dihydroxyphenylalanine PET/MR image fusion in pediatric supratentorial infiltrative astrocytomas: a prospective pilot study. J Nucl Med. 2014;55:718–723.

5

Genetic Alterations of Glioblastoma

Romana Richterová and Branislav Kolarovszki

Abstract

The current research in oncology is focused on genetics and molecular oncology in order to obtain better understanding of the etiology of tumor disease. Detailed knowledge of oncogenesis mechanisms could lead to invention of effective therapeutic tools against cancer. Under healthy conditions, cell cycle is regulated by oncogenes and tumor suppressor genes, which should be in strict balance. Genesis of tumor is a consequence of the accumulation of genetic alterations, which help the cell to escape normal cellular regulatory mechanisms and destruction by immune system. Glioblastoma (GBM) is a highly malignant primary brain tumor occurring mostly in population of adults. Patients suffering from GBM have very poor prognosis. Despite development in radiology methods promising earlier diagnosis and development of clinical and radiation oncology with newer treatment regimes, the effect of therapy remains limited and prognosis of patients has not improved as expected. Target of GBM research are genes involved in response to oxidative stress and DNA damage, genes regulating cell cycle, genes determining immune response, growth factors, and others. Genetic alterations are studied in connection to their possible relationship to susceptibility of brain tissue for tumor formation, to sensitivity of brain tissue for various environmental etiology factors, to effect of anticancer treatment or resistance of tumor tissue to therapy, to overall survival, and progression-free interval.

Keywords: glioblastoma, genes, alteration, mutations, genetic pathways

1. Introduction

Glioblastoma (GBM) is a brain tumor of neuroectodermal origin. It is a second most common primary brain neoplasm and the most common from malignant brain tumors. This tumor arises from neural stem cells (NSCs), progenitor cells, dedifferentiated mature neural cells or neuroepithelial stem cells that transform into cancer stem cells (CSCs) or glioblastoma stem (GSC) or stem-like cells [1]. Stem cells have a high potential of self-renewal and differentiation. GBM is a tumor with highest degree of anaplasia within gliomas. It is classified as grade IV according to the WHO classification of brain tumors from 2007. This lesion has a rapid growth, is unbounded, infiltrates surrounding brain tissue, but rarely metastasizes. When metastases occur, it is usually within the central nervous system. Typical histopathological features of this tumor are cells of recognizably astrocyte origin, but displaying cellular pleomorphism with multinucleation, frequent mitoses, and areas of necrosis surrounded by palisading nuclei (increased tumor cell density) and endothelial proliferation as a manifestation of cellular hyperplasia with numerous clusters of blood vessels forming so-called glomeruloid formations. GBM cells spread along tracts in white matter infiltrate cerebrospinal fluid and vessels between meningeal layers. Invasion of GBM cells begins with the degradation of surrounding matrix proteins by proteases and proteinases. Movement of tumor cells through surrounding brain tissue requires receptor turnover, formation and degradation of focal adhesion molecules and rearrangement of cytoskeleton components. These changes are consequences of genetic alterations, such as overexpression, amplification, deletion or mutation in focal adhesion kinase and phosphatidylinositol 3-kinase (PI3K) pathways [2] and mainly caused by activation of growth factors and their receptors (integrins and protein deleted in colorectal cancer (DCC), hyaluron receptors CD44, RHAMM, BEHAB, ontogenetic protein SPARC, receptors for platelet-derived growth factor (PDGF), transforming growth factor (TGF)-α, epidermal growth factor (EGF), and basic fibroblast growth factor (bFGF)). Some components of extracellular matrix such as laminin or fibronectin are overexpressed in GBM and their silencing reduces invasiveness of GBM cells [3]. Besides microscopic characteristics, GBM is connected with a huge amount of genetic alterations causing higher proliferation, migration, and invasiveness of tumor cells. The intrinsic ability of GBM cells to invade normal brain tissue impedes complete surgical resection and predictably results in early local recurrence and mortality. Thoroughgoing explanation of GBM genetic pathways with their gene alterations is necessary for choosing of more suitable therapy and in predicting patient prognosis. This chapter offers an overview of the most common genetic alterations occurring in GBM.

2. Classification of GBM

According to the WHO classification of brain tumors based on histopathological origin, GBM is a primary brain tumor of neuroepithelial, glial origin. Ranking of GBM in clinical and prognostic significance is within the highest grade IV. GBM could also be classified according to mode of occurrence, as it could be a result of progression from less malignant glial tumor (so-called secondary type) or it could occur de novo (primary type). Another specific type is pediatric GBM. The most common is primary type. Primary, secondary, and pediatric GBMs have their own specific genetic and epigenetic alterations occurring in their gliomagenesis (see **Figure 1**). As diagnosis of GBM presents with heterogeneity of altered genetic pathways evidenced by The Cancer Genome Atlas Research Network's study, classification based on gene expression profile distinguishes a classical, mesenchymal, proneural, and neural type of GBM. Classical type typically harbors no TP53 mutations, but very high rate of epidermal growth factor receptor (EGFR) mutations. This type has a slightly better survival. Mesenchymal type displays frequent mutations of neurofibromatosis gene 1 (NF1), TP53, and PTEN genes and aggressive anticancer therapy brings a significant increase in survival of these patients. Third, proneural subtype presents with highest mutation rate of TP53, PDGFRA, and isocitrate dehydrogenase (IDH) and usually affects younger adults. Last, neural type occurs more often in older population and contains several gene mutations at an average rate [4]. These classifications show high heterogeneity of genetic profile, aggressiveness, clinical characteristics, and expected prognosis of GBM patients with a strong need of definite uniform classification of subtypes leading to more specific treatment for each GBM subtype.

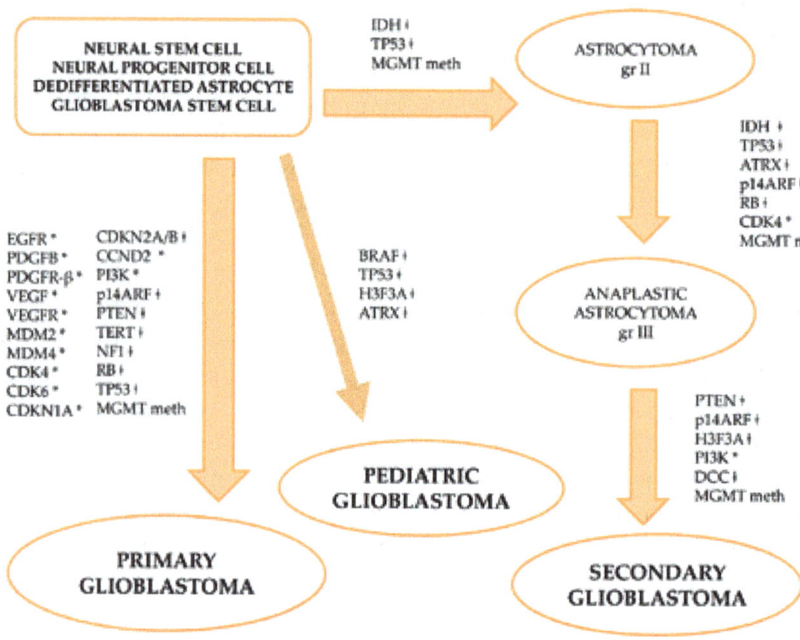

Figure 1. Genes involved in genesis of primary, secondary, and pediatric glioblastoma. *Gain of function through amplification or mutation; *homozygous deletion or mutation.

3. Most frequent genetic alterations of GBM

As mentioned above, alterations of oncogenes and tumor suppressor genes could deflect cell from normal cell cycle. Accumulation of genetic alterations of these genes initiates oncogenesis. In oncogenes, lesion of one allele is sufficient to cause mutation. Activation of oncogene causes avoidance of apoptosis and cell further proliferates. Amplification and activating mutation are the most common genetic alteration of oncogenes. On the other hand, lesion of both alleles is required to evoke mutation in tumor suppressor genes. These genes and their protein products when activated inhibit cell proliferation. Frequently observed alterations are deletion and inhibitory mutation.

During years of genetic research, there have been established three critical genetic pathways whose alterations lead to the formation of GBM: inactivation of p53 and retinoblastoma (RB) pathways (see **Figure 2**), activation of the PI3K pathway, and deregulation of growth factor (receptor tyrosine kinase—RTK) signaling (see **Figure 3**). TP53 signaling pathway is altered in 87% of GBMs, mostly affecting p53, murine double minute-2 (MDM2), MDM4, and cyclin-dependent kinase (CDK)N2A genes. Approximately 78% of GBMs harbor RB signaling disruption with most frequently altered genes: RB1, CDK4, CDK6, CCND2, and cyclin-dependent kinase inhibitor 2 (CDKN2) family. Finally, RTK/RAS/PI3K activation was found in 88% of tumors, affecting usually NF1, PIK3R1, and PIK3CA genes.

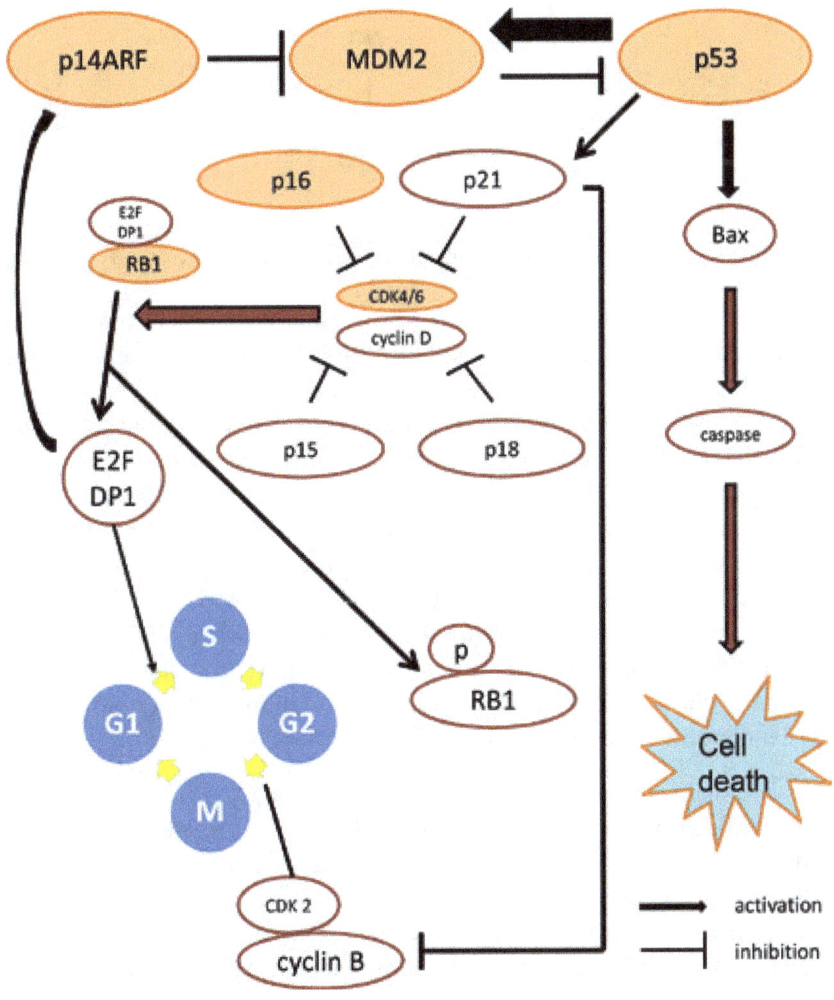

Figure 2. p53 and RB cell cycle and cell death signaling pathway. Proteins marked with full color are most frequently altered in glioblastoma.

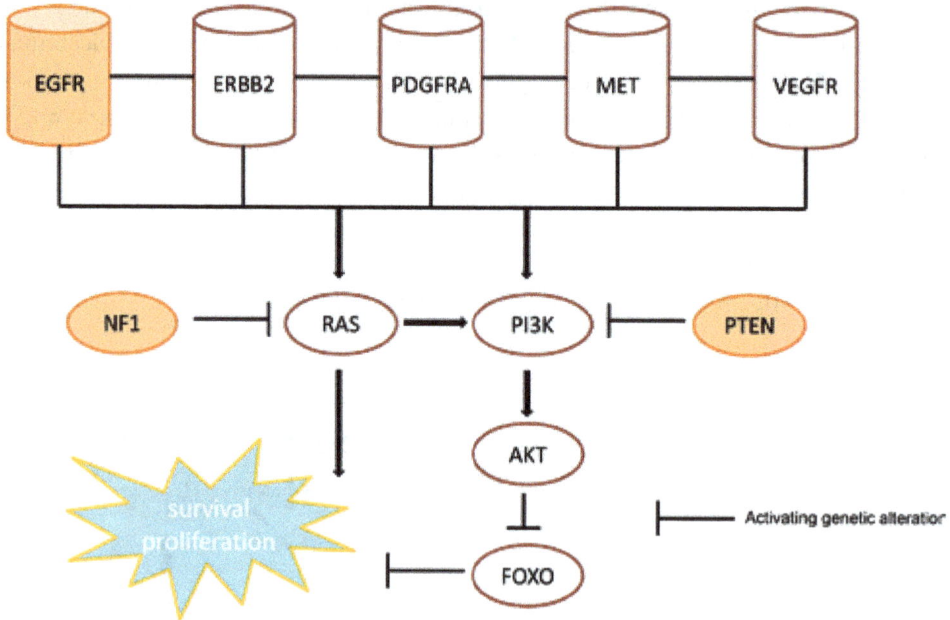

Figure 3. RTK/RAS/PI3K pathway. Proteins marked with full color are most frequently altered in glioblastoma.

GBM is classified as primary or secondary according to altered genes. Primary GBM is a tumor with de novo formation. On the other hand, GBM as a result of malignant transformation of lower-grade glial tumor is called secondary [1]. Also, clinical manifestation and age of diagnosis vary within these two types. Typical for primary GBM is very short anamnesis and age over 50. On the contrary, patients with secondary GBM usually have previous anamnesis of lower grade glioma and younger age depending on the age at the time of diagnosis of preexisting lower grade glioma. Both – primary and secondary GBM – have their own specific gene alterations occurring in their gliomagenesis (see **Figure 1**). Typical alterations for primary GBM are homozygous deletion or mutation of *EGFR, PDGFRα, MDM2, CDK4,* and *PI3K* genes, and amplification or mutation of *CDKN2A/B, PTEN, NF1,* and *RB* genes. Secondary GBM also has some typical alterations, which are mutation of *IDH* and *TP53* genes and 9p deletion. The best-known prognostic factor of GBM, hypermethylation of methylguanin-O-methyltransferase *(MGMT)* gene promoter, occurs in both primary and secondary GBM.

Gene **TP53** is a crucial tumor suppressor gene located on 17p13.1. It is one of the most frequently mutated genes in human tumor cells [5]. Protein p53 restricts cell proliferation and growth, modulates cell reaction to DNA damage, activates DNA repair, causes cell arrest in G1/S regulation point, and induces apoptosis, senescence, and autophagy. TP53 also regulates neovascularization and cell differentiation [6]. Suppression of pluripotency and inhibition of self-renewal of stem cells belong to the most recently discovered functions of TP53 [7]. TP53-mediated apoptosis is almost not present in glioma cells. Dysfunction of TP53 disrupts the p14ARF pathway, what delays apoptosis and that further promotes genome instability. [8]. High incidence of alterations is in p53-binding domain, mainly codons 175, 248, and 273.

Polymorphism Arg72Pro is under suspicion of higher susceptibility to GBM, but this relationship is not yet definitely confirmed. Mutation or deletion of TP53 is found in 35% of GBM cases, but is more frequent in astrocytomas grade II [6, 9] and plays a role in their progression to secondary GBM. On the other hand, it is present in only about 10% of primary GBM [10].

Oncogene **MDM2** is located on 12q14.3-q15. Protein product of this oncogene is E3 ubiquitin ligase which acts like transcriptional factor. This ligase has five forms and two of them have the ability to interact with p53. The function of this protein is suppression of cell cycle arrest and apoptosis by negative effect on p53 and promotion of cell growth and renewal [11]. The effect of MDM2 is repression of transcriptional activity of p53 and amplification or overexpression of this oncogene completely excludes p53 from having an effect on cell cycle. MDM2 overexpression plays an important role in genesis of glioma, but it seems that they are not involved in glioma progression into higher grade [12]. This overexpression is present in about 10–14% of GBM and is always connected with the presence of wild type TP53. It is an alternative mechanism to disrupt p53 pathway in tumor genesis [6]. This alteration is typical for primary GBM [12].

MDM4 is located on 1q32. MDM4 encodes mdm2-related protein, which has p53-binding domain and RING finger domain. MDM4 binds p53 protein and so inhibits p53-mediated transcriptional transactivation. It also binds MDM2 protein via RING finger domain. Overexpression and amplification of MDM4 occur in GBM, though it is not common (7%). MDM4 alterations do not occur together with p53 or MDM2 alteration. It is an alternative mechanism by which a small part of GBMs escapes p53-regulated growth control. This oncoprotein may inhibit oncogenesis. Ubiquitin-specific protease 2a (USP2A) binds to MDM4, stabilizes it and protects against degradation. USP2–MDM4 interaction could be a determinant of malignant potential. MDM4 and USP2a are highly expressed in GBMs from patients with longer survival [13].

RB gene located on 13q14.2 has a protein product RB, which controls cell cycle, and acts as a gatekeeper to S-phase entry. RB protein is an end point of kinase activities of CDK4/6-cyclin D complexes. Transcription factor E2F binds to RB protein, which is normally not phosphorylated. Complex RB–E2F is a silencing complex restricting access to transcription factors. Phosphorylation of RB leads to release of E2F and such conformation allows CDK2 to access cell cycle during S-phase and this promotes another phosphorylation and that further inhibits the binding of E2F to RB protein [14]. Mutation of this gene has the same effect on cell cycle as the amplification of CDK4/CDK6 or mutation of CDKN2A/CDKN2B, but these alterations are never present together. This means that gliomagenesis proceeds by only one of these alternative genetic pathways. RB pathway is frequently altered in GBM and has a huge role in gliomagenesis [15]. Alterations of RB pathway are present almost universally in human cancers. It is very common in primary GBM, and is present in about 80% [4, 16]. Impaired RB1 expression is associated with increased tumor proliferation and decreased survival; however, more direct correlation with prognosis is in astrocytomas grade II and III than in GBM [17]. Mutation or deletion of RB1 is present in 11% of GBM [16].

CDKN1A gene encodes protein p21 and is located on chromosome 6p. Protein p21 is a member of kinase inhibitor protein family (KIP). Level of p53 protein regulates transcription of p21.

Apoptosis and cell cycle arrest mediated by p53 induce transcription of p21. This protein controls cell proliferation by regulatory binding to complexes of CDK. It negatively effects complexes of cyclin E/CDK2 and cyclin A/CDK2 and activates cyclin D/CDK. CDKN1A amplification is frequent in GBM [18].

Gene **CDKN1B** is localized on 12p13.1-p12. Its protein product is p27, which is also a member of KIP family. This protein also binds to CDK complexes, inhibits cyclin E/CDK2 and cyclin A/CDK2, and it activates cyclin D/CDK. In proliferating cells, p27 was found in complex with cyclin D/CDK and in G_1 – arrested cells, p27 was bound to cyclin E/CDK2. Very low levels of expression [19] are typical of GBM.

On 9p21 are located genes **CDKN2A** (protein product p16) and **CDKN2B** (product p15). These proteins are inhibitors of CDK and they inhibit phosphorylation of RB1 protein by binding to cyclin D, what prevents their interaction with CDK4/6. Regulation of p16/p14ARF pathway is determining the susceptibility to the only proved environmental risk factor of gliomagenesis – ionizing radiation [20]. Higher risk of glioma formation was observed in patients with CDKN2A and CDKN2B mutations [21, 22]. Homozygous deletion of CDKN2A is present in almost 50% of gliomas and is connected with poor prognosis [14]. But polymorphisms of *CDKN2A/CDKN2B* genes are not proved to be connected with tumor grade and prognosis [23].

Protein **p14ARF** is an alternate reading frame product of CDKN2A locus on 9p21. This protein has tumor suppressor activity, regulates cell cycle, initiates p53-dependent cell cycle arrest and apoptosis [20] and is induced by mitogenic stimulation. It inhibits MDM2 and so promotes p53. The finding of p14ARF loss in conjunction with p53 gene loss suggests that the protein may have other p53-independent tumor suppressor functions. P14ARF mediates antiangiogenic effects by upregulating expressions of tissue inhibitor of metalloproteinase-3 in p53-independent fashion. About 60–80% of high-grade gliomas show loss of tumor suppressor p14ARF activity by homozygous mutation [24].

CDKN2C gene has locus on 1p32, encodes protein p18, interacts with CDK4 and CDK6 and prevents their activation. It functions as a cell growth regulator that controls G1 cell cycle progression and also suppresses tumorigenesis. Homozygous deletion is a most common cause of CDKN2C inactivation. This deletion occurs in tumors harboring also CDKN2A deletions. Expression of CDKN2C is almost absent in 43% of GBMs. It is suggested that p16 deletion occurs as an early event in tumorigenesis and p18 inactivation should happen later in tumor formation [25].

Genes **CDK4** (12q14) and **CDK6** (7q21-22) have protein products CDK4 and CDK6 with catalytic kinase activity. Their inhibitors are proteins p15 and p16. CDK4 and CDK6 proteins make complexes with cyclin D. Gene CDK6 is an oncogene, which is required for proliferation of tumor cells and its viability [16]. Overexpression of CDK proteins inhibits the function of their inhibitors – proteins p15 and p16. Amplification of CDK4 is observed in 18% and CDK6 in 1% of GBMs [16].

CCND2 gene (cyclin D2), locus 12p13, encodes a protein of cyclin family that function as regulators of CDK kinases. Cyclin D2 makes a complex with CDK4 and CDK6 and works as a regulatory subunit of this complex, which is required for G1/S cell cycle transition. Association of cyclin D2 and CDK4/6 leads to phosphorylation of RB and RB-related proteins that allows cell to enter S phase of cell cycle. Deregulation of this cell cycle transition often causes formation of tumor and is frequently seen in GBM. Amplification of CCND2 occurs in 2% of GBM cases. Study on *in vitro* GSC showed high expression levels of cyclin D2 and suppression of its expression led in experimental model to G1 arrest. This suggests an important role of cyclin D2 in cell cycle progression and in tumorigenicity of GSC [26].

PIK3CA gene (phosphatidylinositol-4, 5-bisphosphate 3-kinase catalytic subunit alpha) located on 3q26.3 encodes ATP-dependent IA PI3K alpha catalytic subunit of phosphatidylinositol 3-kinase. This gene is a part of PI3K pathway, which plays a role in proliferation, cellular metabolism, apoptosis, differentiation, migration, and survival [27]. Binding of RTK to its receptor activates regulatory units of PI3K pathway, this activates catalytic subunits, which phosphorylates phosphatidylinositol 4, 5-bisphosphate (PIP2), converts it to phosphatidylinositol 3, 4, 5-triphosphate (PIP3). PIP3 activates downstream signaling cascades as the AKT and mTOR pathways, which are involved in proliferation and cell survival [28]. Hyperactivation of these pathways contributes to tumor progression. Mutations of this gene constitutively activate the PI3K catalytic activity and drive the GBM formation and progression [29]. Treatment of GBM with PI3K-targeted agents is promising [28]. PIK3CB gene (phosphatidylinositol-4, 5-bisphosphate 3-kinase catalytic subunit beta) located on 3q22.3 encodes IA PI3K beta catalytic subunit of phosphatidylinositol 3-kinase. This gene was identified as a marker predicting recurrence and prognosis of GBM [30].

PIK3R1 gene (phosphatidylinositol-3-kinase regulatory subunit 1) located on 5q13.1 is also part of PI3K pathway. Mutations and amplifications of these genes also occur in GBM [29]. PIK3R1 mutations act through the catalytic subunit by binding to it and inhibiting its activity [31]. Result of such PIK3R1 mutation is no inhibition of catalytic subunit and so constant activity of whole pathway leading to invasion and migration of tumor cells. Experimental knockdown of PIK3CA and PIK3R1 leads to decrease in proliferation, migration, and invasion of GBM cell lines [32].

Gene phosphatase and tensin homology – **PTEN** located on 10q23.3 is a tumor suppressor gene. PTEN protein, product of this gene, is a lipid phosphatase counteracting the effect of PI3K signaling. PTEN regulates this pathway by converting PIP3 to PIP2. After exposure to ionizing radiation, PTEN acts as a critical determinant of cell fate between the senescence and apoptosis [33]. Germ line mutations of PTEN were described in some autosomal hereditary diseases, such as Cowden disease, Bannayan-Zonana syndrome, etc. Monosomy of chromosome 10 is frequently present in GBM and rarely in low-grade astrocytoma. Inactivation of this tumor suppressor gene is present in both primary and secondary GBM [6]. PTEN gene is mutated or lost in 60–70% of GBM and this condition is associated with poor prognosis [18].

Signal transducer and activator of transcription 3 – **STAT3** gene (locus 17q21.31) encodes a protein member of STAT family. In response to growth factors or cytokines, this protein becomes phosphorylated and acts as a transcription factor. STAT3 regulates cell growth, nervous system development, stem cell differentiation, apoptosis, and is commonly activated in tumors. It also regulates growth and self-renewal of GBM stem cells. STAT3 has an antiapoptotic role, is activated in high percentage of GBM, and is required for maintaining of multipotency of tumor cells [34].

Oncogene **AKT3** (v-akt murine thymoma viral oncogene homolog 3) located on 1q44 codes a protein, member of serine/threonine protein kinase family (AKT). These AKT kinases are regulators of processes such as cell proliferation, differentiation, apoptosis, tumorigenesis, glycogen synthesis, and glucose uptake and their overexpression induces cell survival and malignant transformation. Enhanced DNA repair can allow damaged or mutated cells to survive, contributing to resistance and tumor recurrence [35]. Inhibition of AKT kinases activity leads to apoptosis. AKTs have three isoforms AKT1, AKT2, AKT3, being one of the major downstream effectors of PI3K. AKT pathway is activated in 70% of gliomas and is usually associated with PTEN mutations [36]. AKT3 is also essential for normal brain development [37] and is stimulated by PDGF, insulin, and insulin-like growth factor (IGF)1. AKT1 protein does not seem to be overexpressed in GBM, level of AKT2 increases with the malignancy grade and AKT3 expression decreases. It seems that AKT3 protein is affected by the negative feedback caused by AKT2 overexpression. Even though ATK3 is downregulated, it exhibits high kinase activity and retained the functional capacity as an oncoprotein and so may inhibit the growth of malignant cells. AKT3 is often amplified in GBM [35]. AKT2 and AKT3 isoform-specific knockdown inhibits cell growth and induces apoptosis [38] and thus is a potential target for therapy of AKT pathway-altered GBM.

NF1 (locus 17q11.2) codes tumor suppressor protein neurofibromin 1, Ras GTPase-activating protein, which was first found to be mutated in a genetic neurodevelopmental disease neurofibromatosis. Neurofibromin negatively regulates Ras and m-TOR signaling in astrocytes. Approximately 23% of GBM harbor inactivating mutation of NF1, typically mesenchymal subtype. NF1 inactivation could be due to genetic loss or mutation or to extensive proteasomal degradation [39].

MYC oncogene (v-myc avian myelocytomatosis viral oncogene homolog) has locus on 8q24.21. Its protein product is a nuclear phosphoprotein and transcriptional factor with various functions in cell cycle progression, cellular transformation, and apoptosis. Oncogenic activation is achieved by mutation, amplification, overexpression, and chromosomal translocation. This gene is an important target for the cooperative actions of p53 and PTEN in the regulation of normal and malignant cell differentiation, self-renewal, and tumorigenic potential. Overexpression of MYC is present in up to 70% of GBM [40] and surprisingly is highly correlated with better overall survival, what could be a result of enhancement of the proapoptotic effect of upregulated MYC [41]. Moreover, a direct relationship was found between MYC overexpression and MGMT methylation, so that MYC overexpression can be considered a good indicator of response to temozolomide treatment [42].

BMI1 – polycomb ring finger oncogene (10p11.23) is a transcriptional epigenetic repressor of genes governing self-renewal, differentiation, and proliferation, which is directly regulated by MYC. It plays a role in the development of the cerebellum and is required for self-renewal of stem cells in the hematopoietic, epithelial, and nervous system [43]. Overexpression of BMI1 is frequently present in GBM and is concurrent with MYC activation and MYC directly induces upregulation of BMI1 [41, 44].

Isocitrate dehydrogenase system comprises two genes: IDH1 located on 2q33.3 and IDH2 located on 15q26.1. Their products are enzymes (IDH1, IDH2, and IDH3) involved in citric acid cycle. The function of IDHs in this basic metabolic pathway is to catalyze oxidative decarboxylation of isocitrate to α-ketoglutarate and reducing NADP+ to NADPH (NAD+ to NADH in case of IDH3). Crucial effect on interaction of an enzyme with a substrate has arginine 132 (R132) in IDH1 and R172 in IDH2. Mutations of these important areas lead to significant reduction of enzyme activity [45, 46]. Mutations of IDH genes are common in patients with secondary GBM, but rare in primary and pediatric (11%) GBM [47, 48]. The fact that IDH mutations are found in a wide spectrum of histologic tumor types indicates that they occur as an early alteration in tumorigenesis [49]. Only 3–7% of primary GBM shows IDH mutations, but is often found in astrocytoma grade II and III and secondary GBM [50]. Though IDH mutations in primary GBM are rare, they create a prognostically favorable subgroup [21]. Also, IDH2 mutation, which is much less frequent than IDH1 mutation, occurs in gliomas [51], but only in about 6% of secondary GBMs [52]. There is also a possible association between the presence of IDH1 mutation and longer overall survival in patients with GBM [53, 54]. Furthermore, IDH mutation appears to be a significant marker of positive chemosensitivity in secondary GBM. Patients with this mutation show a higher response rate to temozolomide, which is widely used in chemotherapy of malignant gliomas. This makes IDH mutation an independent favorable prognostic factor for overall survival with comparable importance to hypermethylation of MGMT promotor [52]. Patients having both IDH mutation and MGMT promoter methylation seem to have best response to therapy and progression-free survival. Mechanism leading to increased effect of chemotherapy is not clearly known, it is possible that IDH mutation promotes treatment-induced apoptosis by inhibiting the cell-protective mechanisms against oxidative stress [55]. Prolonged survival of secondary GBM patients with IDH mutation was proved in patients with tumors of astrocytic, but not oligodendroglial origin [56]. Tumors with IDH mutation often show also the presence of TP53 mutation; on the other hand, tumors with wild type IDH often have alteration typical for primary GBM (*PTEN, EGFR, CDKN2A*, or *CDKN2B*). This fact confirms the existence of separate genetic pathways for primary and secondary GBM [50]. IDH mutations are novel and very important and useful prognostic factor of gliomas [21]. An inhibitor of IDH1 significantly retards GBM growth through inducing differentiation [57].

DCC gene with locus on 18q21.3 has product DCC protein. This protein is highly expressed in the nervous system. DCC is a transmembrane protein and creates part of the receptor for netrin 1. Netrins play a role in direct cell and axon migration during neural development. Their expression is also detectable in adult tissue, but their function is not yet clear [58]. DCC induces apoptosis and cell cycle arrest in G2 phase. Also plays a role in chemo-attraction to netrin-1 slowing the rate of spontaneous cell migration. DCC has probably anti-oncogenic function, although if disruption of netrin signaling contributes to tumorigenesis is not yet understood [59]. According to immunohistochemical examination, expression of DCC decreases in many malignancies including GBM and also decreases during progression from low-grade astrocytomas to GBM. This points out the connection of DCC with the formation of secondary, but not with primary GBM [59].

Paternally expressed gene 3 – **PEG3**, located on 19.chromosome, is an imprinted gene expressed mainly during embryogenesis, but also in some adult tissues – ovary, testis, muscle, and brain [60]. Overexpression is frequent in oligodendrogliomas, for GBM very low expression is typical. Deregulation of PEG3 induces the formation of gliomas [61].

GST genes – glutathione S-transferases genes: GSTP1 (location 11q13), GSTM1 (1p13.3), GSTT1 (22q11.23), and GSTO1 (10q25.1). Proteins of these genes are phase II biotransformation enzymes, which detoxify a wide range of exogenous agents including carcinogens. GSTs are responsible for glutathion conjugation of alkylators and scavenging of free radicals generated by radiation [62]. These enzymes provide enzymatic and nonenzymatic functions. GSTs also have important roles in cellular processes as cell proliferation, apoptosis, oncogenesis, tumor progression, drug resistance, and cell response to stress [63]. Genetic variations of GST genes determine the response to carcinogens. Polymorphisms of these genes result in absent or altered enzyme activity and are associated with survival rate in cancer patients. The relationship between these polymorphisms and brain tumor risk is not clear, although there have been some results referring to possible association between GSTM1 null genotype and brain tumor incidence [64]. Patients with brain tumors and GST polymorphisms have higher risk of adverse effects of chemotherapy with nitrosourea alkylating agents.

EGF gene is located on 4q25. EGF is a ligand for its receptor (EGFR), inducing a dimerization of one or several members of the EGFR family (ErbB1-4). This activates several tyrosine kinases and other downstream signal molecules promoting transcription in the cell nucleus [65]. These molecules are important for cell proliferation, survival, migration, and differentiation. EGF polymorphism 61G/A on the promoter part of this gene is associated with glioma susceptibility and with the degree of malignancy [66]; however, results of studies are controversial, probably due to diverse distribution of EGF gene frequencies among the different ethnic groups. EGF 61G/A polymorphism is also probably associated with the survival time of glioma patients [67].

EGFR gene, located on 7p12, encodes EGFR protein, which is a transmembrane receptor responsible for communication with its extracellular ligands – EGF and TGF-α and for transmission of their signalization within the cell. EGFR has an effect on cell apoptosis, angiogenesis, tumor proliferation, and ability to metastasize and is connected to sensitivity to therapy and drug resistance. EGFR is the most frequently amplified gene in astrocytomas, mainly in GBM. Expression of EGFR is higher in high-grade and poorly differentiated GBMs. Both overexpression and amplification of EGFR are correlated with tumor progression. Over 50% of GBM have mutations of EGFR. Presence of EGFR mutation is associated with early relapses and poor prognosis [68]. These mutations exist in three variations: EGFRvIII, δEGFR, and de2-7EGFR (deletion, loss of exons 2-7 of mRNA strand). δEGFR promotes tumorigenesis of GBM by increasing cellular proliferation, decreasing apoptosis, and promoting tumor cell invasiveness. Amplification and de2-7EGFR-specific mutation is typical for primary GBM, in which monosomy of chromosome 10 is also simultaneously present. Amplification of EGFR is mostly associated with CDKN2A deletion, but usually occurs without homozygote deletion or mutation of PTEN. Alteration of EGFR alone is probably not sufficient to cause tumorigenesis, but another alteration in RB1 pathway is required.

PDGF exists in five types of dimers consisting of four types of polypeptides, each encoded by a different gene – A, B, C, and D. PDGFA (7p22), PDGFB (22q13.1), PDGFC (4q32), and PDGFD (8q11). This system comprises two receptors: PDGFR-α (gene PDGFRA, 4q11-q13) and PDGFR-β (gene PDGFRB, 5q31-q32). PDGF system is involved in cell cycle regulation, cell migration, and chemotaxis and has also developmental functions – also in glial development [69]. PDGFR-α is expressed only in subset of GBMs. PDGFR-β is more commonly expressed in GBM by self-renewing GBM stem cells. PDGF pathway aberrations are mostly associated proneural and mesenchymal subtypes of GBM [70]. Overexpression of PDGF and its receptors is often found also in low-grade gliomas, suggesting this alteration as an early oncogenic event and if often found in secondary GBM [71].

IGF system is composed of two ligands: IGF1 (gene IGF1, 12q23.2), IGF2 (also called somatomedin A, gene IGF2, 11p15.5), their receptors: IGF1R (15q26.3) and IGF2R (6q26), six binding proteins (IGFBP 1-6), and various IGFBP-related peptides. IGF has a role in regulation of cell processes. IGF1 is a major physiological mediator of the growth hormone and has a huge influence on cell proliferation and differentiation. It inhibits apoptosis by blocking the initiation of the apoptotic pathway. IGF1R is involved in malignant transformation processes. IGF-binding proteins modulate interactions between IGF and IGFR. IGFBP3 (located on 7p13-p12) acts as an apoptotic agent and inhibits the activity of IGF1 and has growth-promoting effects [72]. Amplification of IGF1, IGF2, and IGF1R genes occurs in gliomas and other cancers. No association between IGF polymorphism and GBM risk has been found.

FGF system is a family of factors involved in various cellular processes, such as developmental, mitogen, cytoprotective, and angiogenic functions. System comprises 18 ligands and four FGF receptors and FGF-binding protein, which increases FGF2-dependent proliferation of fibroblast cells and may have an important role in oncogenesis. FGF2 (bFGF, 4q27-q25), known as a pro-angiogenic factor for vessel formation and wound repair, is a potential oncoprotein in GBM. Upregulated FGF2–FGFR1 signaling is implicated in the pathogenesis of GBM. Overexpression of FGF2 promotes GBM cell proliferation and also exerts an anti-apoptotic function by upregulating of anti-apoptotic genes BCL-2 and BCL-X and thus making tumor resistant to chemotherapy [73]. FGF2 also modulates apoptosis and thus promotes survival via resistance to radiation-induced cell death [74].

Vascular endothelial growth factor – **VEGF** system is the most potent angiogenesis- and vasculogenesis-promoting system. There are known six VEGF ligands and three receptors (VEGFR1, locus 13q12, VEGFR2, locus 4q11-q12, VEGFR3, locus 5q34-q35). VEGF system stimulates endothelial cell migration, growth, proliferation, and survival, also acts as microvascular permeability factor and increases extravasation of plasma proteins [75]. Activation of endothelial nitric oxide (NO) synthase leads to generation of NO and thus further activates angiogenesis. The main angiogenic effect of this system is mediated by interaction of VEGF (VEGFA) with VEGFR2. Angiogenesis is crucial for tumor formation, growth, and maintenance of blood supply. As the tumor develops, it may activate secondary angiogenic pathways, such as bFGF, TGF, and PDGF. GBMs exhibit high levels of VEGF [76]. Higher vascular permeability leads also to radiologic postcontrast enhancement. GBMs with high levels of VEGF are more likely to exhibit ring-like enhancement, what makes relatively clear border on postcontrast imaging. In such tumors, the gross total resection is easier to obtain. High expression of VEGF is associated with poor prognosis, but there are other factors determining prognosis, such as the extent of resection [76].

TGFβ superfamily is involved in morphogenesis, embryonic development, adult stem cell differentiation, immune reaction, wound healing, and inflammation [77]. This superfamily comprises over 30 proteins divided into two branches: TGFβ subfamily and the bone morphogenetic protein-like (BMP-like) group. The TGFβ subfamily contributes to carcinogenesis and makes tumors more aggressive and BMP-like group has a tumor suppression effect [78]. TGFβ subfamily is composed of three isoforms coded by three different genes – TGFBI (19q13), TGFBII (1q41), and TGFBIII (14q24). This subfamily regulates cell proliferation, differentiation, and extracellular matrix production [79]. All three isoforms are widely expressed in GBM, but TGFβ expression is increased in mesenchymal GBM [80].

Proto-oncogene **MET** (7q31) codes hepatocyte growth factor receptor with tyrosine kinase activity and belongs to RTK family. This receptor is usually expressed in epithelial cells. MET after binding with its ligand hepatocyte growth factor (HGF) plays a role in various cellular signaling pathways involved in proliferation, motility, migration, invasion, and tissue homeostasis by activating the RAS, PI3K, STAT, beta-catenin, and NOTCH signal transduction pathways [81]. It is aberrantly activated in many cancers (lung, pancreas, ovary, salivary gland, and breast cancers) as well as in GBM via mutation, amplification, or overexpression. Mutation of MET in GBM is rare [4]. Amplification is present in 5% and overexpression in 13% of GBM [82]. Overexpression and amplification of MET are not perfectly concordant. This abnormal activation of MET promotes malignancy and is partially associated with the aggressiveness as it was found only in grade IV, not in grade II or III gliomas, but relationship to prognosis is not clear [82, 83]. Amplification of EGFR could be associated with aberrant MET expression [4]. Under research are MET inhibitors in GBM treatment. Moreover, targeting the MET pathway potentiates the responsiveness of GBM to γ-radiation [82].

HGF gene (7q21.1) codes for HGF protein, a pleiotropic factor and cytokine, promoting cell proliferation, survival, motility, scattering, differentiation, and morphogenesis [84]. It is usually expressed by mesenchymal cells, but could be secreted also by tumor cells. In addition, HGF has a protective function in several diseases, including liver cirrhosis and promotes tissue regeneration. It also stimulates mobility and invasiveness of tumor cells and induces angiogenesis [81]. GBM with autocrine activation of HGF has also activated MET signaling and that predicts sensitivity to MET inhibitors in treatment [85]. HGF serum levels serve as biomarkers of responsiveness to such therapy. HGF levels in serum and cerebrospinal fluid correlate with prognosis, and are associated with higher mortality and recurrence rates [86].

Gene **ATRX** (α-thalassemia/mental-retardation-syndrome-X-linked), located at Xq21.1, was discovered as a gene responsible for rare developmental disorder characterized by α-thalassemia and intellectual impairment. It also has a role in the regulation of transcription, heterochromatin structure, and genome stability and is frequently deregulated in human cancer [87]. ATRX alterations are commonly present together with IDH and TP53 mutations. They are detected in 80% of secondary GBMs, but only in 7% of primary [88]. Mutations of ATRX gene are frequent also in pediatric GBM [89].

The B-Raf proto-oncogene serine/threonine kinase – **BRAF** gene, located on 7q34, is a member of Raf kinase family and serves as a strong activator of the extracellular signal-regulated kinase/mitogen-activated protein kinase 1 and 2 (Erk 1/2) signal transduction cascade which modulates cell growth, proliferation, migration, differentiation, and apoptosis. Mutations of BRAF gene usually occur at codon 600, which is a site of activation loop of the kinase domain. Consequence of this BRAF V600E mutation is a protein with increased kinase activity. This mutation is usually present in lower-grade gliomas, but was found in 54% of epithelioid GBM [90], in 7% of giant cell GBM [91]. Within classical GBM types, BRAF mutation was present in 8% of adult and in 12% of pediatric GBM cases. These GBMs were all classified as primary. In adults, they create a group of tumors that are present in younger age (mean age of 39 years), none of these tumors harbored IDH mutation and seem to have slightly longer survival [92]. GBMs with BRAF V600E mutation may represent a small, but more favorable subgroup. In such patients, BRAF/MEK inhibitor treatment may be beneficial in combination with other therapies [93].

H3 histone, family 3A – **H3F3A** gene, located on 1q42.12, encodes replication-independent histone H3.3. Histones are basic nuclear proteins responsible for the nucleosome structure of the chromosomal fiber. ATRX and DAXX genes are encoding subunits of a chromatin remodeling complex required for H3.3 incorporation at pericentric heterochromatin and telomeres [94]. The histone H3.3 mutations result in amino acid substitution at K27 or G34 – two critical positions within the histone tail involved in key regulatory posttranslational modifications. H3F3A mutations are often seen in tumors with somatic TP53 mutation, within histological grades are specific for GBM and are highly prevalent in children and young adults, and they are present in one-third of pediatric GBMs [95]. Interestingly, K27-mutated tumors were predominantly seen in midline structures – thalamus, pons (diffuse intrinsic pontine gliomas), and spinal cord and have potentially poor prognosis. G34-mutated GBMs have better overall survival [96].

Telomerase reverse transcriptase –**TERT** gene is located on 5p15.33. This gene encodes the enzymatic core of telomerase. Telomeres are repeated sequences of DNA at the ends of chromosomes. Under physiological conditions, as the cell divides, telomeres become progressively shorter. Telomerase counteracts the shortening of telomeres by adding small segments of DNA at the end of chromosome after each cell division. Enhanced telomerase activity facilitates cellular immortality and promotes oncogenesis. Mutations of TERT promoter unmask binding sites for transcription factors, upregulate TERT expression and cellular telomerase activity [97]. TERT mutations are much more common in primary GBM and are inversely correlated with IDH mutations. Primary GBMs with TERT mutation exhibit significantly shorter overall survival than TERT-wild type tumors [98]. This unfavorable prognosis was absent after gross total resection and temozolomide therapy, what may indicate that TERT mutation makes tumor more susceptible to chemotherapy.

Tumor suppressor **PARK2** gene (parkin RBR E3 ubiquitin protein ligase) has locus on 6q25.2-q27. The exact function of this gene is still to be explored. It codes an E3 ubiquitin ligase mediating the targeting of substrate proteins for proteasome degradation. Germ line mutations of this gene cause Parkinson's disease, somatic mutations contribute to cancer. PARK2 is one of the most commonly inactivated tumor suppressor genes in GBM [99]. Deletion or inactivating mutation of this gene causes inability of PARK2 to promote ubiquitination and results in cyclin E deregulation, which can promote tumor cell growth. Low expression of PARK2 is associated with poor survival [100].

MGMT gene encodes a protein with alkyltransferase activity. MGMT is a DNA repair enzyme, which is responsible for tumor resistance to alkylating and methylating agents. Activity of this enzyme is regulated by this promoter area. This promoter, when methylated, causes inactivation of MGMT. Approximately 44% of GBM has MGMT promoter methylation [21]. Methylation status of MGMT is clinically the most relevant molecular parameter to predict sensitivity of gliomas do DNA alkylating chemotherapeutics [101]. This methylation is associated with prolonged progression-free survival and overall survival in patients with GBM treated with alkylating agents, such as temozolomide. [102]. Expression of MGMT is not associated with tumor grade [68].

4. Conclusion

GBM is the most aggressive and devastating primary brain tumor with very grim prognosis. The patient's survival rarely exceeds a year and a half with all accessible therapy used. Only 3% of GBM patients have survival over 5 years. This fact makes this tumor a very severe diagnosis directly affecting life expectancy of the patient and quality of his/her life. Explanation of its genesis could bring us closer to invention of effective treatment and genetic profile of concrete GBM tissue would help to design the individualized therapy management for each patient. Understanding the genetic and epigenetic characterization could help to distinguish various GBM subgroups, indistinguishable by histological appearance, but classified according to molecular and genetic alterations. This could lead to establishment of GBM classification with clinical impact, subgroup-specific treatment, and better design of future trials. The aim was to achieve prolonged progression-free interval and overall survival with maintaining satisfactory quality of life. It is very important if concrete genetic alteration is connected to tumor formation or if it is prognostic factor. Other factors influencing prognosis are histological type and tumor grade, age of patient, Karnofsky performance score at the time of diagnosis, extend of surgical resection, tumor localization, and appropriate therapeutic management. Tumor localization and extend of its surgical resection influence progression-free interval as well as overall survival. Detailed and complete explanation and discovery of altered genes and whole genetic pathways of GBM is the basis for new distinctive GBM classification. Such a new tumor division could bring us closer to routine genetic examination of frequently altered genetic pathways from tumor sample and aiming of therapy directly against specific genetic and epigenetic targets. Such individualized therapy could decrease the number of adverse effects, but first of all, hopefully, would finally ameliorate survival and life quality of patients, suffering from this severe disease.

Acknowledgements

This work was supported by projects: Competence Center for Research and Development in the diagnosis and therapy of oncological diseases, ITMS 26220220153 and The application of PACS (Picture Archiving and Communication System) in the reasearch and development, ITMS 26210120004.

Author details

Romana Richterová* and Branislav Kolarovszki

*Address all correspondence to: romana.richterova@gmail.com

Department of Neurosurgery, Jessenius Faculty of Medicine in Martin, Comenius University in Bratislava, Martin, Slovakia

References

[1] Ricard D, Idbaih A, Ducray F, Lahutte M, Hoang-Xuan K, Delattre JY: Primary brain tumours in adults. Lancet. 2012;379:1984–1996. DOI: 10.1016/S0140-6736(11)61346-9

[2] Michael KE, Dumbauld DW, Burns KL, Hanks SK, Garcia AJ: Focal adhesion kinase modulates cell adhesion strengthening via integrin activation. Mol Biol Cell. 2009;20:2508–2519. DOI: 10.1091/mbc.E08-01-0076

[3] Sengupta SNS, Hindi ES, Wainwright DA, Han Y, Lesniak MS: Short hairpin RNA-mediated fibronectin knockdown delays tumor growth in a mouse glioma model. Neoplasia. 2010;12:837–847.

[4] Cancer Genome Atlas Research Network: Comprehensive genomic characterization defines human GBM genes and core pathways. Nature. 2008;455:1061–1068. DOI: 10.1038/nature07385

[5] Iacob G, Dinca EB: Current data and strategy in GBM multiforme. J Med Life. 2009;2:386–393.

[6] Hede SM, Nazarenko I, Nistér M, Lindström MS: Novel perspectives on p53 function in neural stem cells and brain tumors. J Oncol. 2011;2011:852970. DOI: 10.1155/2011/852970

[7] Zhao Z, Xu Y: p53 and stem cells: new developments and new concerns. Trends Cell Biol. 2010;20:170–175. DOI: 10.1016/j.tcb.2009.12.004

[8] Krakstad C, Chekenya M: Survival signaling and apoptosis resistance in GBMs: opportunities for targeted therapeutics. Mol Cancer. 2010;9:135–149. DOI: 10.1186/1476-4598-9-135

[9] Wade M, Wang YV, Wahl GM: The p53 orchestra: Mdm2 and Mdmx set the tone. Trends Cell Biol. 2010;20:299–309. DOI: 10.1016/j.tcb.2010.01.009

[10] Furnari FB, Fenton T, Bachoo RM, Mukasa A, Stommel JM, Stegh A, Hahn WC, Ligon KL, Louis DN, Brennan C, Chin L, DePinho RA, Cavenee WK: Malignant astrocytic glioma: genetics, biology, and paths to treatment. Genes Dev. 2007;21:2683–2710. DOI: 10.1101/gad.1596707

[11] Thomasova D, Mulay SR, Bruns H, Anders HJ: p53-independent roles of MDM2 in NF-κB signaling: implications for cancer therapy, wound healing, and autoimmune diseases. Neoplasia. 2012;14:1097–1101.

[12] Wang AL, Liu ZX, Li G, Zhang LW: Expression and significance of P53 protein and MDM-2 protein in human gliomas. Chin Med J (Engl). 2011;124:2530–2533.

[13] Wang CL, Wang JY, Liu ZY, Ma XM, Wang XW, Jin H, Zhang XP, Fu D, Hou LJ, Lu YC: Ubiquitin-specific protease 2a stabilizes MDM4 and facilitates the p53-mediated intrinsic apoptotic pathway in GBM. Carcinogenesis. 2014;35:1500–1509. DOI: 10.1093/carcin/bgu015

[14] Goldhoff P, Clarke J, Smirnov I, Berger MS, Prados MD, James CD, Perry A, Phillips JJ: Clinical stratification of GBM based on alterations in retinoblastoma tumor suppressor protein (RB1) and association with the proneural subtype. J Neuropathol Exp Neurol. 2012;71:83–89. DOI: 10.1097/NEN.0b013e31823fe8f1

[15] Chow LM, Endersby R, Zhu X, Rankin S, Qu C, Zhang J, Broniscer A, Ellison DW, Baker SJ: Cooperativity within and among Pten, p53, and Rb pathways induces high-grade astrocytoma in adult brain. Cancer Cell. 2011;19:305–316. DOI: 10.1016/j.ccr.2011.01.039

[16] Wiedemeyer WR, Dunn IF, Quayle SN, Zhang J, Chheda MG, Dunn GP, Zhuang L, Rosenbluh J, Chen S, Xiao Y, Shapiro GI, Hahn WC, Chin L: Pattern of retinoblastoma pathway inactivation dictates response to CDK4/6 inhibition in GBM. Proc Natl Acad Sci USA. 2010;107:11501–11506. DOI: 10.1073/pnas.1001613107

[17] Kim CS, Jung S, Jung TY, Jang WY, Sun HS, Ryu HH: Characterization of invading glioma cells using molecular analysis of leading-edge tissue. J Korean Neurosurg Soc. 2011;50:157–165. DOI: 10.3340/jkns.2011.50.3.157

[18] Walker C, Baborie A, Crooks D, Wilkins S, Jenkinson MD: Biology, genetics and imaging of glial cell tumours. Br J Radiol. 2011;84:90–106. DOI: 10.1259/bjr/23430927

[19] Yue WY, Sai K, Wu QL, Xia YF, Yu SH, Chen ZP: Long-term molecular changes in WHO grade II astrocytomas following radiotherapy. Chin J Cancer. 2012;31:159–165. DOI: 10.5732/cjc.011.10149

[20] Liu Y, Shete S, Hosking FJ, Robertson LB, Bondy ML, Houlston RS: New insights into susceptibility to glioma. Arch Neurol. 2010;67:275–278. DOI: 10.1001/archneurol.2010.4

[21] Weller M, Felsberg J, Hartmann C, Berger H, Steinbach JP, Schramm J, Westphal M, Schackert G, Simon M, Tonn JC, Heese O, Krex D, Nikkhah G, Pietsch T, Wiestler O, Reifenberger G, von Deimling A, Loeffler M: Molecular predictors of progression-free and overall. Survival in patients with newly diagnosed GBM: a prospective translational study of the German glioma network. J Clin Oncol. 2009;27:5743–5750. DOI: 10.1200/JCO.2009.23.0805

[22] Shete S, Hosking FJ, Robertson LB, Dobbins SE, Sanson M, Malmer B, Simon M, Marie Y, Boisselier B, Delattre JY, Hoang-Xuan K, El Hallani S, Idbaih A, Zelenika D, Andersson U, Henriksson R, Bergenheim AT, Feychting M, Lönn S, Ahlbom A, Schramm J, Linnebank M, Hemminki K, Kumar R, Hepworth SJ, Price A, Armstrong G, Liu Y, Gu X, Yu R, Lau C, Schoemaker M, Muir K, Swerdlow A, Lathrop M, Bondy M, Houlston RS: Genome-wide association study identifies five susceptibility loci for glioma. Nat Genet. 2009;41:899–904. DOI: 10.1038/ng.407

[23] Simon M, Hosking FJ, Marie Y, Gousias K, Boisselier B, Carpentier C, Schramm J, Mokhtari K, Hoang-Xuan K, Idbaih A, Delattre JY, Lathrop M, Robertson LB, Houlston RS, Sanson M: Genetic risk profiles identify different molecular etiologies for glioma. Clin Cancer Res. 2010;16:5252–5259. DOI: 10.1158/1078-0432.CCR-10-1502

[24] Zerrouqi A, Pyrzynska B, Febbraio M, Brat DJ, Van Meir EG: P14ARF inhibits human GBM-induced angiogenesis by upregulating the expression of TIMP3. J Clin Invest. 2012;122:1283–1295. DOI: 10.1172/JCI38596

[25] Solomon DA, Kim JS, Jenkins S, Ressom H, Huang M, Coppa N, Mabanta L, Bigner D, Yan H, Jean W, Waldman T: Identification of p18 INK4c as a tumor suppressor gene in GBM multiforme. Cancer Res. 2008;68:2564–2569. DOI: 10.1158/0008-5472.CAN-07-6388

[26] Koyama-Nasu R, Nasu-Nishimura Y, Todo T, Ino Y, Saito N, Aburatani H, Funato K, Echizen K, Sugano H, Haruta R, Matsui M, Takahashi R, Manabe E, Oda T, Akiyama T: The critical role of cyclin D2 in cell cycle progression and tumorigenicity of GBM stem cells. Oncogene. 2013;32:3840–3845. DOI: 10.1038/onc.2012.399

[27] Courtney KD, Corcoran RB, Engelman JA: The PI3K pathway as drug target in human cancer. J Clin Oncol. 2010;28:1075–1083. DOI: 10.1200/JCO.2009.25.3641

[28] Wen PY, Lee EQ, Reardon DA, Ligon KL, Alfred Yung WK: Current clinical development of PI3K pathway inhibitors in GBM. Neuro Oncol. 2012;14:819–829. DOI: 10.1093/neuonc/nos117.

[29] Parsons DW, Jones S, Zhang X, Lin JC, Leary RJ, Angenendt P, Mankoo P, Carter H, Siu IM, Gallia GL, Olivi A, McLendon R, Rasheed BA, Keir S, Nikolskaya T, Nikolsky Y, Busam DA, Tekleab H, Diaz LA Jr, Hartigan J, Smith DR, Strausberg RL, Marie SK, Shinjo SM, Yan H, Riggins GJ, Bigner DD, Karchin R, Papadopoulos N, Parmigiani G,

Vogelstein B, Velculescu VE, Kinzler KW: An integrated genomic analysis of human GBM multiforme. Science. 2008;321:1807–1812. DOI: 10.1126/science.1164382

[30] Varghese RT, Liang Y, Guan T, Franck CT, Kelly DF, Sheng Z: Survival kinase genes present prognostic significance in glioblastoma. Oncotarget. 2016;7:20140-20151. DOI: 10.18632/oncotarget.7917

[31] Sun MHP, Hofmann BT, Hart JR, Vogt PK: Cancer derived mutations in the regulatory subunit p85alpha of phosphoinositide 3-kinase function through the catalytic subunit p110alpha. Proc Natl Acad Sci USA. 2010;107:15,547–15,552. DOI: 10.1073/pnas.1009652107

[32] Weber GL, Parat MO, Binder ZA, Gallia GL, Riggins GJ: Abrogation of PIK3CA or PIK3R1 reduces proliferation, migration, and invasion in GBM multiforme cells. Oncotarget. 201;2:833–849.

[33] Lee JJ, Kim BC, Park MJ, Lee YS, Kim YN, Lee BL, Lee JS: PTEN status switches cell fate between premature senescence and apoptosis in glioma exposed to ionizing radiation. Cell Death Differ. 2011;18:666–677. DOI: 10.1038/cdd.2010.139

[34] Sherry MM, Reeves A, Wu JK, Cochran BH: STAT3 is required for proliferation and maintenance of multipotency in GBM stem cells. Stem Cells. 2009;27:2383–2392. DOI: 10.1002/stem.185

[35] Turner KM, Sun Y, Ji P, Granberg KJ, Bernard B, Hu L, Cogdell DE, Zhou X, Yli-Harja O, Nykter M, Shmulevich I, Yung WK, Fuller GN, Zhang W: Genomically amplified Akt3 activates DNA repair pathway and promotes glioma progression. Proc Natl Acad Sci USA. 2015;112:3421–3426. DOI: 10.1073/pnas.1414573112

[36] Omuro AM, Faivre S, Raymond E: Lessons learned in the development of targeted therapy for malignant gliomas. Mol Cancer Ther. 2007;6:1909–1919.

[37] Easton RM, Cho H, Roovers K, Shineman DW, Mizrahi M, Forman MS, Lee VM, Szabolcs M, de Jong R, Oltersdorf T, Ludwig T, Efstratiadis A, Birnbaum MJ: Role for Akt3/protein kinase Bgamma in attainment of normal brain size. Mol Cell Biol. 2005;25:1869–1878.

[38] Mure H, Matsuzaki K, Kitazato KT, Mizobuchi Y, Kuwayama K, Kageji T, Nagahiro S: Akt2 and Akt3 play a pivotal role in malignant gliomas. Neuro Oncol. 2010;12:221–232. DOI: 10.1093/neuonc/nop026

[39] Verhaak RG, Hoadley KA, Purdom E, Wang V, Qi Y, Wilkerson MD, Miller CR, Ding L, Golub T, Mesirov JP, Alexe G, Lawrence M, O'Kelly M, Tamayo P, Weir BA, Gabriel S, Winckler W, Gupta S, Jakkula L, Feiler HS, Hodgson JG, James CD, Sarkaria JN, Brennan C, Kahn A, Spellman PT, Wilson RK, Speed TP, Gray JW, Meyerson M, Getz G, Perou CM, Hayes DN; Cancer Genome Atlas Research Network: Integrated genomic analysis identifies clinically relevant subtypes of GBM characterized by abnormalities in PDGFRA, IDH1, EGFR and NF1. Cancer Cell. 2010;17:98–110. DOI: 10.1016/j.ccr.2009.12.020

[40] Faria MH, Gonçalves BP, do Patrocínio RM, de Moraes-Filho MO, Rabenhorst SH: Expression of Ki-67, topoisomerase II alpha and c-MYC in astrocytic tumors: correlation with the histopathological grade and proliferative status. Neuropathology. 2006;26:519–527.

[41] Cenci T, Martini M, Montano N, D'Alessandris QG, Falchetti ML, Annibali D, Savino M, Bianchi F, Pierconti F, Nasi S, Pallini R, Larocca LM: Prognostic relevance of c-Myc and BMI1 expression in patients with glioblastoma. Am J Clin Pathol. 2012;138:390–396. DOI: 10.1309/AJCPRXHNJQLO09QA

[42] De Salvo M, Maresca G, D'agnano I, Marchese R, Stigliano A, Gagliassi R, Brunetti E, Raza GH, De Paula U, Bucci B: Temozolomide induced c-Myc-mediated apoptosis via Akt signaling in MGMT expressing glioblastoma cells. Int J Radiat Biol. 2011;87:518–533. DOI: 10.3109/09553002.2011.556173

[43] Shakhova O, Leung C, Marino S: Bmi1 in development and tumorigenesis of the central nervous system. J Mol Med. 2005;83:596–600.

[44] Guo WJ, Datta S, Band V, Dimri GP: Mel-18, a polycomb group protein, regulates cell proliferation and senescence via transcriptional repression of Bmi-1 and c-Myc oncoproteins. Mol Biol Cell. 2007;18:536–546.

[45] Pusch S, Sahm F, Meyer J, Mittelbronn M, Hartmann C, von Deimling A: Glioma IDH1 mutation patterns off the beaten track. Neuropathol Appl Neurobiol. 2011;37:428–430. DOI: 10.1111/j.1365-2990.2010.01127.x

[46] Zhao S, Lin Y, Xu W, Jiang W, Zha Z, Wang P, Yu W, Li Z, Gong L, Peng Y, Ding J, Lei Q, Guan KL, Xiong Y: Glioma-derived mutations in IDH1 dominantly inhibit IDH1 catalytic activity and induce HIF-1alpha. Science. 2009;324:261–265. DOI: 10.1126/science.1170944

[47] Toedt G, Barbus S, Wolter M, Felsberg J, Tews B, Blond F, Sabel MC, Hofmann S, Becker N, Hartmann C, Ohgaki H, von Deimling A, Wiestler OD, Hahn M, Lichter P, Reifenberger G, Radlwimmer B: Molecular signatures classify astrocytic gliomas by IDH1 mutation status. Int J Cancer. 2011;128:1095–1103. DOI: 10.1002/ijc.25448

[48] Kim W, Liau LM: IDH mutations in human glioma. Neurosurg Clin N Am. 2012;23:471–480. DOI: 10.1016/j.nec.2012.04.009

[49] Yan H, Parsons DW, Jin G, McLendon R, Rasheed A, Yuan W, Kos I, Batinic-Haberle I, Jones S, Riggins GJ, Friedman H, Friedman A, Reardon D, Herndon J, Kinzler KW, Velculescu VE, Vogelstein B, Bigner DD: IDH1 and IDH2 mutations in gliomas. N Engl J Med. 2009;360:765–773. DOI: 10.1056/NEJMoa0808710

[50] Ichimura K, Pearson DM, Kocialkowski S, Bäcklund LM, Chan R, Jones DT, Collins VP: IDH1 mutations are present in the majority of common adult gliomas but rare in primary GBMs. Neuro Oncol. 2009;11:341–347. DOI: 10.1215/15228517-2009-025

[51] Reitman ZJ, Yan H: Isocitrate dehydrogenase 1 and 2 mutations in cancer: alterations at a crossroads of cellular metabolism. J Natl Cancer Inst. 2010;102:932–941. DOI: 10.1093/jnci/djq187

[52] SongTao Q, Lei Y, Si G, YanQing D, HuiXia H, XueLin Z, LanXiao W, Fei Y: IDH mutations predict longer survival and response to temozolomide in secondary GBM. Cancer Sci. 2012;103:269–273. DOI: 10.1111/j.1349-7006.2011.02134.x

[53] Nobusawa S, Watanabe T, Kleihues P, Ohgaki H: IDH1 mutations as molecular signature and predictive factor of secondary GBMs. Clin Cancer Res. 2009;15:6002–6007. DOI: 10.1158/1078-0432.CCR-09-0715

[54] Beiko J, Suki D, Hess KR, Fox BD, Cheung V, Cabral M, Shonka N, Gilbert MR, Sawaya R, Prabhu SS, Weinberg J, Lang FF, Aldape KD, Sulman EP, Rao G, McCutcheon IE, Cahill DP: IDH1 mutant malignant astrocytomas are more amenable to surgical resection and have a survival benefit associated with maximal surgical resection. Neuro-Oncology. 2014;16:81–91. DOI: 10.1093/neuonc/not159

[55] Reitman ZJ, Yan H: Isocitrate dehydrogenase 1 and 2 mutations in cancer: alterations at a crossroads of cellular metabolism. J Natl Cancer Inst. 2010;102:932–941. DOI: 10.1093/jnci/djq187

[56] Takahashi Y, Nakamura H, Makino K, Hide T, Muta D, Kamada H, Kuratsu J: Prognostic value of isocitrate dehydrogenase 1, O6-methylguanine-DNA methyltransferase promoter methylation, and 1p19q co-deletion in Japanese malignant glioma patients. World J Surg Oncol. 2013;11:284. DOI: 10.1186/1477-7819-11-284

[57] Rohle D, Popovici-Muller J, Palaskas N, Turcan S, Grommes C, Campos C, Tsoi J, Clark O, Oldrini B, Komisopoulou E, Kunii K, Pedraza A, Schalm S, Silverman L, Miller A, Wang F, Yang H, Chen Y, Kernytsky A, Rosenblum MK, Liu W, Biller SA, Su SM, Brennan CW, Chan TA, Graeber TG, Yen KE, Mellinghoff IK: An inhibitor of mutant IDH1 delays growth and promotes differentiation of glioma cells. Science. 2013;340:626–630. DOI: 10.1126/science.1236062

[58] Rajasekharan S, Kennedy TE: The netrin protein family. Genome Biol. 2009;10:239. DOI: 10.1186/GBM-2009-10-9-239

[59] Jarjour AA, Durko M, Luk TL, Marçal N, Shekarabi M, Kennedy TE: Autocrine netrin function inhibits glioma cell motility and promotes focal adhesion formation. PLoS One. 2011;6:e25408. DOI:10.1371/journal.pone.0025408

[60] Jiang X, Yu Y, Yang HW, Agar NY, Frado L, Johnson MD: The imprinted gene PEG3 inhibits Wnt signaling and regulates glioma growth. J Biol Chem. 2010;285:8472–8480. DOI: 10.1074/jbc.M109.069450

[61] Otsuka S, Maegawa S, Takamura A, Kamitani H, Watanabe T, Oshimura M, Nanba E: Aberrant promoter methylation and expression of the imprinted PEG3 gene in glioma. Proc Jpn Acad Ser B. 2009;85:157–165. DOI: 10.2183/pjab.85.157

[62] Kilburn L, Okcu F, Wang T, Cao Y, Renfro-Spelman A, Aldape KD, Gilbert MR, Bondy M: Glutathione S-transferase polymorphism are associated with survival in anaplastic glioma patients. Cancer. 2010;116:2242–2249. DOI: 10.1002/cncr.25006

[63] Lo H, Ali-Osman F: Genetic polymorphism and function of glutathione S-transferases in tumor drug resistance. Curr Opin Pharmacol. 2007;7:367–374. DOI: 10.1016/j.coph.2007.06.009

[64] Schwartzbaum JA, Ahlbom A, Lönn S, Warholm M, Rannug A, Auvinen A, Christensen HC, Henriksson R, Johansen C, Lindholm C, Malmer B, Salminen T, Schoemaker MJ, Swerdlow AJ, Feychting M: An international casecontrol study of glutathione transferase and functionally related polymorphisms and risk of primary adult brain tumors. Cancer Epidemiol Biomarkers Prev. 2007;16:559–565. DOI: 10.1158/1055-9965.EPI-06-0918

[65] Sjöström S, Anderson U, Liu Y, Brännström T, Broholm H, Johansen C, Collatz-Laier H, Henriksson R, Bondy M, Melin B: Genetic variation in EGF and EGFR and GBM outcome. Neuro-Oncol. 2010;12:815–821. DOI: 10.1093/neuonc/noq018

[66] Chen X, Yang G, Zhang D, Zhang W, Zou H, Zhao H, Zhang X, Zhao S: Association between the epidermal growth factor +61 G/A polymorphism and glioma risk: a meta-analysis. PLoS One. 2014;9:e95139. DOI: 10.1371/journal.pone.0095139

[67] Pinto GR, Yoshioka FK, Clara CA, Santos MJ, Almeida JR, Burbano RR, Rey JA, Casartelli C: Association study of an epidermal growth factor gene functional polymorphism with the risk and prognosis of gliomas in Brazil. Int J Biol Markers. 2009;24:277–281.

[68] Hu X, Miao W, Zou Y, Zhang W, Zhang Y, Liu H: Expression of p53, epidermal growth factor receptor, Ki-67 and O6-methylguanine-DNA methyltransferase in human gliomas. Oncol Lett. 2013;6:130–134.

[69] Ozawa T, Brennan CW, Wang L, Squatrito M, Sasayama T, Nakada M, Huse JT, Pedraza A, Utsuki S, Yasui Y, Tandon A, Fomchenko EI, Oka H, Levine RL, Fujii K, Ladanyi M, Holland EC: PDGFRA gene rearrangements are frequent genetic events in PDGFRA-amplified GBMs. Genes Dev. 2010;24:2205–2218. DOI: 10.1101/gad.1972310

[70] Kim Y, Kim E, Wu Q, Guryanova O, Hitomi M, Lathia JD, Serwanski D, Sloan AE, Weil RJ, Lee J, Nishiyama A, Bao S, Hjelmeland AB, Rich JN: Platelet-derived growth factor receptors differentially inform intertumoral and intratumoral heterogeneity. Genes Dev. 2012;26:1247–1262. DOI: 10.1101/gad.193565.112

[71] Westermark B: Platelet-derived growth factor in GBM-driver or biomarker? Ups J Med Sci. 2014;119:298–305. DOI: 10.3109/03009734.2014.970304

[72] Lönn S, Rothman N, Shapiro WR, Fine HA, Selker RG, Black PM, Loeffler JS, Hutchinson AA, Inskip PD: Genetic variation in insulin-like growth factors and brain tumor risk. Neuro-Oncol. 2008;10:553–559. DOI: 10.1215/15228517-2008-026

[73] Pardo OE, Wellbrock C, Khanzada UK, Aubert M, Arozarena I, Davidson S, Bowen F, Parker PJ, Filonenko VV, Gout IT, Sebire N, Marais R, Downward J, Seckl MJ: FGF-2 protects small cell lung cancer cells from apoptosis through a complex involving PKCepsilon, B-Raf and S6K2. The EMBO Journal. 2006;25:3078–3088.

[74] Haley EM, Kim Y: The role of basic fibroblast growth factor in GBM multiforme and GBM stem cells and in their in vitro culture. Cancer Lett. 2014;346:1–5. DOI: 10.1016/j.canlet.2013.12.003

[75] Desjardins A, Friedman HS: Bevacizumab therapy for GBM: a passionate discussion. CNS Oncol. 2014;3:1–3. DOI: 10.2217/cns.13.53

[76] Wang K, Wang YY, Wang JF, Ma J, Jiang T, Dai JP: Radiologic features and expression of vascular endothelial growth factor stratify survival outcomes in patients with GBM. AJNR Am J Neuroradiol. 2016;37:629-635. DOI:10.3174/ajnr.A4567

[77] Santibanez JF, Quintanilla M, Bernabeu C: TGF-beta/ TGF-beta receptor system and its role in physiological and pathological conditions. Clin Sci (Lond). 2011;121:233–251. DOI: 10.1042/CS20110086

[78] Weiss A, Attisano L: The TGFbeta superfamily signaling pathway. Wiley Interdisciplinary Reviews. Developmental Biol. 2013;2:47–63. DOI: 10.1002/wdev.86

[79] Kaminska B, Kocyk M, Kijewska M: TGF beta signaling and its role in glioma pathogenesis. Adv Exp Med Biol. 2013;986:171–187. DOI: 10.1007/978-94-007-4719-7_9

[80] Frei K, Gramatzki D, Tritschler I, Schroeder JJ, Espinoza L, Rushing EJ, Weller M: Transforming growth factor-β pathway activity in GBM. Oncotarget. 2015;6:5963–5977.

[81] Organ SL, Tsao MS: An overview of the c-MET signaling pathway. Ther Adv Med Oncol. 2011;3:7–19. DOI: 10.1177/1758834011422556

[82] Kwak Y, Kim SI, Park CK, Paek SH, Lee ST, Park SH: C-MET overexpression and amplification in gliomas. Int J Clin Exp Pathol. 2015;8:14932–14938.

[83] Kong DS, Song SY, Kim DH, Joo KM, Yoo JS, Koh JS, Dong SM, Suh YL, Lee JI, Park K, Kim JH, Nam DH: Prognostic significance of c-Met expression in GBMs. Cancer. 2009;115:140–148. DOI: 10.1002/cncr.23972

[84] Basilico C, Arnesano A, Galluzzo M, Comoglio PM, Michieli P: A high affinity hepatocyte growth factor-binding site in the immunoglobulin-like region of Met. J Biol Chem. 2008;283:21,267–21,277. DOI: 10.1074/jbc.M800727200

[85] Xie Q, Bradley R, Kang L, Koeman J, Ascierto ML, Worschech A, De Giorgi V, Wang E, Kefene L, Su Y, Essenburg C, Kaufman DW, DeKoning T, Enter MA, O'Rourke TJ, Marincola FM, Vande Woude GF: Hepatocyte growth factor (HGF) autocrine activation predicts sensitivity to MET inhibition in GBM. Proc Natl Acad Sci USA. 2012;109:570–575. DOI: 10.1073/pnas.1119059109

[86] Garcia-Navarrete R, Garcia E, Arrieta O, Sotelo J: Hepatocyte growth factor in cerebrospinal fluid is associated with mortality and recurrence of GBM, and could be of prognostic value. J Neurooncol. 2010;97:347–351. DOI: 10.1007/s11060-009-0037-8

[87] Watson LA, Goldberg H, Bérubé NG: Emerging roles of ATRX in cancer. Epigenomics. 2015;7:1365–13678. DOI: 10.2217/epi.15.82

[88] Liu XY, Gerges N, Korshunov A, Sabha N, Khuong-Quang DA, Fontebasso AM, Fleming A, Hadjadj D, Schwartzentruber J, Majewski J, Dong Z, Siegel P, Albrecht S, Croul S, Jones DT, Kool M, Tonjes M, Reifenberger G, Faury D, Zadeh G, Pfister S, Jabado N: Frequent ATRX mutations and loss of expression in adult diffuse astrocytic tumors carrying IDH1/IDH2 and TP53 mutations. Acta Neuropathol. 2012;124:615–625. DOI: 10.1007/s00401-012-1031-3

[89] Appin CL, Brat DJ: Molecular pathways in gliomagenesis and their relevance to neuropathologic diagnosis. Adv Anat Pathol. 2015;22:50–58. DOI: 10.1097/PAP.0000000000000048

[90] Kleinschmidt-DeMasters BK, Aisner DL, Birks DK, Foreman NK: Epithelioid GBMs show a high percentage of BRAF V600E mutation. Am J Surg Pathol. 2013;37:685–698. DOI: 10.1097/PAS.0b013e31827f9c5e

[91] Schindler G, Capper D, Meyer J, Janzarik W, Omran H, Herold-Mende C, Schmieder K, Wesseling P, Mawrin C, Hasselblatt M, Louis DN, Korshunov A, Pfister S, Hartmann C, Paulus W, Reifenberger G, von Deimling A: Analysis of BRAF V600E mutation in 1320 nervous system tumors reveals high mutation frequencies in pleomorphic xanthoastrocytoma, ganglioglioma and extra-cerebellar pilocytic astrocytoma. Acta Neuropathol. 2011;121:397–405. DOI: 10.1007/s00401-011-0802-6

[92] Gutmann DH: BRAF-V600E mutation in pediatric and adult GBM. Neuro-Oncology. 2014;16:318–319. DOI: 10.1093/neuonc/not146

[93] Takahashi Y, Akahane T, Sawada T, Ikeda H, Tempaku A, Yamauchi S, Nishihara H, Tanaka S, Nitta K, Ide W, Hashimoto I, Kamada H: Adult classical GBM with a BRAFV600E mutation. World J Surg Oncol. 2015;13:100. DOI: 10.1186/s12957-015-0521-x

[94] Lewis PW, Elsaesser SJ, Noh KM, Stadler SC, Allis CD: Daxx is an H3.3-specific histone chaperone and cooperates with ATRX in replication-independent chromatin assembly at telomeres. Proc Natl Acad Sci USA. 2010;107:14,075–14,080. DOI: 10.1073/pnas.1008850107

[95] Schwartzentruber J, Korshunov A, Liu XY, Jones DTW, Pfaff E, Jacob K, Sturm D, Fontebasso AM, Quang DA, Tonjes M, Hovestadt V, Albrecht S, Kool M, Nantel A, Konermann C, Lindroth A, Jäger N, Rausch T, Ryzhova M, Korbel JO, Hielscher T, Hauser P, Garami M, Klekner A, Bognar L, Ebinger M, Schuhmann MU, Scheurlen W, Pekrun A, Frühwald MC, Roggendorf W, Kramm C, Dürken M, Atkinson J, Lepage P, Montpetit A, Zakrzewska M, Zakrzewski K, Liberski PP, Dong Z, Siegel P, Kulozik AE,

Zapatka M, Guha A, Malkin D, Felsberg J, Reifenberger G, von Deimling A, Ichimura K, Collins VP, Witt H, Milde T, Witt O, Zhang C, Castelo-Branco P, Lichter P, Faury D, Tabori U, Plass C, Majewski J, Pfister SM, Jabado N: Driver mutations in histone H3.3 and chromatin remodelling genes in paediatric GBM. Nature. 2012;482:226–231. DOI: 10.1038/nature10833

[96] Sturm D, Witt H, Hovestadt V, Khuong-Quang DA, Jones DT, Konermann C, Pfaff E, Tönjes M, Sill M, Bender S, Kool M, Zapatka M, Becker N, Zucknick M, Hielscher T, Liu XY, Fontebasso AM, Ryzhova M, Albrecht S, Jacob K, Wolter M, Ebinger M, Schuhmann MU, van Meter T, Frühwald MC, Hauch H, Pekrun A, Radlwimmer B, Niehues T, von Komorowski G, Dürken M, Kulozik AE, Madden J, Donson A, Foreman NK, Drissi R, Fouladi M, Scheurlen W, von Deimling A,Monoranu C, Roggendorf W, Herold-Mende C, Unterberg A, Kramm CM, Felsberg J, Hartmann C, Wiestler B, Wick W, Milde T, Witt O, Lindroth AM, Schwartzentruber J, Faury D, Fleming A, Zakrzewska M, Liberski PP, Zakrzewski K, Hauser P, Garami M, Klekner A, Bognar L, Morrissy S, Cavalli F, Taylor MD,van Sluis P, Koster J, Versteeg R, Volckmann R, Mikkelsen T, Aldape K, Reifenberger G, Collins VP, Majewski J, Korshunov A, Lichter P, Plass C, Jabado N, Pfister SM: Hotspot mutations in H3F3A and IDH1 define distinct epigenetic and biological subgroups of GBM. Cancer Cell. 2012;22:425–437. DOI: 10.1016/j.ccr.2012.08.024

[97] Huang FW, Hodis E, Xu MJ, Kryukov GV, Chin L, Garraway LA: Highly recurrent TERT promoter mutations in human melanoma. Science. 2013;339:957–959. DOI: 10.1126/science.1229259

[98] Simon M, Hosen I, Gousias K, Rachakonda S, Heidenreich B, Gessi M, Schramm J, Hemminki K, Waha A, Kumar R: TERT promoter mutations: a novel independent prognostic factor in primary GBMs. Neuro Oncol. 2015;17:45–52. DOI: 10.1093/neuonc/nou158

[99] Veeriah S, Taylor BS, Meng S, Fang F, Yilmaz E, Vivanco I, Janakiraman M, Schultz N, Hanrahan AJ, Pao W, Ladanyi M, Sander C, Heguy A, Holland EC, Paty PB, Mischel PS, Liau L, Cloughesy TF, Mellinghoff IK, Solit DB, Chan TA: Somatic mutations of the Parkinson's disease-associated gene PARK2 in glioblastoma and other human malignancies. Nat Genet. 2010;42:77–82. DOI: 10.1038/ng.491

[100] Lin DC, Xu L, Chen Y, Yan H, Hazawa M, Doan N, Said JW, Ding LW, Liu LZ, Yang H, Yu S, Kahn M, Yin D, Koeffler HP: Genomic and Functional Analysis of the E3 Ligase PARK2 in Glioma. Cancer Res. 2015;75:1815–1827. DOI: 10.1158/0008-5472.CAN-14-1433

[101] Von Deimling A, Korshunov A, Hartmann C: The next generation of glioma biomarkers: MGMT methylation, BRAF fusions and IDH1 mutations. Brain Pathol. 2011;21:74–87. DOI: 10.1111/j.1750-3639.2010.00454.x

[102] Glas M, Happold C, Rieger J, Wiewrodt D, Bähr O, Steinbach JP, Wick W, Kortmann RD, Reifenberger G, Weller M, Herrlinger U: Long-term survival of GBM patients treated with radiotherapy and lomustine plus temozolomide. J Clin Oncol. 2009;27:1257–1261. DOI: 10.1200/JCO.2008.19.2195

6

The Roles of MicroRNAs in Glioblastoma Biology and Biomarker

Takashi Sasayama, Kazuhiro Tanaka and Eiji Kohmura

Abstract

MicroRNAs (miRNAs) are small, noncoding RNAs transcribed from DNA that are 18–24 nucleotides in length. A single miRNA has the capacity to regulate a large number of target messenger RNAs (mRNAs), and the main function of miRNAs is to downregulate gene expression. A large set of miRNAs is overexpressed or downregulated in various human cancers compared with normal tissues, and gene silencing by miRNAs enhances tumor malignancies.

In glioblastomas (GBMs), a number of miRNAs are reported to display aberrant expression patterns, and miRNAs have been shown to strongly influence cell viability, cell proliferation, invasiveness, angiogenesis, metabolism, and microenvironment. Since early findings, the number of studies published on this subject has steadily increased, elucidating numerous interesting miRNA-mediated mechanisms in the tumorigenesis of GBM.

A number of studies have recently suggested that circulating miRNAs could be potential biomarkers for cancer diagnosis. Not only the role of miRNAs in glioma development but also their specificity makes them important candidate biomarkers that could provide important characteristic information about a tumor and improve treatment and prognosis. This review summarizes current progress and future directions in this exciting and steadily expanding field.

Keywords: glioblastoma, microRNA, hallmarks, biomarker, circulating

1. Introduction

Glioblastomas (GBMs) are the most common and intractable primary neoplasms of the central nervous system (CNS). Gross total surgical excision followed by radiotherapy up to a total dose of 60 Gy was the only accepted GBM management for decades because no chemotherapeutic agents significantly improved the survival of patients with GBM until the introduction of temozolomide, an oral alkylating agent (1). Despite aggressive treatments, recurrence is inevitable and fatal in GBMs. In a recent clinical study, the median survival was up to approximately 20 months and the two-year survival rate was approximately 30~40% (2, 3). Therefore, more efforts need to be made to change the poor prognosis of patients with GBM.

MicroRNAs (miRNAs) are small (18–24 nt), noncoding RNAs that are transcribed from the intergenic or intronic regions of DNA. miRNAs regulate the expression levels or translational levels of messenger RNAs (mRNAs) post-transcriptionally and affect to various biological processes, such as cell proliferation, cell survival, differentiation, and metabolism (4). Primary miRNAs (pri-miRNAs), transcribed from DNA and have short stem-loop structures (SLSs), are processed into premature miRNAs (pre-miRNAs) and then finally processed into mature miRNAs (5). A single miRNA has many targets of mRNAs, binding its target sites mostly in the 3′ untranslated region (3′-UTR) of the mRNA. The main function of miRNAs is to down-regulate gene expression, and miRNAs can function either as tumor suppressors or as oncogenes (6).

A number of miRNAs are reported to display aberrant expression patterns in GBMs (7). In 2005, the first miRNA dysregulation was identified in GBMs (8). miR-21 detected by northern blot was overexpressed in GBM tissues when compared with non-neoplastic control tissues. On the other hand, a systemic screen for miRNA aberrations by miRNA microarray in GBM was performed by other researchers (7). Using miRNA microarray analysis, we previously reported that miR-10b, miR-21, miR-183, miR-92b, and miR-106b are highly expressed in GBMs compared with normal brain tissue (9). Several other reports have also identified these miRNAs as being upregulated in GBMs (8). Recently, we reported that the expression of miR-183 involved in HIF-1α expression and its downstream molecules (10). Since then, it has been documented that miRNA dysregulation could play an important role in development and progression.

2. MicroRNA expression in glioblastoma

Similar to other malignant tumors, GBM has the hallmarks of cancer: biological capabilities of sustaining proliferative signaling, inducing angiogenesis, evading growth suppressors, resistance to apoptosis, activating invasion and metastasis, genomic instability, reprogramming energy metabolism, limitless replicative potential, and evading immune destruction. It is generally accepted that hallmark features of GBM are not only a reflection of genetic abnormalities and aberrant signal transition but also the dysregulation of miRNA-mediated translational control. The miRNA-mRNA interactions transform the short "nonsense" sequences into endogenous oncogenes or tumor suppressors. miRNA expression patterns could define a tumor type, implying that certain changes in miRNAs might drive the malignant transformation to a particular tumor. Therefore, whether a miRNA acts as an oncomiR or tumor suppressor-miRNA depends on the regulated genes and cellular context.

The first report on altered miRNA expression in GBMs was published in 2005 (8). In this report, miR-21 was shown to be highly upregulated and to have antiapoptotic capabilities in GBM cells. These findings suggest that overexpressed miR-21 may function as an oncogene in GBMs by blocking expression of key apoptosis-enabling genes (8). In the same year, Ciafre et al. analyzed the global expression levels of 245 microRNAs in both GBM cell lines and patient biopsies (7). A systemic screen for miRNA aberrations by microarray identified a set of dysregulated miRNAs in GBM tissues, including the upregulation of miR-10b, miR-21, and miR-25 and downregulation of miR-128 and miR-181a/181b-/181c (7). Since then, miRNA expression in GBMs has been evaluated in several profiling studies. We previously reported that miR-10b, miR-21, miR-183, miR-92b, and miR-106b are highly expressed in GBMs compared with normal brain tissue, and miR-134, miR-302c, miR-324, miR-379, and miR-368-3p are downregulated in GBMs (9). In 2008, Silber et al. reported 13 miRNAs to be downregulated and three miRNAs to be upregulated in anaplastic astrocytomas and GBMs (11). Furthermore, they revealed that expression levels of miRNA-124 and miRNA-137 were significantly decreased compared with non-neoplastic brain tissue, and both of them induce differentiation of adult neural stem cells. Another study carried out by Godlewski et al. found 8 microRNAs to be upregulated and 11 downregulated when analyzing 245 microRNAs in the setting of GBM (12). A microarray-based study by Rao et al. analyzing 756 microRNAs identified another 55 upregulated and 29 downregulated microRNAs in primary and secondary GBMs and anaplastic astrocytoma compared with controls (13). This study not only validated the role of several deregulated microRNAs but also provided data for the development of a 23 microRNA signature pattern for distinguishing between anaplastic astrocytoma and GBM (13).

3. Hallmarks of glioblastoma and microRNAs

3.1. Growth signal activation and microRNAs

Cell proliferation in GBM could be triggered by somatic alterations within the receptor tyrosine kinase (RTK)-signaling pathways. The most important pathways in GBM are the phosphatidylinositide 3-kinase (PI3K)/AKT and RAS/mitogen-activated protein kinase (MAPK) pathways (14). Abnormally augmented signals downstream from RTKs enable tumor cells to sustain proliferation that is under tight control in normal cells. At least 90% of GBM cases harbor genetic alterations in RTK pathways. Epidermal growth factor receptor (EGFR), platelet-derived growth factor receptor alpha polypeptide (PDGFRA), MET proto-oncogene (MET), and fibroblast growth factor receptor (FGFR) are among the most commonly dysregulated RTKs in GBM (15). EGFR and PDGFRA are well-established oncogenes in GBM (16), and thus, identification of their miRNA regulators following the discovery of functional implications of miRNAs in GBMs is warranted.

miR-7 is a common regulator of the PI3K/ATK and MAPK pathways, both of which are launched by EGFR through its two direct targets, the transcription factors PI3K and Raf-1, respectively (17). Human EGFR mRNA 3′-untranslated region contains three miR-7 target sites (18). Transient expression of miR-7 in GBM cells strongly inhibited *in vivo* GBM xenograft growth (17). Decreased expression of miR-128 correlates with aggressive human glioma subtypes, and miR-128 represses growth and mediates differentiation by targeting oncogenic EGFR and PDGFRA (19). The authors demonstrated that miR-128 suppresses glioma formation in a glioma mouse model, suggesting miR-128 as a glioma tumor suppressor that targets RTK signaling to repress gliomagenesis. miR-218 targets multiple components of RTK-signaling pathways, including the EGFR pathway, and miR-218 repression increases the abundance and activity of multiple RTK effectors (20). The expression of miR-218 is significantly decreased in the mesenchymal subtype of GBM, and the miR-218-RTK-HIF2α-signaling axis promotes GBM cell survival and tumor angiogenesis (20). A large-scale, genomewide miRNA expression analysis revealed miR-219 was downregulated in GBM, and exogenous overexpression of miR-219 in glioma cells inhibited proliferation and soft agar colony formation (21). In addition, overexpression of miR-219-5p reduced the activity of PI3 kinase and MAP kinase in glioma cell lines by targeting to EGFR (21). Moreover, overexpression of miR-133 decreased GBM cell growth and increased cell apoptosis, whereas depletion of miR-133 increased cell growth (22). The protein translation inhibition of EGFR by miR-133 was confirmed by a dual luciferase reporter assay (22). miR-340 overexpression suppressed several oncogenes, including EGFR (23). miR-340 induces glioma cells toward terminal differentiation and regulates glioma cell development by downregulating ROCK1 expression (23). miR-491 directly targets EGFR, CDK6, and Bcl-xL (24). Importantly, miR-491 is commonly codeleted with its adjacent CDKN2A on chromosome 9p21.3 in GBM. As a negative regulator of EGFR expression, miR-491 is a tumor suppressor gene. On the other hand, miR-148a expression was elevated in GBM specimens compared with normal human brain and astrocytes (25). miR-148a is a prognostic onco-miRNA that targets MIG6 and BIM to regulate EGFR and apoptosis in GBM (25). By inhibiting MIG6 expression, miR-148a reduced EGFR trafficking to Rab7-expressing compartments, including late endosomes and lysosomes. This process coincided with reduced degradation and elevated expression and activation of EGFR (25). Furthermore, the protein expression of EGFR decreased in cells with forced overexpression of miR-34a (26). Yin et al. reported that both deletion of miR-34a and amplification of EGFR were associated with significantly decreased overall survival of patients with GBM (26).

PDGFRA is a direct target of miR-34a, a downregulated miRNA in the proneural subtype compared with the mesenchymal subtype of GBM (27, 28). miR-34a specifically affects the growth of proneural glioma cells *in vitro* and *in vivo* (28). miR-34a repression in proneural gliomas is only modestly dependent on p53. Derepression of PDGFRA by the downregulation of miR-34a in the proneural subtype that results in a more proliferative phenotype may be responsible for the difference in response to clinical treatment for GBM. Gene mutation or amplification in MET is a relatively rare event in GBM (29). However, miR-34a expression inhibited c-Met reporter activities in glioma cells. In addition, miR-34a levels in human gliomas were inversely correlated with c-Met levels. Transient transfection of miR-34a into gliomas strongly inhibited cell proliferation, cell cycle progression, cell survival, and cell invasion (30).

MET is highly expressed in the mesenchymal subtype of GBM (31). miR-182 sensitized glioma cells to TMZ-induced apoptosis, promoted glioma initiating cell (GIC) differentiation, and reduced tumor cell proliferation via knockdown of c-Met, Bcl2L12, and HIF2A (32). miR-144-3p specifically bound to the MET 3′-untranslated region (3′ UTR) and inhibited its expression. miR-144 strongly repressed GBM cell proliferation and invasion by suppressing MET *in vitro* and *in vivo* (33).

RAS signaling, upstream of MAP kinase, is reported to be regulated by miRNAs. Although only 1% of GBMs have a RAS mutation or amplification, 10% of GBMs contain neurofibromin 1 (NF1) inactivating genetic alterations that lead to hyperactive RAS activity by enhancing the intrinsic GTPase activity (29). Two recent reports focused on miRNAs targeting RAS in GBMs and showed that miR-143 directly targets N-RAS (34) and that let-7a directly targets K-RAS (35). Low expression of let-7a was correlated with a poor prognosis of primary GBM patients (35). In addition, miR-124 governs glioma growth and angiogenesis and enhances chemosensitivity by targeting R-RAS and N-RAS (36). In addition, miR-124 inhibits the MAP kinase pathway by repressing SOS1 mRNA (37). Moreover, these miRNAs are all downregulated in GBM specimens, underlying the malignant transformation.

Phosphatase and tensin homolog (PTEN) and NF1 are the most important negative regulators of cell proliferative pathways. The inactivated genetic mutations of NF1 and PTEN are found in 10 and 41% of GBM cases, respectively (29). NF1 is targeted by miR-9, which is an miRNA upregulated in GBM and promotes the proliferation and migration of glioma cells (38, 39). In addition, NF1 is a direct target of miR-514a, and over-expression of miR-514a inhibited NF1 expression, which correlated with increased survival cells (40). The protein phosphatase activity of PTEN is involved in cell proliferation, preventing cells from growing. miR-26a, frequently amplified at the DNA level in human gliomas, is identified as a direct regulator of PTEN expression (41). miR-26a-mediated PTEN repression in a murine glioma model enhances *de novo* glioma formation (41). Overexpression of miR-26a in PTEN-competent and PTEN-deficient GBM cells promoted tumor growth *in vivo* and further increased growth in cells overexpressing CDK4 or CENTG1 (42). Guo et al. reported that c-Myc modulates genes associated with oncogenesis in GBM through deregulation of miRNAs via the c-Myc-miR-26a-PTEN-signaling pathway (43). CREB, a proto-oncogenic transcription factor that is overexpressed in gliomas, can promote gliomagenesis by modulating the expression of oncogenic miR-23a, which represses PTEN directly (44). miR-23a-mediated suppression of PTEN led to the activation of AKT/ERK pathways and epithelial-mesenchymal transition (EMT) (45). miR-17-5p (46), and miRNA-1908 (47) directly target PTEN in GBMs. Overexpression of miR-17 prolongs GBM cell survival and increases cell motility, and induces HIF-1α activation in response to stress by targeting PTEN. (46). miR-1908 promotes proliferation, invasion, and sphere formation in GBM cells by targeting PTEN, and PTEN levels are inversely correlated with miR-1908 levels in GBM tissues (47). The expression of PTEN-targeting miR-17-5p, miR-19a, miR-19b, miR-21, miR-130b, miR-221, and miR-222 was significantly higher in irradiated glioma cells than in nonirradiated cells, and the PTEN expression levels were lower in the irradiated glioma cells than in the nonirradiated cells (48).

In recent years, molecular target therapy-targeting RTK pathways has been one of the most exciting developments in cancer therapy, and certain molecular targeted drugs have been clinically validated. However, for GBMs, no effective molecular targeted drug has yet been developed. By understanding the roles of miRNAs in growth signal activation, miRNA-based treatments should also be taken into consideration either alone or in combination.

3.2. Sustained angiogenesis and microRNAs

New growth in the vascular network is important because the proliferation, as well as metastatic spread, of tumor cells depends on an adequate supply of oxygen and nutrients and the removal of waste products. GBMs have a strong angiogenetic property because GBMs possess glomeruloid microvascular proliferation, a hallmark of GBMs (49). GBMs stimulate new blood vessel formation through processes driven primarily by vascular endothelial growth factor A (VEGF-A), the most established proangiogenic protein in the VEGF family. The overexpression of VEGF-A, and subsequent activation of its receptors, is an important event during glioma progression (50).

miRNA-205, an miRNA significantly downregulated in GBMs, can specifically suppress expression of VEGF-A directly (51). Moreover, miRNA-205 induces apoptosis and depresses the invasion of glioma cells *in vitro* (51). VEGF-A upregulation can be induced by hypoxia inducible factor 1 alpha subunit (HIF-1α), which is negatively regulated by the von Hippel-Lindau (VHL) tumor suppressor (52). HIF-1α levels were upregulated in glioma cells following transfection with miR-183 mimic RNA, and VEGF-A and glucose transporter 1 (GLUT1), which are downstream molecules of HIF-1α, were upregulated in cells transfected with miR-183 (10). miR-21, miR-23b, and miR-566 are reported to target VHL and decrease the production of the VHL protein, upregulating VEGF-A expression. miR-21 directly targets VHL and peroxisome-proliferator-activated receptor a (PPARa), and miR-21 regulates EGFR/AKT signaling through VHL/β-catenin and the PPARa/AP-1 axis (53). miR-21 significantly colocalized with the hypoxia- and angiogenesis-associated markers HIF-1α and VEGF (54). Downregulation of miR-23b triggered growth inhibition, induced apoptosis, and suppressed invasion of glioma *in vitro* (55). miR-23b deletion decreased HIF-1α/VEGF expression and suppressed β-catenin/Tcf-4 transcription activity by targeting VHL (55). Inhibition of miR-566 expression increases the expression levels of VHL, decreases the expression levels of VEGF, and inhibits the invasive and migratory abilities of GBM cells (56). Moreover, miR-7 downregulates the expression of O-linked *N*-acetylglucosamine transferase (OGT) involved in the VEGF-signaling pathway, leading to a profound reduction in vascularization, similar to the antiangiogenic drug sunitinib (57).

miR-101 is downregulated in GBMs and targets EZH2, a histone methyltransferase affecting gene expression profiles in an epigenetic manner. Inhibition of EZH2 by miR-101 attenuated GBM cell growth, migration, and GBM-induced endothelial tubule formation (58). Ectopic expression of miR-137 inhibited angiogenesis in a SCID mouse xenograft model. EZH2 was identified as a direct target of miR-137, and EZH2 overexpression can rescue the inhibitory effect of miR-137 on cell proliferation and angiogenesis (59). A key step in angiogenesis is the upregulation of growth factor receptors on endothelial cells. miR-296 level is increased in primary tumor endothelial cells isolated from GBM tissues (60). Overexpressed miR-296 enhances angiogenesis by directly targeting the hepatocyte growth factor-regulated tyrosine kinase substrate (HGS), results in upregulation of the VEGF receptoe-2 and PDGF receptor-β (60). miR-93 promotes angiogenesis by suppressing integrin-β8 (61). *In vivo* studies revealed that miR-93-expressing cells induced blood vessel formation, allowing blood vessels to extend to tumor tissues in high densities (61). Angiogenesis promoted by miR-93 in return facilitated cell survival, resulting in enhanced tumor growth. miR-17~92 promotes angiogenesis and tumor growth by downregulation of clusterin (62). Specifically, miR-17-5p and miR-20 reduce the expression of the type-II TGFβ receptor and miR-18 limits the expression of Smad4, namely miR-17~92 attenuates the TGFβ-signaling pathway to shut down clusterin expression, thereby stimulating angiogenesis and tumor cell growth.

Because angiogenesis is a hallmark of GBM, targeting therapies against angiogenesis using the VEGF antibody was previously considered to be promising in GBM. However, recently, two phase-III studies revealed that the addition of the VEGF antibody bevacizumab to radiotherapy-temozolomide did not improve survival in patients with GBM, although improved progression-free survival and maintenance of baseline quality of life and performance status were observed with bevacizumab (2, 3). Therefore, new therapeutic targets or strategies need to be developed. To make progress, a better understanding of the miRNAs contributing to angiogenesis will lead to more effective antiangiogenic therapy for patients with GBM.

3.3. Insensitivity to antigrowth signals and microRNAs

To proliferate without limit, GBM cells must circumvent biologically programmed pathways that negatively regulate cell proliferation. There are two major tumor suppressor genes, retinoblastoma 1 (RB1) and tumor protein p53. Similarly, a better understanding of the dysfunction of the RB1 and p53 pathways should also implicate the roles of dysregulated miRNAs. The mutation of p53 results in the inability to stop further cell-cycle progression triggered by oncogenic signals (63). miR-10b, one of the most studied miRNAs in GBMs, is highly upregulated in human GBM and pleiotropically regulates invasion, angiogenicity, and apoptosis of GBM cells. The pleiotropic effect of miR-10b is caused by its suppression of multiple tumor-suppressive genes, including p53 (7, 64, 65). miR-10b directly targets p53 in GBM, giving the tumors a way to evade growth control and enable persistent cell proliferation by perturbing the miRNAs expression.

Moreover, p53 signaling is under the precise control of the negative regulator mouse double minute 2 (MDM2). MDM2 regulates the ubiquitin-dependent degradation and transcriptional activity of p53 (66). MDM2 mRNA is upregulated in both GBM cell lines and samples (67), and the upregulation could be a consequence of the downregulation of miR-17, miR-181b, miR-25, or miR-32, which directly target MDM2 gene expression (46, 67, 68). It is worth noting that miR-25 and miR-32 are two miRNAs repressed by p53, suggesting a feedback circuit between p53 and MDM2 mediated by miRNAs (67). The feedback circuit can explain the overexpression of miR-25 in GBM reported by several separate studies, in which the miRNA is meant to be downregulated to increase MDM2 expression and thus inactivate p53 (7, 39, 69). In addition, miR-181b is downregulated in GBM samples, further indicating that miRNA contributes to the complexity of the pathological progression of gliomas (68).

Another key tumor suppressive is p16INK4a, an important inhibitor of RB pathway (70), namely p16INK4a can bind specifically to CDK4/6 and inhibit the catalytic activity of CDK4/6-cyclin D complexes (71). Approximately, 80% of GBMs have one or more alterations affecting the RB1 function. In addition to targeting p53 in GBMs, miR-10b also targets p16INK4a, and the inhibition of miR-10b leads to cell cycle arrest (65). miR-26a also targets RB1 in GBMs. Additionally, CDK-cyclin complex-mediated phosphorylation is one of the main mechanisms by which RB1 protein is inactivated (72). The frequent gain-of-function mutations on CDK4/6-cyclin D complexes underscore their importance and potential in the development and progression of GBM. miR-124 is reported to radiosensitize human glioma cells by downregulating CDK4 (73), whereas CDK6 is a direct target of miR-138 (74) and miR-491-3p/5p (24). miR-195 inhibited glioma cell proliferation by downregulating expression of cyclin D1 and cyclin E1, via directly targeting cyclin D1 and cyclin E1 mRNA (75). Notably, those miRNAs that target cyclin-CDK complexes are all downregulated in GBM samples (69).

3.4. Invasion in the brain and microRNAs

The invasive propensity of glioma cells remains the major obstacle to improving the poor outcomes of patients with GBM. GBM cells prefer to migrate through the tortuous extracellular spaces of the brain. Therefore, it is supposed that the interaction of invading glioma cells with the extracellular matrix (ECM) is crucial in the initiation of invasion and migration. Generally, cell attachment is mediated by interactions between cell-cell and cell-ECM receptors, including integrins and cadherins, and degradation of ECM components by metalloproteinases is essential for cell detachment (76). The matrix metalloproteinases (MMPs) and a disintegrin and metalloproteinases (ADAMs) are two distinct types of metalloproteinases secreted by glioma cells to overcome the dense matrix, and the proteolytic activity can be blocked by endogenous metalloproteinase inhibitors, such as tissue inhibitors of metalloproteinase (TIMPs) and reversion-inducing-cysteine-rich protein with kazal motifs (RECK) (76).

miR-218 expression has been found to be significantly downregulated in GBM tissue samples (77). Several studies have shown that miR-218 is a negative regulator of invasion in GBM through various pathways (77, 78). miR-218 has been reported to target the mRNA of Lef1, the transcription factor that is upregulated by β-catenin (77). Suppression of Lef1 leads to the reduction of MMP-2, MMP-7, and MMP-9 activity and inhibition of invasion *in vitro* (79). Another mechanism through which miR-218 negatively regulates GBM invasion is targeting IKKβ mRNA along with reducing the transcription of NF-kB. NF-kB is a transcription factor that is important in many cellular processes and has been strongly linked to the migration and invasion of various cancer cells (78). NF-kB's target genes include MMP-9; therefore, its inhibition by miR-218 causes a decrease in invasion.

MMP-9 is a direct target of miR-491-5p, which is upregulated in GBM (24). miR-491-5p expression has been reported to reduce cell proliferation and invasion by targeting MMP9 (80). miR-491-3p also reduces the invasiveness of GBM cells by targeting the mRNA of insulin-like growth factor-binding protein 2 (IGFBP2). MMP-9 is also a direct target of miR-211 (81). MMP-3 is targeted by miR-152 (82). Additionally, ADAM17, a non-MMP, is under the direct regulation of miR-145 (83). It is clear that if glioma cells lose the control of MMPs and ADAMs by miRNAs, ECM homeostasis is compromised and the combined activity of these proteases remodels the ECM to favor tumor invasion. miR-101 is a tumor suppressor that is downregulated in GBM, as well as other cancers. (58). It has been shown to downregulate the invasion of glioma cells, as well as proliferation and migration, by targeting the transcription factor Kruppel-like factor 6 (KLF6). This suppression of KLF6 reduced the expression of chitinase-3-like protein 1 (CHI3L1) and inactivated MEK1/2 and PI3K signaling (72). miR-101 downregulation has been shown to result in EZH2-induced proliferation, migration, and angiogenesis in GBM (74).

Similarly, miR-152 is a tumor suppressor that is often downregulated in cancers, including in GBM. It was shown to suppress the invasion of glioma stem cells, as well as cell proliferation, migration, invasion, and apoptosis. It has been reported that miR-152 exerts its tumor-suppressing effects by targeting the transcription factor Kruppel-like factor 4 (KLF4). This suppression of KLF4 causes the transcriptional downregulation of galectin-3 (LGALS3) and the inactivation of MEK1/2 and PI3K signaling (75).

Because the MMPs and ADAMs each comprises more than 20 members, targeting a single target appears to be nonessential in cancerous diseases, which provides miR-21 with an opportunity to broadly inhibit metalloproteinase function. miR-21 regulates multiple genes associated with glioma cell migration and invasion, including the RECK and TIMP3 genes, which are inhibitors of matrix metalloproteinases (84).

In addition, interactions with the ECM are mostly mediated by integrins, which enable cells to sense the extracellular environment and adjust their behavior to environmental cues. miR-124, frequently downregulated in GBM, targets β1 integrin and is shown to affect glioma cell migration and invasion *in vitro* (85). PPP1R13L (protein phosphatase 1, regulatory subunit 13 like), an inhibitory member of the apoptosis-stimulating protein of p53 family (IASPP), was found to be a direct target of miR-124 in GBM cells. miR-124-mediated PPP1R13L regulates invasion of GBM cells (86). Cai et al. found that miR-542-3p expression was decreased in GBM cells, and miR-542-3p suppressed GBM cell invasion by not only targeting AKT1 but also directly downregulating its two important upstream regulators, ILK (integrin-linked kinase) and PIK3R1 (87). miR-181 family is downregulated in GBM and is inversely correlated with activities of NF-kB-targeting genes. Furthermore, miR-181b was shown to suppress epithelial-mesenchymal transition (EMT) by targeting KPNA4 (88). miR-181c overexpression inhibits TGF-β signaling by downregulating TGFBR1 (transforming growth factor, beta receptor 1), TGFBR2 and TGFBRAP1 (transforming growth factor, beta receptor-associated protein 1) expression. miR-181c expression levels are correlated with poor prognosis of patients with GBM.

miR-125a are downregulated in GBMs and directly target the 3′-UTR of podoplanin (PDPN) and inhibit invasion, apoptosis, and proliferation of GBMs. In addition, miR-125a inhibits Nrg1, one of the most active members of the EGF-like family, and suppresses the proliferation and migration of GBM cells *in vitro* and *in vivo* (89). miR-203 expression is decreased in anaplastic astrocytoma and GBM tissues. Forced expression of miR-203 was shown to suppress glioma cell proliferation, migration, and invasion, by disrupting the Robo1/ERK/MMP-9-

signaling axis (90). In addition, miR-203 inhibits the proliferation and invasion by directly targeting phospholipase D2 (PLD2) (91). miR-29b expression, downregulated in GBMs, was inversely proportional to that of BCL2-like 2 (BCL2L2) mRNA or protein (92). Interestingly, BCL2L2 mRNA is highly expressed in the mesenchymal type of GBM. BCL2L2 repression is of central importance to miR-29b antitumor activity in migration, invasion, and angiogenesis. Moreover, miR-29b regulates PDPN, which promotes glioma invasion.

miR-10b is overexpressed in GBM and induces glioma cell invasion by modulating expression of RhoC, MMP-14, and uPAR (urokinase-type plasminogen activator receptor) via HOXD10 (93). Multifocal lesions of malignant gliomas were associated with higher expression levels of miR-10b (9). Dong et al. reported that not only miR-10b inhibition but also miR-21 inhibition could exert synergistic inhibition of the invasion of glioma cells. miR-10b pleiotropically regulates invasion, angiogenicity, and apoptosis of glioma cells by the suppression of multiple tumor suppressors, including p53, FOXO3, HOXD10, and NOTCH1 (64). miR-155 has been identified to be an oncomiR and is highly expressed in several solid cancers, including GBM. Knockdown of miR-155 sensitizes glioma cells to the chemotherapy of temozolomide by targeting p38 isoforms of mitogen-activated protein kinase 13 (MAPK13) and MAPK14 (94).

In sum, the roles of miRNAs in glioma cell invasion or migration further our understanding of the genesis of the aggressive glioma phenotype. Some of these miRNAs have been discovered, whereas more still remain to be found. The blockade of excessive pro-invasive miRNAs or the restoration of weakened anti-invasive miRNAs will provide extra treatment options for advanced-stage gliomas that are marked by poor prognoses for decades (**Table 1**).

Hallmarks of glioblastoma	miRNAs	Targets	Expression	Function	Ref
Growth signal activation	miR-7	EGFR, PI3K, Raf-1	down	downregulate PI3K/ATK and MAPK pathways	Liu (17), Webster (18)
	miR-128	EGFR, PDGFRA	down	downregulate PI3K/ATK and MAPK pathways	Papagiannakopoulos (19)
	miR-218	EGFR	down	downregulate PI3K/ATK and MAPK pathways	Mathew (20)
	miR-219	EGFR	down	downregulate PI3K/ATK and MAPK pathways	Rao (21)
	miR-133	EGFR	down	downregulate PI3K/ATK and MAPK pathways	Xu (22)
	miR-340	EGFR	down	induce terminal differentiation	Huang (23)

Hallmarks of glioblastoma	miRNAs	Targets	Expression	Function	Ref
	miR-491	EGFR, CDK6, Bcl-xL	down	inhibit cell proliferation, negative regulator of EGFR	Li (24)
	miR-148a	MIG6, BIM	up	reduce EGFR trafficking	Kim (25)
	miR-34a	PDGFRA	down	inhibit cell proliferation and cell cycle progression inhibit cell survival invasion	Genovese (27), Silber (28)
	miR-182	MET, Bcl2L12, HIF2A		promote glioma initiating cell differentiation	Kouri (32)
	miR-144-3p	MET	down	repress GBM cell proliferation and invasion	Lan (33)
	let-7a	K-RAS	down	downregulate PI3K/ATK and MAPK pathways	Wang (35)
	miR-143	N-RAS	down	inhibit cell proliferation	Wang (34)
	miR-124	SOS1, R-RAS	down	inhibit cell proliferation	Shi (36), Lv (37)
	miR-9	NF1	up	inhibit cell proliferation	Tan (38)
	miR-26a	PTEN	up	promote tumor growth	Huse (41)
	miR-23a	PTEN	up	activate of AKT/ERK pathways and EMT	Tan (44), Tian (45)
	miR-17-5p	PTEN	up	formation of colonies and neurospheres	Li (46)
	miRNA-1908	PTEN	up	promote the tumor forming potential and anchorage-independent growth	Xia (47)
	miR-19a	PTEN	up	promote tumor growth	Tokudome (48)
	miR-19b	PTEN	up	promote tumor growth	Tokudome (48)
	miR-21	PTEN	up	promote tumor growth	Tokudome (48)
	miR-130b	PTEN	up	enhance stem cell-like phenotype	Tokudome (48)
	miR-221	PTEN	up	promote tumor growth	Tokudome (48)
	miR-222	PTEN	up	promote tumor growth	Tokudome (48)
Sustained angiogenesis	miR-205	VEGF-A	down	inhibit expression of VEGF-A induce apoptosis and depress the invasion	Yue (51)
	miR-183	IDH2	up	increase HIF1 expression	Tanaka (10)
	miR-21	VHL, PPARa	up	regulate EGFR/AKT signaling	Harmansen (54)

Hallmarks of glioblastoma	miRNAs	Targets	Expression	Function	Ref
	miR-23b	VHL	up	inhibit tumor growth and invasion, induce apoptosis	Chen (55)
	miR-566	VHL	up	inhibit invasion and migration	Xiao (56)
	miR-7	OGT	down	reduce vascularization	Babae (57)
	miR-101	EZH2	down	attenuate GBM growth and migration/invasion	Smits (58)
	miR-137	EZH2	down	inhibit cell proliferation and angiogenesis	Sun (59)
	miR-93	Integrin-β8	up	promote tumor growth and angiogenesis	Fang (61)
Insensitivity to antigrowth signals	miR-10b	p53, p16INK4a	up	promote cell cycle	Gabriely (65)
	miR-17-3p	MDM2		inhibit tumor progression	Li (46)
	miR-181b	MDM2	down	inhibit tumor progression	Suh (67)
	miR-25-3p	MDM2, p53	up	inhibit cellular proliferation	Suh (67)
	miR-32-5p	MDM2, p53	up	inhibit cellular proliferation	Suh (67)
	miR-26a	RB1	up	promote cell proliferation	Lundberg (72)
	miR-124	CDK4	down	cell cycle arrest	Deng (73)
	miR-138	CDK6	down	cell cycle arrest	Qiu (74)
	miR-491-3p/5p	CDK6	down	cell cycle arrest	Li (24)
	miR-195	cyclin D1, cyclin E1	down	cell cycle arrest	Hui (75)
Invasion and metastasis	miR-218	IKKβ, Lef1	down	inhibit cell invasion	Liu (77), Song (78)
	miR-491	IGFBP2, MMP9	down	reduce cell proliferation and invasion	Yan (80)
	miR-211	MMP9	down	reduce cell invasion	Asuthkar (81)
	miR-101	KLF6, EZH2	down	reduce invasion of glioma stem cells	Smits (58), Qiu (74)
	miR-152	MMP3, KLF4	down	reduce cell invasion and angiogenesis suppress invasion of glioma stem cells	Zheng (82), Hui (75)

Hallmarks of glioblastoma	miRNAs	Targets	Expression	Function	Ref
	miR-145	ADAM17	down	reduce glioma cell invasion and angiogenesis	Lu (83)
	miR-21	TIMP3, RECK	up	promote cell invasion	Gabriely (84), Zhao (86)
	miR-124	β1 integrin, IASPP	down	suppress cell migration and invasion	Fowler (85)
	miR-542-3p	AKT1	down	suppress cell invasion	Cai (87)
	miR-181b	KPNA4	down	inhibit cell invasion and proliferation	Wang (88)
	miR-181c	TGFBR1, TGFBR2, TGFBRAP1	down	inhibit cell invasion and proliferation	Wang (88)
	miR-125a	PDPN, Nrg1	down	inhibit invasion and proliferation	Yin (89)
	miR-203	PLD2	down	suppress cell proliferation and invasion,disrupt the Robo1/ERK/MMP-9 signaling axis	Dontula (90), Chen (91)
	miR-29b	BCL2L2, PDPN	down	inhibit glioma invasion	Chung (92)
	miR-10b	HOXD10, FOXO3, NOTCH1	up	induce glioma cell invasion	Sun (93)
	miR-155	MAPK13, MAPK14	up	regulates glioma cells invasion and chemosensitivity	Liu (94)
Antiapoptosis	miR-21	PDCD4, HNRPK, TP53BP2, p63	up	antiapoptosis	Corsten (95), Gaur (96)
	miR-92a	BCL2L11	up	antiapoptosis	Papagiannakopoulos (97)
	miR-92b	NLK	up	antiapoptosis	Niu (98)
	miR-93	ITGB8	up	antiapoptosis	Fang (61)
	miR-221	p27, p57	up	antiapoptosis	Medina (100)
	miR-222	p27, p57	up	antiapoptosis	Medina (100)
Genome instability and mutation	miR-106a		up	DNA replication and mitosis	Liu (101)
	miR-106b	RBL1, RBL2	up	DNA replication and mitosis	Liu (101)

Hallmarks of glioblastoma	miRNAs	Targets	Expression	Function	Ref
	miR-17-92		up	DNA replication and mitosis	Liu (101)
	miR-20			DNA replication and mitosis	Liu (101)
	miR-221	p27	up	Cell cycle chechpoint regulation	Gillies (103)
	miR-222	p27	up	Cell cycle chechpoint regulation	Gillies (103)
	miR-155	MLH1, MSH2, MSH6	up	DNA mismatch repair	Liu (94)
	miR-125b	p53, MXD1	down	cell cycle arrest to repair damaged DNA spindle assembly checkpoint	Wan (104), Le (105)
	miR-29	PIK3R1, CDC42	down	upregulate p53	Park (106)
	miR-34	CCND1, CCNE2, CDK4, MET, MYC, SNAI1, and SIRT1	down	DNA damage response upregulate p53 downstream molecules	He (107)
	miR-101	ATM, PRKDC	down	DNA repair regulate non-homologous end joining of DNA double strand breaks	Yan (109)
					Li (111)
Tumor-promoting inflammation	miR-21	LRRFIP1	up	regulate NF-kB signaling pathway	
	miR-146a	TRAF6, IRAK1		regulate NF kB activation	Taganov (112), Park (113)
	miR-124		down	inhibit STAT3 pathway	Wei (117)
Reprogramming energy metabolism	miR-451	CAB39	up	regulate LKB1/AMPK signaling activity	Godlewski (124)
	mir-145	c-Myc, Sox9, ADD3	down	reduce Lin28/Lin28b transcription	Rani (130), Gan (132)
	miR-34c	c-Myc		regulate c-Myc mRNA stability and translation	Masui (134)

Hallmarks of glioblastoma	miRNAs	Targets	Expression	Function	Ref
	let-7	RAS, Myc, CCND1, LIN28, HMGA2	down	regulate glucose metabolism	Boyerinas (135)
	let-7a	K-ras	down	regulate glucose metabolism	Boyerinas (135)
	miR-326	PKM2, NOB1	down	regulate glucose metabolism RNA metabolism	Kefas (136), Zhou (137)
Evading immune destruction	miRs-29b		down	differentiation of tumor-associated macrophage	Graff (140)
	miR-125a		down	differentiation of tumor-associated macrophage	Graff (140)
	miR-146a		down	differentiation of tumor-associated macrophage	Graff (140)
	miR-155	C/EBPβ	up	lead to and inversion of M2 into M1 macrophages	Graff (140)
	miR-221	STAT1,2	up	phosphorylation of STAT1 and STAT2	Zhang (143)
	miR-222	STAT1,2	up	phosphorylation of STAT1 and STAT2	Zhang (143)
	miR-20a	NKG2DL	up	immune evasion of glioma cells at the level of the NKG2D recognition pathway	Codo (146)
	miR-93	NKG2DL	up	immune evasion of glioma cells at the level of the NKG2D recognition pathway	Codo (146)
	miR-106b	NKG2DL	up	immune evasion of glioma cells at the level of the NKG2D recognition pathway	Codo (146)
	miR-138	CTLA-4, PD1	down	tumor regression	Wei (147)

Table 1. Hallmarks of glioblastoma and microRNAs.

3.5. Antiapoptosis and microRNAs

Among the tumor-associated miRNAs, miR-21 is frequently overexpressed in various types of tumors, including GBMs (7, 9), and plays a critical role in cell death and apoptosis. Knock-down of miR-21 in cultured GBM cells triggered activation of caspases and led to increased apoptotic cell death (8). miR-21 knockdown disrupts glioma growth *in vivo* and displays synergistic cytotoxicity when combined with the agent tumor necrosis factor-related apoptosis (s-TRAIL), leading to an increase in caspase activity (95). In particular, it was reported that the downregulation of miR-21 in GBM-derived cell lines resulted in an increased expression of a specific target, PDCD4 (programmed cell death 4), a known tumor suppressor gene, with a consequent decrease in proliferation and increase in apoptosis (96). Furthermore, miR-21 regulated a network of p53, TGF-b, and mitochondrial apoptosis tumor suppressor genes in GBM cells, targeting HNRPK (heterogeneous nuclear ribonucleoprotein K), TP53BP2 (tumor protein p53-binding protein 2), and p63, a member of the p53 family of genes (97).

miR-92a and miR-92b, upregulated in glioma, target BCL2L11 (98) and NLK (99), respectively. Their inhibition promotes tumor-suppressive phenotypes through the induction of apoptosis. In addition, miR-93 was found to be upregulated in glioma specimens and resulted in an enhancement in cell survival, promoting sphere formation, and augmenting tumor growth by suppressing the expression of ITGB8 target (61).

miR-221 and 222 were extensively investigated in glioma. These miRNAs were found to be upregulated in this cancer, and both were reported to target the cell growth-suppressive cyclin-dependent kinase inhibitors p27 and p57 (100).

3.6. Genome instability and microRNAs

Genomic instability is defined as a high frequency of mutations within the genome, including changes in nucleic acid sequences, chromosomal rearrangements, or aneuploidy. The stability of the human genome is maintained by multiple mechanisms such as the cell cycle checkpoint, DNA damage response, and mitotic separation machinery. Defects in the DNA damage response could cause genomic DNA mutations, deletions, insertions, or gross chromosomal gains and losses upon cell division and subsequently lead to cancer. Genomic instability is present in GBM and affects the prognosis of patients.

Several members of the miR-106b-25 cluster and its paralog miR-17-92 cluster were associated with DNA replication and mitosis. Overexpression of miR-106b-5p in glioma tumor cells significantly promoted cell proliferation, suggesting a role of this miRNA in cell cycle regulation (101). A mechanistic study revealed that two target genes, retinoblastoma-like 1 (RBL1) and RBL2, were involved in miR-106b-5p's regulation of cell proliferation (101). RBL proteins were involved in genomic instability, coinciding with decreased DNA methylation and increased acetylation of histone H3.

p27, one of the cyclin-dependent kinase inhibitor, inhibits cell cycle progression at the G1 phase by blocking the activation of cyclin-CDK complexes (102). The downregulation of p27 expression by miRNAs could abrogate the cell cycle checkpoints and could increase DNA damages in GBM cells. The regulatory effect of miR-221/222 on p27 and the subsequent effect on cell proliferation were also demonstrated in GBM cells (103). Moreover, p27 inhibition abrogated the growth advantage of cells with miR221/miR-222 downregulation (103).

DNA mismatch repair (MMR) is a system for recognizing and correcting insertions, deletions, and misincorporated bases at DNA replication and recombination. Deficiency of MMR system can be a cause for the development and progression of GBMs. There are two essential members of the DNA MMR genes, MutS homologs and MutL homologs. Computational algorithms predicted, and subsequently *in vitro* studies confirmed, several essential MMR genes, including MLH1, MSH2, and MSH6, as potential binding sites for miR-155. miR-155 is known to elevate its expression levels in primary and secondary GBMs (94).

As an important sensor in the DNA damage response, p53 functions to block the cell cycle to repair damaged DNA. Several miRNAs affect p53 or p53-regulated genes via different mechanisms. For instance, miR-125b, which has been shown to play a potential role in the development of glioma stem cells (104), directly targets p53 by binding to 3′-UTR of p53 and negatively regulates p53 expression (105). In addition, miR-125b negatively regulates MXD1 expression, an adaptor protein for MAD2L2 in the spindle assembly checkpoint. Moreover, miR-29, commonly downregulated in GBMs, indirectly upregulates p53 by targeting PIK3R1 and CDC42 (106). Previous studies have shown that miR-34 is directly regulated by p53 and represses various oncogenes, such as CCND1, CCNE2, CDK4, MET, MYC, SNAI1, and SIRT1. However, these miR-34-targeting oncogenes are upregulated in GBM, because miR-34 is usually downregulated (107). Several studies have shown that miR-34 is indispensable for the DNA damage response, and miR-34a-regulated genes are strongly related with DNA repair and apoptosis (108).

Ataxia telangiectasia mutated (ATM) is an important mediator in connecting DNA damage signals to downstream events, including damage repair. miR-101, a miRNA downregulated in GBM, could directly target ATM via the canonical action mechanism (109). In addition, miR-101 also targets PRKDC (protein kinase, DNA activated, catalytic polypeptide) to regulate nonhomologous end joining of DNA double-strand breaks (109).

3.7. Tumor-promoting inflammation and microRNAs

NF-kB is a transcription factor with pleiotropic activity owing to its central roles in inflammatory processes. A critical regulator of NF-kB activation is the IkB kinase (IKK-β) complex (110). Ectopic expression of miR-218, which is downregulated in GBM, reduced NF-kB activity, whereas inhibition of miR-218 enhanced the transcriptional activity of NF-kB (78). miR-218 could inactivate NF-kB signaling by directly targeting the 3′-UTR of the IKK-β (78). miR-21 was revealed as another regulator involved in the NF-kB-signaling pathway in GBM. Li et al. confirmed LRRFIP1 (leucine-rich repeat interacting protein 1) as a direct target of miR-21 (111). LRRFIP1 is a transcriptional repressor that preferentially binds to the GC-rich consensus sequence and regulates expression of TNF, EGFR, and PDGFA signaling. miR-21 contributes to drug resistance through the depression of LRRFIP1 expression, leading to the reduction of cytotoxicity of chemotherapeutic drugs through the activation of the NF-kB pathway (111).

miR-146a is known as miRNA associated with the innate immune response to microbial infection (112). Promotor analysis revealed that miR-146a is a NF-kB-dependent miRNAs (112). miR-146a has complementary sequences in the mRNA of the TNF receptor-associated factor 6 (TRAF6) and IL-1 receptor-associated kinase 1 (IRAK1), key adaptor molecules downstream of toll-like and cytokine receptors (113). miR-146a overexpression enhanced apoptosis and suppressed NF-kB activation in TMZ-treated GBM cells (114). Increased expression of miR-146a was observed in glioneuronal lesions (115), and miR-146a expression in human glial cells was strongly induced by IL-1β (115). miR-146a expression by transfection in astrocytes regulated many mRNA expression levels, including those of IRAK-1, IRAK-2, and TRAF-6. In addition, the expression of IL-6 and COX-2 was suppressed by miR-146a (115).

Recent evidence suggests that the signal transducer and activator of transcription (STAT) family proteins play a crucial role in selectively inducing and maintaining a procarcinogenic inflammatory microenvironment, both upon the initiation of malignant transformation and during cancer progression (116). Upon upregulating miR-124, a miRNA downregulated in GBM, specifically in glioma cancer stem cells (gCSC), the STAT3 pathway was inhibited, and miR-124 reversed gCSC-mediated immunosuppression of T cell proliferation and induction of regulatory T cells (Treg) (117). Systemic administration of miR-124-transfected T cell transfers exerted potent antiglioma therapeutic effects in murine models of GBM (117).

Human glioma immune activation is potently elicited by a cytokine combination. Cytokines such as IL-1β and TNFα induce the expression of miR-155 and miR-155*, the miRNAs crucial in immunity and inflammation-induced oncogenesis, and this expression is dose dependently suppressed by IRF3. Importantly, IRF3 also inhibits glioma proliferation, migration, and invasion (118).

3.8. Reprogramming energy metabolism and microRNAs

Cellular metabolism of malignant tumor is considerably different from that of normal cell, because of limitless proliferation and motility. (119). GBM cells uptake a large amount of glucose, and aerobic glycolysis generates various substrates, such as fatty acids and nucleotides that are required for rapidly proliferating cells, and is associated with a survival advantage in the tumor cells (Warburg effect). MR spectroscopy analyses have shown that as much as 90% of the glucose converts into lactate by aerobic glycolysis in GBM cells. Clinically, it is known that the levels of lactate are elevated in GBM tissue compared with those in contralateral normal brain tissue. In addition, lactate was shown to be high-grade gliomas than for low-grade gliomas, and glutamate levels were significantly elevated for GBMs. Pretreatment F^{18}-2-fluoro-2-deoxy-D-glucose (FDG)-PET provides significant additional prognostic information in high-grade gliomas (120).

In normal cells, the 5′-adenosine monophosphate-activated protein kinase (AMPK) pathway is the major cellular sensor of energy availability (121), but its function in cancer is not clear. AMPK is activated by metabolic stress to promote energy conservation and glucose uptake, allowing cells to survive periods of low-energy availability. Allosteric interaction with elevated intracellular AMP, which acts to inhibit dephosphorylation of AMPK (122), and phosphorylation at Thr172 by the protein kinase LKB1 are necessary for AMPK activation under conditions of bioenergetic stress (123).

Godlewski et al. identified miR-451 as a glioma-expressed miRNA that regulates the balance of proliferation and migration in glioma cells in response to changes in glucose levels (124). miR-451 regulates LKB1 activity through direct targeting of CAB39, a component of the active LKB1 complex. Glucose deprivation was shown to reduce miR-451 levels (124). Thus, miR-451 plays an essential role in LKB1/AMPK signaling in glioma cells. When glucose is sufficient, elevated miR-451 levels lead to reduced LKB1/AMPK pathway activation, which facilitates cell proliferation by allowing unrestrained mTOR activity and reducing apoptosis. In contrast, when glucose is limiting, miR-451 levels decline, allowing for increased CAB39 expression and activation of AMPK by LKB1-mediated phosphorylation. This effect promotes cell survival in response to metabolic stress and activates pathways involved in glioma motility.

Previous reports indicate that Myc is frequently upregulated or amplified in gliomas. As a transcriptional factor, Myc interacts with many tumor-related oncogenes in glioma cells, such as SPARC (125), GAS1 (126), and VEGF (127). c-Myc has been shown to stimulate glutamine metabolism by increasing the expression of amino acid transporters and glutaminase (128). Mechanistically, c-Myc expression has been shown to be suppressed by miR-145, which results in reduced Lin28/Lin28b transcription (129). miR-145 is one of the miRNAs significantly downregulated during malignant transformation in GBMs (130). miR-145 overexpression suppresses the activity of oncogenic proteins Sox9, leading to reduction of cell proliferation and invasion of GBM cells (130). Reduced levels of miR-145 may lead to metabolic remodeling in glioma cells via Sox9, because Sox9 is known as a regulator of c-myc.

mTORC2 regulates c-Myc and glycolysis through FoxO acetylation, and mTORC2 controls FoxO acetylation through class IIa HDACs, independently of Akt. FoxOs antagonize c-Myc (131) by increasing the expression of miR-145 (132) and miR-34c (133), limiting c-Myc mRNA stability and translation. In GBM cells, miR-34c levels were suppressed by FoxO1/FoxO3 knockdown, and miR-34c regulated c-Myc levels in GBM cells (134). The let-7 family has nine members, and previous studies have identified the let-7 miRNA as a tumor suppressor that regulates many important target genes during tumor development (135), such as RAS, Myc, CCND1, LIN28, and HMGA2, which are involved in cell cycle progression and cell stemness. The majority of let-7a miRNA functions in glioma malignancy are believed to involve K-Ras, suggesting that let-7a-mediated manipulation of K-Ras may also be involved in regulating glucose metabolism and GBM cell growth. The M2 isoform of pyruvate kinase (PK) is upregulated in most cancers, including GBM. The regulation of PKM2 was shown to occur via miR-326 (136). There are four isoforms of PK in mammals, and PKM2 is highly expressed in undifferentiated tissues and tumors. Because PKM2 is regulated by tyrosine phosphorylation and is overexpressed in malignant tumors, PKM2 is considered as key molecule of aerobic glycolysis. In addition, Zhou et al. reported that the human Nin one binding protein (NOB1), which is required for the biogenesis and function of the 26S proteasome and plays a role in RNA metabolism, is a direct target of miR-326 (137).

3.9. Evading immune destruction and microRNAs

In the past, the infiltration of innate and adaptive immune cells into the tumor microenvironment was considered an immune attack against tumors. However, now, it is widely accepted that immune cells also promote tumor initiation, progression, and metastasis (138). Tumor-associated macrophages (TAMs) control the majority of immunological processes within tumors exerting both regressive (M1) and progressive (M2) effects on tumor development (139). However, the majority of TAMs exhibit an M2-like phenotype. Remarkably, miRs-29b, miR-125a, miR-146a, and miR-155 are involved in the differentiation of TAMs (140). Overexpression of miRNA-155 was shown to attenuate the production of cytokines (IL-6 and TNF-α) by suppressing C/EBPβ expression, which led to an inversion of M2 into M1 macrophages (141). M2 TAMs are capable of releasing anti-inflammatory cytokines such as the immunosuppressive cytokine IL-10, which promotes tumor growth (142).

Natural killer T (NKT) cells are a subfraction of T cells. A large number of published studies have demonstrated that NKT cells have miscellaneous functions in immune regulation, one of which is that NKT cells are tumor cell killers, based on the production of antitumor cytokines. In addition to contributing to immune protection, NKT cells are involved in immune tolerance in the body. Tang et al. showed that glioma cells can induce immune-tolerant IL-6+ and IL-10+ NKT cells via miR-92a.

Another study revealed miR-221 and miR-222 as possible regulators of IFN pathways. Type-I IFN receptor activation triggers the JAK-mediated tyrosine phosphorylation of STAT family proteins. Zhang et al. found that STAT1 and STAT2 expression and phosphorylation were upregulated after repression of miR-221/222 in U251 cells (143). Upregulation of STAT pathway is controlled by the IFN-α activation after knockdown of miR-221/222 cluster in U251 glioma cells (143).

NKG2D is one of the major activating receptors of natural killer (NK) cells and binds to several ligands (NKG2DL). NKG2D recognizes different MHC class I-homologous ligands (NKG2DL), including the MHC class I-chain-related molecules A (MICA) and B (MICB) and the UL16- binding proteins (ULBP)1-6 (144), which are also present on the surface of glioma cells (145). Codo et al. reported that miR-20a, miR-93 or miR-106b regulates NKG2DL expression in glioma cells (146), suggesting that the expression of miRNA-targeting NKG2DL may contribute to the immune evasion of glioma cells at the level of the NKG2D recognition pathway.

In addition, miRNA regulates immunocheckpoint molecules. miR-138 could bind the 3′-UTR of CTLA-4 and PD-1, and transfection of human CD4+ T cells with miR-138 suppressed expression of CTLA-4 and PD-1 (147). *In vivo* treatment in immunocompetent mice using miR-138 revealed marked tumor regression and prolonged survival time. Moreover, inoculated tumors showed decrease in intratumoral regulatory T cell, CTLA-4, and PD-1 expression (147). miR-138 exerts antiglioma efficacy by targeting immune checkpoints that may have rapid translational potential as novel immunotherapeutic agents.

On the other hand, miRNA expression is transcriptionally regulated by various cytokines. Ohno et al. analyzed the effect of IFN-β treatment on miR-21 expression in glioma cells and intracranial glioma xenografts (148). Systematic delivery of IFN-β markedly reduced the level of miR-21 in glioma cells 6 hours after the addition of IFN-β.

4. Circulating microRNA in glioma patients

In 2008, Chim et al. firstly demonstrated the existence of placental miRNAs in maternal plasma (149). In the same year, several miRNAs were detected in the serum of the tumor patients. Quantitative real-time polymerase chain reaction (RT-PCR) analyses revealed sera levels of miR-155, miR-210, and miR-21 are higher in diffuse large B-cell lymphoma patient sera than healthy controls (150). To prevent degradation in the circulation, miRNAs are released by cells in both exosomes and miRNA/protein complexes. Exosomes are lipid vesicles ranging between 50 and 100 nm in size and contain a range of molecules, including mRNA, miRNA, DNA, and proteins. The detection of biomarkers within serum is attractive because of the relatively non-invasive process of collection (**Figure 1**).

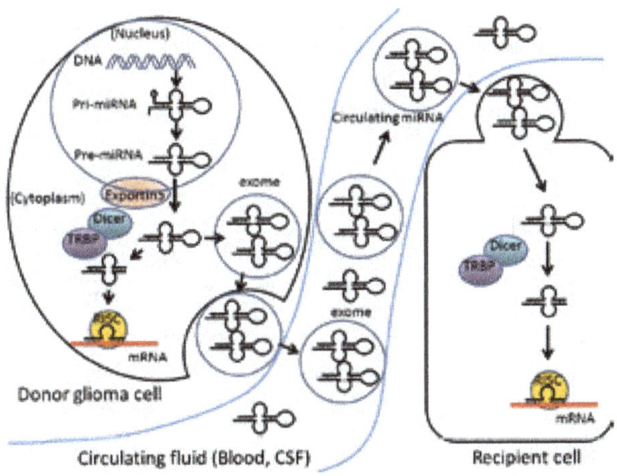

Figure 1. Cell-cell communication through circulating microRNAs. MicroRNAs contained in exosomes are released from glioma cells where they can enter the blood-stream or CSF-stream and circulate through the body to distant sites. These exosomal miRNAs are taken up by recipient cells, where the miRNAs can then suppress target genes in the recipient cells. Circulating miRNAs released by glioma cells may involve in growth signal, angiogenesis, anti-apoptosis, tumor metabolism, and immunoregulation.

Over the past few years, researchers have investigated the capability of using miRNAs as blood biomarkers for the diagnosis of tumors. Circulating miRNAs can be isolated from serum or plasma, but recent studies have indicated plasma to be a more adequate source for miRNA extraction (150). However, depending on plasma preparation, the level of circulating miRNA can be altered. Cheng et al. showed that processing differences resulted in a variation in residual platelet contamination in plasma and significant differences in miRNA abundance (151). Consequently, supplementary centrifugation, the refusal of samples with platelet counts above a certain limit and the quantification of hemolysis are mandatory in accurately determining miRNA levels in plasma.

Cerebrospinal fluid (CSF) is another useful biofluid and is in direct contact with the extracellular fluid of the brain. CSF has various functions, such as protecting the brain, transporting biological substances, and excreting toxic and waste substances. Although the composition of CSF reflects that of the blood plasma, active transport and secretions from the brain tissues contribute to the composition of CSF. Therefore, the analyses of CSF can suggest biological brain processes and is indispensable for understanding disorders of brain (152).

Clinically, histopathological examinations have been widely used to diagnose glioma, but they are invasive because microsurgical resection or stereotactic biopsy is needed to acquire specimens. In this context, it is of great interest to develop novel biomarkers for glioma. Currently, several miRNAs have been identified as noninvasive biomarkers for the diagnosis of cancers, including breast, lung, and gastric cancer. Previous studies have reported that miRNAs can be detected in circulating exosomes in the serum or CSF of glioma, suggesting that miRNAs might be useful biomarkers for glioma diagnosis. However, to effectively apply these findings to clinical detection, further studies must be conducted (**Table 2**).

No.	Authors	Year	Source	Number of glioma	Number of control	microRNA
Blood						
1	Skog	2008	serum	2 (GBM)	none	let-7a, miR-15b, miR-16, miR-19b, miR-21, miR-26a, miR-27a, miR-92, miR-93, miR-320, miR-20
2	Roth	2011	blood	20 (GBM)	20 (Healthy controls)	miR-128(↑), miR-342-3p(↓)
3	Wang	2012	plasma	50 (GBM)	10 (Healthy controls)	miR-21(↑), miR-128(↓), miR-342-3p(↓)
4	Yang	2013	serum	122 (Astro cytoma)	123 (Healthy controls)	miR-15b*(↓), miR-23a(↓), miR-133a(↓), miR-150*(↓),miR-197(↓), miR-497(↓), miR-548b-5p(↓)
5	Dong	2014	serum	3 (GBM)	3 (Healthy controls)	miR-576-5p(↑), miR-340(↑), miR-626(↑), miR-320(↓), let-7g-5p(↓), miR-7-5p(↓)
6	Manterola	2014	serum	25 (GBM)	25 (Healthy controls)	miR-320(↑), miR-574-3p(↑)
7	Shao	2015	plasma	70 (Glioma)	70 (Healthy	miR-454-3p(↑)

No.	Authors	Year	Source	Number of glioma	Number of control	microRNA
					controls)	
8	Wu	2015	serum	83 (Glioma)	69 (Healthy controls)	miR-29b(↓)
9	Liu	2015	serum	120 (Glioma)	120 (Healthy controls)	miR-29b(↓)
10	Lai	2015	blood	136 (GBM)	50 (Healthy controls)	miR-210(↑)
11	Sun	2015	serum	151 (Glioma)	53 (Healthy controls),52 (Meningioma)	miR-128(↓)
12	Yue	2016	serum	20 (Glioma)	5 (Healthy controls)	miR-205(↓)
13	Wei	2016	serum	33 (Glioma)	33 (Healthy controls)	miR-125b(↓)
Cerebrospinal fluid (CSF)						
1	Baraniskin	2012	CSF	10 (Glioma)	10 (Neurologic disorders), 23 (CNS lymphoma), 7 (Metastatic tumor)"	miR-15b(↑), miR-21(↑)
2	Teplyuk	2012	CSF	19 (GBM)	15 (Non-neoplastic control),44 (Metastatic tumor), "	miR-10b(↑), miR-21(↑), miR-200 family(↑)
3	Akers	2013	CSF	13 (GBM)	13 (Non-neoplastic control)	miR-21(↑)
4	Shi	2015	CSF	8 (Astro cytoma), 25 (Epen dymoma), 45 (GBM)	none	miR-21(↑)

Table 2. Circulating microrna in glioma patients.

4.1. Serum and plasma

The first analysis of exosomes in serum identified the presence of 11 miRNAs in the samples from two different patients with primary GBM in 2008 (153). However, the levels were generally lower in exosomes but correlated well with the tumor profile (153). In 2011, Roth et al. analyzed miRNA profiles from the blood of 20 patients with GBM and 20 matched healthy controls (154). Among 1158 tested miRNAs, 52 were significantly deregulated, and of these, two candidates, miR-128 (upregulated) and miR-342-3p (downregulated), remained the most significant miRNAs. The altered expression of these two miRNAs was confirmed in a validation cohort by RT-PCR. In this model, the discrimination between blood samples of patients with GBM and healthy controls reached an accuracy of 81%, specificity of 79%, and sensitivity of 83%. In 2012, Wang et al. determined the plasma miRNA levels of 50 patients with glioma and 10 healthy donors using RT-PCR (155). The plasma level of miR-21 was increased and the levels of miR-128 and miR-342-3p were significantly decreased in the patients with glioma compared with those in normal controls. These miRNAs were able to discriminate patients with glioma from healthy controls with high specificity and sensitivity. However, there were not significant differences between patients with glioma and other brain tumors such as meningioma or pituitary adenoma. Yang et al. performed genomewide serum miRNA analysis using serum samples of 122 untreated astrocytoma patients and 123 normal controls (156). The seven-miRNA panel (miR-15b*, miR-23a, miR-133a, miR-150*, miR-197, miR-497, and miR-548b-5p) demonstrated a high sensitivity (88.00%) and specificity (97.87%) for malignant astrocytoma prediction (156). These identified miRNAs also exhibited a global decrease in tumor tissues relative to normal tissues. Interestingly, these miRNAs in serum were markedly elevated after tumor removal.

In miRNA microarray analysis of the serum of patients with GBM and normal controls, 115 miRNAs were upregulated in the GBM group and 24 miRNAs were downregulated (157). In these microRNAs, a six-membered serum miRNA expression profile (upregulated miRs; miR-576-5p, miR-340, and miR-626, downregulated miRs; miR-320, let-7g-5p, and miR-7-5p) could serve as a noninvasive biomarker for GBM diagnosis (157). Manterola et al. found that the serum expression levels of miR-320 and miR-574-3p were significantly altered in the patients with GBM (158). In addition, small noncoding RNA (RNU6-1) was an independent predictor of a diagnosis of GBMs. Shao et al. compared the expression levels of miR-454-3p between preoperative plasmas from 70 patients with glioma and 70 healthy controls and between these preoperative and postoperative plasmas (159). The expression levels of miR-454-3p in plasma in patients with glioma were significantly higher, and the area under receiver operating characteristic (ROC) curve (AUC) of the expression of miR-454-3p for glioma diagnosis was 0.9063. In addition, the expression levels of miR-454-3p in the postoperative plasmas were significantly downregulated relative to the preoperative plasmas. Wu et al. analyzed serum from 83 patients with glioma and 69 healthy controls and evaluated the availability of the serum miR-29 family in the screening of glioma (160). The predictive value of the serum miR-29 family for glioma was moderate (AUC = 0.74), but that in high-grade glioma detection was sufficient (AUC = 0.81). Another study also showed that the expressions of miR-29b in blood were significantly different compared with those of a healthy control (161).

miR-125b is widely considered a tumor suppressor-miRNA and an ideal biomarker for clinical diagnosis in various human cancers. The study of serum miR-125b from 33 gliomas and 33 healthy controls revealed that the serum miR-125b level was significantly lower in patients with glioma (162). The ROC curve analysis yielded an AUC value of 0.839 (162). Furthermore, a meta-analysis was conducted to assess the diagnostic accuracy of miR-125b in cancer diagnosis, and the results revealed that employing miR-125b as a biomarker for cancer detection achieved a sensitivity of 82% and a specificity of 77% (162).

miR-210 is reported to be another potentially useful biomarker in the serum of patients with glioma. Lai et al. analyzed blood samples collected from patients with glioma (n=136) and healthy controls (n=50) and revealed that an approximately sevenfold increase in miR-210 expression was detected in serum samples from patients with GBM relative to healthy controls (163). miR-210 has been found to be upregulated in a variety of other solid tumor types and potentially influences cellular function through diverse pathways; the miRNA has also been correlated with hypoxia (164). A number of targets of miR-210 have been reported, including VEGF (165), BCL2 (166), and E2F transcription factor 3 (167). Sun et al. analyzed the expression levels of miR-128 in serum samples from 151 gliomas, 52 meningiomas, and 53 normal donors and showed that miR-128 expression was significantly decreased in glioma preoperative serum compared with others. ROC analyses showed that serum miR-128 levels were reliable in distinguishing patients with glioma from normal controls and patients with meningioma, with AUC values of 0.9095 and 0.8283, respectively (168). Although the mechanism has not yet been clarified, the study demonstrated that serum miR-128 expression was significantly elevated after surgery. miR-128 functions as a vital suppressor of tumorigenesis in glioma cells and is reported to downregulate p70S6K1 and its downstream signaling molecules, including VEGF and HIF-1. Another study showed that serum miR-205 expression was significantly lower in patients with glioma than in healthy controls ($p < 0.001$) (169). Interestingly, serum miR-205 expression levels were inversely correlated with pathological grades (169).

4.2. Cerebrospinal fluid

Baraniskin et al. (170) reported the first investigation of microRNA expression in CSF from patients with glioma in 2012. The results demonstrated that miR-15b and miR-21 were differentially expressed in CSF samples from patients with glioma compared with control subjects with various neurologic disorders, including CNS lymphoma and carcinomatous brain metastases. The combination of miR-15b and miR-21 resulted in increased diagnostic accuracy, with 90% sensitivity and 100% specificity in distinguishing patients with glioma from control subjects. Interestingly, miR-15 levels were significantly higher in glioma than in CNS lymphoma or metastatic tumor; however, miR-21 levels were significantly lower in glioma than in CNS lymphoma or metastatic tumor.

Teplyuk et al. (171) determined the CSF levels of several cancer-associated miRNAs for 118 patients diagnosed with different types of brain cancers. The levels of miR-10b and miR-21 were significantly increased in the CSF of patients with GBM and brain metastasis of breast and lung cancer compared with non-neoplastic conditions. Members of the miR-200 family were useful markers for discriminating between GBM and metastatic brain tumors. In addition, quantification of as few as seven microRNAs in CSF (miR-10b, miR-21, miR-125b, miR-141, miR-200a, miR-200b, and miR-200c) enabled differential recognition of GBM and metastatic brain tumor with high accuracy (91%–99%) (171).

Akers et al. analyzed extracellular vesicles (EVs) containing miRNAs in the CSF from patients with GBMs. The EV fraction was isolated by differential centrifugation. Although the analytic algorithm for quantitatively assessing EV miRNA remains underdeveloped, the authors showed that the CSF miR-21 levels of patients with GBM were 10-fold higher than those in the CSF of nononcologic patients (172).

Recently, another study reported results to those of Akers and coworkers. Exosomal miR-21 levels in the CSF of patients with glioma were found to be significantly higher than in controls, although no difference was detected in serum-derived exosomal miR-21 expression. Interestingly, the CSF-derived exosomal miR-21 levels correlated with a level of dissemination and a location of recurrence. Therefore, exosomal miR-21 in CSF may be a predictive marker for the early stages of tumor recurrence or metastasis (173).

5. Future prospects

Over the past decade, our understanding of genetic alterations and the tumor-specific signal pathways in glioma has been made, although this knowledge to date has not been translated into the prognosis of the patients with glioma. However, a better understanding of key pathways associated with gliomagenesis and malignant transformation could promise further improvements in glioma therapy. Maximum safe resection followed by radiotherapy up to a total dose of 60 Gy and TMZ-based chemotherapy have been established as a standard therapy, but new molecular targeting drugs, including small-molecule cell cycle inhibitors and biological and immune-based therapies have begun to yield promising results in clinical studies.

Over the past two decades, miRNAs have emerged as molecules central to glioma biology. miRNAs represent an additional layer of complexity in tumor biology and have been further validated as regulators of processes fundamental to glioma. This field is rapidly changing. Herein, we have reviewed the emerging roles of miRNAs as drivers of glioma formation and progression with a focus on glioma hallmarks. miRNAs may be essential in glioma growth, angiogenesis, invasion, genomic instability, tumor-promoting inflammation, and glioma-specific metabolism. In recent years, functions of miRNAs in gliomagenesis and microenvironment have been considerably elucidated, and we have validated the tumor suppressive or oncogenic functions of miRNAs in glioma. Now, we should move toward a next phase involving clinical trials with miRNAs as glioma therapies. For example, miR-34, a tumor-suppressive miRNA that simultaneously downregulates the expressions of MET, PDGFRA, and CDK6 is currently in clinical trials as a directed therapy for advanced solid tumors. In glioma, the restoration of miR-34a can possibly outperform any single targeted agents tailored to those targets. There remain several problems to use miRNAs in glioma therapy. These include not only accumulation of our knowledge of miRNAs' biological functions in glioma, but also the development of new and safe methods for delivery to glioma cells. Although the clinical application of miRNAs in GBM has yet to be realized, we believe the future of glioma therapy could be bright.

In this review, we have also focused on circulating miRNAs of serum, plasma, and CSF in patients with glioma. The use of miRNAs has several limitations, such as the diversity of methodologies that exist for miRNA detection and the small cohort size for the validation steps reported in current studies. Nonetheless, circulating miRNAs may exhibit diagnostic values, the combination of biomarkers may improve the diagnostic accuracy, and the combination of circulating miRNAs and other screening methods may be particularly useful in glioma detection. However, a standard protocol of sample treatment and suitable internal controls should be further established to make the level of detection comparable to that of other methods before miRNA biomarkers are fully utilized in clinical practice.

Author details

Takashi Sasayama*, Kazuhiro Tanaka and Eiji Kohmura

*Address all correspondence to: takasasa@med.kobepu.ac.jp

Department of Neurosurgery, Kobe University Graduate School of Medicine, Kusunoki-cho, Chuo-ku, Kobe, Japan

References

[1] Stupp R, Mason WP, van den Bent MJ, Weller M, Fisher B, Taphoorn MJ, et al. Radiotherapy plus concomitant and adjuvant temozolomide for glioblastoma. The New England Journal of Medicine. 2005;352(10):987–96.

[2] Gilbert MR, Dignam JJ, Armstrong TS, Wefel JS, Blumenthal DT, Vogelbaum MA, et al. A randomized trial of bevacizumab for newly diagnosed glioblastoma. The New England Journal of Medicine. 2014;370(8):699–708.

[3] Chinot OL, Wick W, Mason W, Henriksson R, Saran F, Nishikawa R, et al. Bevacizumab plus radiotherapy-temozolomide for newly diagnosed glioblastoma. The New England Journal of Medicine. 2014;370(8):709–22.

[4] Bartel DP, Chen CZ. Micromanagers of gene expression: the potentially widespread influence of metazoan microRNAs. Nature Review Genetics. 2004;5(5):396–400.

[5] Ambros V, Lee RC. Identification of microRNAs and other tiny noncoding RNAs by cDNA cloning. Methods in Molecular Biology. 2004;265:131–58.

[6] Lu J, Getz G, Miska EA, Alvarez-Saavedra E, Lamb J, Peck D, et al. MicroRNA expression profiles classify human cancers. Nature. 2005;435(7043):834–8.

[7] Ciafre SA, Galardi S, Mangiola A, Ferracin M, Liu CG, Sabatino G, et al. Extensive modulation of a set of microRNAs in primary glioblastoma. Biochemical and Biophysical Research Communications. 2005;334(4):1351–8.

[8] Chan JA, Krichevsky AM, Kosik KS. MicroRNA-21 is an antiapoptotic factor in human glioblastoma cells. Cancer Research. 2005;65(14):6029–33.

[9] Sasayama T, Nishihara M, Kondoh T, Hosoda K, Kohmura E. MicroRNA-10b is overexpressed in malignant glioma and associated with tumor invasive factors, uPAR and RhoC. International Journal of Cancer Journal International du Cancer. 2009;125(6): 1407–13.

[10] Tanaka H, Sasayama T, Tanaka K, Nakamizo S, Nishihara M, Mizukawa K, et al. MicroRNA-183 upregulates HIF-1alpha by targeting isocitrate dehydrogenase 2 (IDH2) in glioma cells. Journal of Neuro-oncology. 2013;111(3):273–83.

[11] Silber J, Lim DA, Petritsch C, Persson AI, Maunakea AK, Yu M, et al. miR-124 and miR-137 inhibit proliferation of glioblastoma multiforme cells and induce differentiation of brain tumor stem cells. BMC Medicine. 2008;6:14.

[12] Godlewski J, Nowicki MO, Bronisz A, Williams S, Otsuki A, Nuovo G, et al. Targeting of the Bmi-1 oncogene/stem cell renewal factor by microRNA-128 inhibits glioma proliferation and self-renewal. Cancer Research. 2008;68(22):9125–30.

[13] Rao SA, Santosh V, Somasundaram K. Genome-wide expression profiling identifies deregulated miRNAs in malignant astrocytoma. Modern Pathology: An Official Journal of the United States and Canadian Academy of Pathology, Inc. 2010;23(10): 1404–17.

[14] Lemmon MA, Schlessinger J. Cell signaling by receptor tyrosine kinases. Cell. 2010;141(7):1117–34.

[15] Cancer Genome Atlas Research N. Comprehensive genomic characterization defines human glioblastoma genes and core pathways. Nature. 2008;455(7216):1061–8.

[16] Furnari FB, Fenton T, Bachoo RM, Mukasa A, Stommel JM, Stegh A, et al. Malignant astrocytic glioma: genetics, biology, and paths to treatment. Genes & Development. 2007;21(21):2683–710.

[17] Liu Z, Jiang Z, Huang J, Huang S, Li Y, Yu S, et al. miR-7 inhibits glioblastoma growth by simultaneously interfering with the PI3K/ATK and Raf/MEK/ERK pathways. International Journal of Oncology. 2014;44(5):1571–80.

[18] Webster RJ, Giles KM, Price KJ, Zhang PM, Mattick JS, Leedman PJ. Regulation of epidermal growth factor receptor signaling in human cancer cells by microRNA-7. The Journal of Biological Chemistry. 2009;284(9):5731–41.

[19] Papagiannakopoulos T, Friedmann-Morvinski D, Neveu P, Dugas JC, Gill RM, Huillard E, et al. Pro-neural miR-128 is a glioma tumor suppressor that targets mitogenic kinases. Oncogene. 2012;31(15):1884–95.

[20] Mathew LK, Skuli N, Mucaj V, Lee SS, Zinn PO, Sathyan P, et al. miR-218 opposes a critical RTK-HIF pathway in mesenchymal glioblastoma. Proceedings of the National Academy of Sciences of the United States of America. 2014;111(1):291–6.

[21] Rao SA, Arimappamagan A, Pandey P, Santosh V, Hegde AS, Chandramouli BA, et al. miR-219-5p inhibits receptor tyrosine kinase pathway by targeting EGFR in glioblastoma. PloS One. 2013;8(5):e63164.

[22] Xu F, Li F, Zhang W, Jia P. Growth of glioblastoma is inhibited by miR-133-mediated EGFR suppression. Tumour biology: The Journal of the International Society for Oncodevelopmental Biology and Medicine. 2015;36(12):9553–8.

[23] Huang D, Qiu S, Ge R, He L, Li M, Li Y, et al. miR-340 suppresses glioblastoma multiforme. Oncotarget. 2015;6(11):9257–70.

[24] Li X, Liu Y, Granberg KJ, Wang Q, Moore LM, Ji P, et al. Two mature products of MIR-491 coordinate to suppress key cancer hallmarks in glioblastoma. Oncogene. 2015;34(13):1619–28.

[25] Kim J, Zhang Y, Skalski M, Hayes J, Kefas B, Schiff D, et al. microRNA-148a is a prognostic oncomiR that targets MIG6 and BIM to regulate EGFR and apoptosis in glioblastoma. Cancer Research. 2014;74(5):1541–53.

[26] Yin D, Ogawa S, Kawamata N, Leiter A, Ham M, Li D, et al. miR-34a functions as a tumor suppressor modulating EGFR in glioblastoma multiforme. Oncogene. 2013;32(9):1155–63.

[27] Genovese G, Ergun A, Shukla SA, Campos B, Hanna J, Ghosh P, et al. microRNA regulatory network inference identifies miR-34a as a novel regulator of TGF-beta signaling in glioblastoma. Cancer Discovery. 2012;2(8):736–49.

[28] Silber J, Jacobsen A, Ozawa T, Harinath G, Pedraza A, Sander C, et al. miR-34a repression in proneural malignant gliomas upregulates expression of its target PDGFRA and promotes tumorigenesis. PloS One. 2012;7(3):e33844.

[29] Brennan CW, Verhaak RG, McKenna A, Campos B, Noushmehr H, Salama SR, et al. The somatic genomic landscape of glioblastoma. Cell. 2013;155(2):462–77.

[30] Li Y, Guessous F, Zhang Y, Dipierro C, Kefas B, Johnson E, et al. MicroRNA-34a inhibits glioblastoma growth by targeting multiple oncogenes. Cancer Research. 2009;69(19): 7569–76.

[31] Verhaak RG, Hoadley KA, Purdom E, Wang V, Qi Y, Wilkerson MD, et al. Integrated genomic analysis identifies clinically relevant subtypes of glioblastoma characterized by abnormalities in PDGFRA, IDH1, EGFR, and NF1. Cancer cell. 2010;17(1):98–110.

[32] Kouri FM, Ritner C, Stegh AH. miRNA-182 and the regulation of the glioblastoma phenotype—toward miRNA-based precision therapeutics. Cell Cycle. 2015;14(24): 3794–800.

[33] Lan F, Yu H, Hu M, Xia T, Yue X. miR-144-3p exerts anti-tumor effects in glioblastoma by targeting c-Met. Journal of Neurochemistry. 2015;135(2):274–86.

[34] Wang L, Shi ZM, Jiang CF, Liu X, Chen QD, Qian X, et al. MiR-143 acts as a tumor suppressor by targeting N-RAS and enhances temozolomide-induced apoptosis in glioma. Oncotarget. 2014;5(14):5416–27.

[35] Wang XR, Luo H, Li HL, Cao L, Wang XF, Yan W, et al. Overexpressed let-7a inhibits glioma cell malignancy by directly targeting K-ras, independently of PTEN. Neuro-oncology. 2013;15(11):1491–501.

[36] Shi Z, Chen Q, Li C, Wang L, Qian X, Jiang C, et al. MiR-124 governs glioma growth and angiogenesis and enhances chemosensitivity by targeting R-Ras and N-Ras. Neuro-oncology. 2014;16(10):1341–53.

[37] Lv Z, Yang L. MiR-124 inhibits the growth of glioblastoma through the downregulation of SOS1. Molecular Medicine Reports. 2013;8(2):345–9.

[38] Tan X, Wang S, Yang B, Zhu L, Yin B, Chao T, et al. The CREB-miR-9 negative feedback minicircuitry coordinates the migration and proliferation of glioma cells. PloS One. 2012;7(11):e49570.

[39] Malzkorn B, Wolter M, Liesenberg F, Grzendowski M, Stuhler K, Meyer HE, et al. Identification and functional characterization of microRNAs involved in the malignant progression of gliomas. Brain Pathology. 2010;20(3):539–50.

[40] Stark MS, Bonazzi VF, Boyle GM, Palmer JM, Symmons J, Lanagan CM, et al. miR-514a regulates the tumour suppressor NF1 and modulates BRAFi sensitivity in melanoma. Oncotarget. 2015;6(19):17753–63.

[41] Huse JT, Brennan C, Hambardzumyan D, Wee B, Pena J, Rouhanifard SH, et al. The PTEN-regulating microRNA miR-26a is amplified in high-grade glioma and facilitates gliomagenesis in vivo. Genes & Development. 2009;23(11):1327–37.

[42] Kim H, Huang W, Jiang X, Pennicooke B, Park PJ, Johnson MD. Integrative genome analysis reveals an oncomir/oncogene cluster regulating glioblastoma survivorship. Proceedings of the National Academy of Sciences of the United States of America. 2010;107(5):2183–8.

[43] Guo P, Nie Q, Lan J, Ge J, Qiu Y, Mao Q. C-Myc negatively controls the tumor suppressor PTEN by upregulating miR-26a in glioblastoma multiforme cells. Biochemical and Biophysical Research Communications. 2013;441(1):186–90.

[44] Tan X, Wang S, Zhu L, Wu C, Yin B, Zhao J, et al. cAMP response element-binding protein promotes gliomagenesis by modulating the expression of oncogenic micro-

RNA-23a. Proceedings of the National Academy of Sciences of the United States of America. 2012;109(39):15805–10.

[45] Tian K, Di R, Wang L. MicroRNA-23a enhances migration and invasion through PTEN in osteosarcoma. Cancer Gene Therapy. 2015;22(7):351–9.

[46] Li H, Yang BB. Stress response of glioblastoma cells mediated by miR-17-5p targeting PTEN and the passenger strand miR-17-3p targeting MDM2. Oncotarget. 2012;3(12): 1653–68.

[47] Xia X, Li Y, Wang W, Tang F, Tan J, Sun L, et al. MicroRNA-1908 functions as a glioblastoma oncogene by suppressing PTEN tumor suppressor pathway. Molecular Cancer. 2015;14:154.

[48] Tokudome T, Sasaki A, Tsuji M, Udaka Y, Oyamada H, Tsuchiya H, et al. Reduced PTEN expression and overexpression of miR-17-5p, -19a-3p, -19b-3p, -21-5p, -130b-3p, -221-3p and -222-3p by glioblastoma stem-like cells following irradiation. Oncology Letters. 2015;10(4):2269–72.

[49] Kleihues P, Burger PC, Scheithauer BW. The new WHO classification of brain tumours. Brain Pathology. 1993;3(3):255–68.

[50] Plate KH, Risau W. Angiogenesis in malignant gliomas. Glia. 1995;15(3):339–47.

[51] Yue X, Wang P, Xu J, Zhu Y, Sun G, Pang Q, et al. MicroRNA-205 functions as a tumor suppressor in human glioblastoma cells by targeting VEGF-A. Oncology Reports. 2012;27(4):1200–6.

[52] Harris AL. Hypoxia—a key regulatory factor in tumour growth. Nature Reviews Cancer. 2002;2(1):38–47.

[53] Zhang KL, Han L, Chen LY, Shi ZD, Yang M, Ren Y, et al. Blockage of a miR-21/EGFR regulatory feedback loop augments anti-EGFR therapy in glioblastomas. Cancer Letters. 2014;342(1):139–49.

[54] Hermansen SK, Nielsen BS, Aaberg-Jessen C, Kristensen BW. miR-21 is linked to glioma angiogenesis: a co-localization study. The Journal of Histochemistry and Cytochemistry: Official Journal of the Histochemistry Society. 2016;64(2):138–48.

[55] Chen L, Han L, Zhang K, Shi Z, Zhang J, Zhang A, et al. VHL regulates the effects of miR-23b on glioma survival and invasion via suppression of HIF-1alpha/VEGF and beta-catenin/Tcf-4 signaling. Neuro-oncology. 2012;14(8):1026–36.

[56] Xiao B, Zhou X, Ye M, Lv S, Wu M, Liao C, et al. MicroRNA566 modulates vascular endothelial growth factor by targeting Von HippelLandau in human glioblastoma in vitro and in vivo. Molecular Medicine Reports. 2016;13(1):379–85.

[57] Babae N, Bourajjaj M, Liu Y, Van Beijnum JR, Cerisoli F, Scaria PV, et al. Systemic miRNA-7 delivery inhibits tumor angiogenesis and growth in murine xenograft glioblastoma. Oncotarget. 2014;5(16):6687–700.

[58] Smits M, Nilsson J, Mir SE, van der Stoop PM, Hulleman E, Niers JM, et al. miR-101 is down-regulated in glioblastoma resulting in EZH2-induced proliferation, migration, and angiogenesis. Oncotarget. 2010;1(8):710–20.

[59] Sun J, Zheng G, Gu Z, Guo Z. MiR-137 inhibits proliferation and angiogenesis of human glioblastoma cells by targeting EZH2. Journal of Neuro-oncology. 2015;122(3):481–9.

[60] Wurdinger T, Tannous BA, Saydam O, Skog J, Grau S, Soutschek J, et al. miR-296 regulates growth factor receptor overexpression in angiogenic endothelial cells. Cancer Cell. 2008;14(5):382–93.

[61] Fang L, Deng Z, Shatseva T, Yang J, Peng C, Du WW, et al. MicroRNA miR-93 promotes tumor growth and angiogenesis by targeting integrin-beta8. Oncogene. 2011;30(7):806–21.

[62] Dews M, Fox JL, Hultine S, Sundaram P, Wang W, Liu YY, et al. The myc-miR-17~92 axis blunts TGF{beta} signaling and production of multiple TGF{beta}-dependent antiangiogenic factors. Cancer Research. 2010;70(20):8233–46.

[63] Kruiswijk F, Labuschagne CF, Vousden KH. p53 in survival, death and metabolic health: a lifeguard with a licence to kill. Nature Reviews Molecular Cell Biology. 2015;16(7):393–405.

[64] Lin J, Teo S, Lam DH, Jeyaseelan K, Wang S. MicroRNA-10b pleiotropically regulates invasion, angiogenicity and apoptosis of tumor cells resembling mesenchymal subtype of glioblastoma multiforme. Cell Death & Disease. 2012;3:e398.

[65] Gabriely G, Yi M, Narayan RS, Niers JM, Wurdinger T, Imitola J, et al. Human glioma growth is controlled by microRNA-10b. Cancer Research. 2011;71(10):3563–72.

[66] Brown CJ, Lain S, Verma CS, Fersht AR, Lane DP. Awakening guardian angels: drugging the p53 pathway. Nature Reviews Cancer. 2009;9(12):862–73.

[67] Suh SS, Yoo JY, Nuovo GJ, Jeon YJ, Kim S, Lee TJ, et al. MicroRNAs/TP53 feedback circuitry in glioblastoma multiforme. Proceedings of the National Academy of Sciences of the United States of America. 2012;109(14):5316–21.

[68] Sun YC, Wang J, Guo CC, Sai K, Wang J, Chen FR, et al. MiR-181b sensitizes glioma cells to teniposide by targeting MDM2. BMC Cancer. 2014;14:611.

[69] Skalsky RL, Cullen BR. Reduced expression of brain-enriched microRNAs in glioblastomas permits targeted regulation of a cell death gene. PloS One. 2011;6(9):e24248.

[70] Burkhart DL, Sage J. Cellular mechanisms of tumour suppression by the retinoblastoma gene. Nature Reviews Cancer. 2008;8(9):671–82.

[71] Serrano M, Hannon GJ, Beach D. A new regulatory motif in cell-cycle control causing specific inhibition of cyclin D/CDK4. Nature. 1993;366(6456):704–7.

[72] Lundberg AS, Weinberg RA. Functional inactivation of the retinoblastoma protein requires sequential modification by at least two distinct cyclin-cdk complexes. Molecular and Cellular Biology. 1998;18(2):753–61.

[73] Deng X, Ma L, Wu M, Zhang G, Jin C, Guo Y, et al. miR-124 radiosensitizes human glioma cells by targeting CDK4. Journal of Neuro-oncology. 2013;114(3):263–74.

[74] Qiu S, Huang D, Yin D, Li F, Li X, Kung HF, et al. Suppression of tumorigenicity by microRNA-138 through inhibition of EZH2-CDK4/6-pRb-E2F1 signal loop in glioblastoma multiforme. Biochim Biophys Acta. 2013;1832(10):1697–707.

[75] Hui W, Yuntao L, Lun L, WenSheng L, ChaoFeng L, HaiYong H, et al. MicroRNA-195 inhibits the proliferation of human glioma cells by directly targeting cyclin D1 and cyclin E1. PloS One. 2013;8(1):e54932.

[76] Nakada M, Nakada S, Demuth T, Tran NL, Hoelzinger DB, Berens ME. Molecular targets of glioma invasion. Cellular and Molecular Life Sciences. 2007;64(4):458–78.

[77] Liu Y, Yan W, Zhang W, Chen L, You G, Bao Z, et al. MiR-218 reverses high invasiveness of glioblastoma cells by targeting the oncogenic transcription factor LEF1. Oncology Reports. 2012;28(3):1013–21.

[78] Song L, Huang Q, Chen K, Liu L, Lin C, Dai T, et al. miR-218 inhibits the invasive ability of glioma cells by direct downregulation of IKK-beta. Biochemical and Biophysical Research Communications. 2010;402(1):135–40.

[79] Li Y, Xu J, Chen H, Bai J, Li S, Zhao Z, et al. Comprehensive analysis of the functional microRNA-mRNA regulatory network identifies miRNA signatures associated with glioma malignant progression. Nucleic Acids Research. 2013;41(22):e203.

[80] Yan W, Zhang W, Sun L, Liu Y, You G, Wang Y, et al. Identification of MMP-9 specific microRNA expression profile as potential targets of anti-invasion therapy in glioblastoma multiforme. Brain Research. 2011;1411:108–15.

[81] Asuthkar S, Velpula KK, Chetty C, Gorantla B, Rao JS. Epigenetic regulation of miRNA-211 by MMP-9 governs glioma cell apoptosis, chemosensitivity and radiosensitivity. Oncotarget. 2012;3(11):1439–54.

[82] Zheng X, Chopp M, Lu Y, Buller B, Jiang F. MiR-15b and miR-152 reduce glioma cell invasion and angiogenesis via NRP-2 and MMP-3. Cancer Letters. 2013;329(2):146–54.

[83] Lu Y, Chopp M, Zheng X, Katakowski M, Buller B, Jiang F. MiR-145 reduces ADAM17 expression and inhibits in vitro migration and invasion of glioma cells. Oncology Reports. 2013;29(1):67–72.

[84] Gabriely G, Wurdinger T, Kesari S, Esau CC, Burchard J, Linsley PS, et al. MicroRNA 21 promotes glioma invasion by targeting matrix metalloproteinase regulators. Molecular and Cellular Biology. 2008;28(17):5369–80.

[85] Fowler A, Thomson D, Giles K, Maleki S, Mreich E, Wheeler H, et al. miR-124a is frequently down–regulated in glioblastoma and is involved in migration and invasion. European Journal of Cancer. 2011;47(6):953–63.

[86] Zhao WH, Wu SQ, Zhang YD. Downregulation of miR-124 promotes the growth and invasiveness of glioblastoma cells involving upregulation of PPP1R13L. International Journal of Molecular Medicine. 2013;32(1):101–7.

[87] Cai J, Zhao J, Zhang N, Xu X, Li R, Yi Y, et al. MicroRNA-542-3p suppresses tumor cell invasion via targeting AKT pathway in human astrocytoma. The Journal of Biological Chemistry. 2015;290(41):24678–88.

[88] Wang H, Tao T, Yan W, Feng Y, Wang Y, Cai J, et al. Upregulation of miR-181s reverses mesenchymal transition by targeting KPNA4 in glioblastoma. Scientific Reports. 2015;5:13072.

[89] Yin F, Zhang JN, Wang SW, Zhou CH, Zhao MM, Fan WH, et al. MiR-125a-3p regulates glioma apoptosis and invasion by regulating Nrg1. PloS One. 2015;10(1):e0116759.

[90] Dontula R, Dinasarapu A, Chetty C, Pannuru P, Herbert E, Ozer H, et al. MicroRNA 203 modulates glioma cell migration via Robo1/ERK/MMP-9 signaling. Genes & Cancer. 2013;4(7–8):285–96.

[91] Chen Z, Li D, Cheng Q, Ma Z, Jiang B, Peng R, et al. MicroRNA-203 inhibits the proliferation and invasion of U251 glioblastoma cells by directly targeting PLD2. Molecular Medicine Reports. 2014;9(2):503–8.

[92] Chung HJ, Choi YE, Kim ES, Han YH, Park MJ, Bae IH. miR-29b attenuates tumorigenicity and stemness maintenance in human glioblastoma multiforme by directly targeting BCL2L2. Oncotarget. 2015;6(21):18429–44.

[93] Sun L, Yan W, Wang Y, Sun G, Luo H, Zhang J, et al. MicroRNA-10b induces glioma cell invasion by modulating MMP-14 and uPAR expression via HOXD10. Brain Research. 2011;1389:9–18.

[94] Liu Q, Zou R, Zhou R, Gong C, Wang Z, Cai T, et al. miR-155 regulates glioma cells invasion and chemosensitivity by p38 isforms in vitro. Journal of Cellular Biochemistry. 2015;116(7):1213–21.

[95] Corsten MF, Miranda R, Kasmieh R, Krichevsky AM, Weissleder R, Shah K. MicroRNA-21 knockdown disrupts glioma growth in vivo and displays synergistic cytotoxicity with neural precursor cell delivered S-TRAIL in human gliomas. Cancer Research. 2007;67(19):8994–9000.

[96] Gaur AB, Holbeck SL, Colburn NH, Israel MA. Downregulation of Pdcd4 by mir-21 facilitates glioblastoma proliferation in vivo. Neuro-oncology. 2011;13(6):580–90.

[97] Papagiannakopoulos T, Shapiro A, Kosik KS. MicroRNA-21 targets a network of key tumor-suppressive pathways in glioblastoma cells. Cancer Research. 2008;68(19):8164–72.

[98] Niu H, Wang K, Zhang A, Yang S, Song Z, Wang W, et al. miR-92a is a critical regulator of the apoptosis pathway in glioblastoma with inverse expression of BCL2L11. Oncology Reports. 2012;28(5):1771–7.

[99] Wang K, Wang X, Zou J, Zhang A, Wan Y, Pu P, et al. miR-92b controls glioma proliferation and invasion through regulating Wnt/beta-catenin signaling via Nemo-like kinase. Neuro-oncology. 2013;15(5):578–88.

[100] Medina R, Zaidi SK, Liu CG, Stein JL, van Wijnen AJ, Croce CM, et al. MicroRNAs 221 and 222 bypass quiescence and compromise cell survival. Cancer Research. 2008;68(8): 2773–80.

[101] Liu F, Gong J, Huang W, Wang Z, Wang M, Yang J, et al. MicroRNA-106b-5p boosts glioma tumorigensis by targeting multiple tumor suppressor genes. Oncogene. 2014;33(40):4813–22.

[102] Polyak K, Lee MH, Erdjument-Bromage H, Koff A, Roberts JM, Tempst P, et al. Cloning of p27Kip1, a cyclin-dependent kinase inhibitor and a potential mediator of extracellular antimitogenic signals. Cell. 1994;78(1):59–66.

[103] Gillies JK, Lorimer IA. Regulation of p27Kip1 by miRNA 221/222 in glioblastoma. Cell Cycle. 2007;6(16):2005–9.

[104] Wan Y, Fei XF, Wang ZM, Jiang DY, Chen HC, Yang J, et al. Expression of miR-125b in the new, highly invasive glioma stem cell and progenitor cell line SU3. Chinese Journal of Cancer. 2012;31(4):207–14.

[105] Le MT, Teh C, Shyh-Chang N, Xie H, Zhou B, Korzh V, et al. MicroRNA-125b is a novel negative regulator of p53. Genes & Development. 2009;23(7):862–76.

[106] Park SY, Lee JH, Ha M, Nam JW, Kim VN. miR-29 miRNAs activate p53 by targeting p85 alpha and CDC42. Nature Structural & Molecular Biology. 2009;16(1):23–9.

[107] He L, He X, Lim LP, de Stanchina E, Xuan Z, Liang Y, et al. A microRNA component of the p53 tumour suppressor network. Nature. 2007;447(7148):1130–4.

[108] Kato M, Paranjape T, Muller RU, Nallur S, Gillespie E, Keane K, et al. The mir-34 microRNA is required for the DNA damage response in vivo in C. elegans and in vitro in human breast cancer cells. Oncogene. 2009;28(25):2419–24.

[109] Yan D, Ng WL, Zhang X, Wang P, Zhang Z, Mo YY, et al. Targeting DNA-PKcs and ATM with miR-101 sensitizes tumors to radiation. PloS One. 2010;5(7):e11397.

[110] Nogueira L, Ruiz-Ontanon P, Vazquez-Barquero A, Moris F, Fernandez-Luna JL. The NFkappaB pathway: a therapeutic target in glioblastoma. Oncotarget. 2011;2(8):646–53.

[111] Li Y, Li W, Yang Y, Lu Y, He C, Hu G, et al. MicroRNA-21 targets LRRFIP1 and contributes to VM-26 resistance in glioblastoma multiforme. Brain Research. 2009;1286:13–8.

[112] Taganov KD, Boldin MP, Chang KJ, Baltimore D. NF-kappaB-dependent induction of microRNA miR-146, an inhibitor targeted to signaling proteins of innate immune responses. Proceedings of the National Academy of Sciences of the United States of America. 2006;103(33):12481–6.

[113] Park H, Huang X, Lu C, Cairo MS, Zhou X. MicroRNA-146a and microRNA-146b regulate human dendritic cell apoptosis and cytokine production by targeting TRAF6 and IRAK1 proteins. The Journal of Biological Chemistry. 2015;290(5):2831–41.

[114] Wu H, Liu Q, Cai T, Chen YD, Wang ZF. Induction of microRNA-146a is involved in curcumin-mediated enhancement of temozolomide cytotoxicity against human glioblastoma. Molecular Medicine Reports. 2015;12(4):5461–6.

[115] Iyer A, Zurolo E, Prabowo A, Fluiter K, Spliet WG, van Rijen PC, et al. MicroRNA-146a: a key regulator of astrocyte-mediated inflammatory response. PloS One. 2012;7(9):e44789.

[116] Yu H, Pardoll D, Jove R. STATs in cancer inflammation and immunity: a leading role for STAT3. Nature Reviews Cancer. 2009;9(11):798–809.

[117] Wei J, Wang F, Kong LY, Xu S, Doucette T, Ferguson SD, et al. miR-124 inhibits STAT3 signaling to enhance T cell-mediated immune clearance of glioma. Cancer Research. 2013;73(13):3913–26.

[118] Tarassishin L, Lee SC. Interferon regulatory factor 3 alters glioma inflammatory and invasive properties. Journal of Neuro-oncology. 2013;113(2):185–94.

[119] Vander Heiden MG, Cantley LC, Thompson CB. Understanding the Warburg effect: the metabolic requirements of cell proliferation. Science. 2009;324(5930):1029–33.

[120] Colavolpe C, Metellus P, Mancini J, Barrie M, Bequet-Boucard C, Figarella-Branger D, et al. Independent prognostic value of pre-treatment 18-FDG-PET in high-grade gliomas. Journal of Neuro-oncology. 2012;107(3):527–35.

[121] Hardie DG. AMP-activated/SNF1 protein kinases: conserved guardians of cellular energy. Nature Reviews Molecular Cell Biology. 2007;8(10):774–85.

[122] Sanders MJ, Ali ZS, Hegarty BD, Heath R, Snowden MA, Carling D. Defining the mechanism of activation of AMP-activated protein kinase by the small molecule A-769662, a member of the thienopyridone family. The Journal of Biological Chemistry. 2007;282(45):32539–48.

[123] Hawley SA, Boudeau J, Reid JL, Mustard KJ, Udd L, Makela TP, et al. Complexes between the LKB1 tumor suppressor, STRAD alpha/beta and MO25 alpha/beta are

upstream kinases in the AMP-activated protein kinase cascade. Journal of Biology. 2003;2(4):28.

[124] Godlewski J, Nowicki MO, Bronisz A, Nuovo G, Palatini J, De Lay M, et al. MicroRNA-451 regulates LKB1/AMPK signaling and allows adaptation to metabolic stress in glioma cells. Molecular Cell. 2010;37(5):620–32.

[125] Guo QM, Malek RL, Kim S, Chiao C, He M, Ruffy M, et al. Identification of c-myc responsive genes using rat cDNA microarray. Cancer Research. 2000;60(21):5922–8.

[126] Zamorano A, Lamas M, Vergara P, Naranjo JR, Segovia J. Transcriptionally mediated gene targeting of gas1 to glioma cells elicits growth arrest and apoptosis. Journal of Neuroscience Research. 2003;71(2):256–63.

[127] Barr LF, Campbell SE, Diette GB, Gabrielson EW, Kim S, Shim H, et al. c-Myc suppresses the tumorigenicity of lung cancer cells and down-regulates vascular endothelial growth factor expression. Cancer Research. 2000;60(1):143–9.

[128] Wang G, Wang J, Zhao H, Wang J, Tony To SS. The role of Myc and let-7a in glioblastoma, glucose metabolism and response to therapy. Archives of Biochemistry and Biophysics. 2015;580:84–92.

[129] Chang TC, Zeitels LR, Hwang HW, Chivukula RR, Wentzel EA, Dews M, et al. Lin-28B transactivation is necessary for Myc-mediated let-7 repression and proliferation. Proceedings of the National Academy of Sciences of the United States of America. 2009;106(9):3384–9.

[130] Rani SB, Rathod SS, Karthik S, Kaur N, Muzumdar D, Shiras AS. MiR-145 functions as a tumor-suppressive RNA by targeting Sox9 and adducin 3 in human glioma cells. Neuro-oncology. 2013;15(10):1302–16.

[131] Dang CV. MYC on the path to cancer. Cell. 2012;149(1):22–35.

[132] Gan B, Lim C, Chu G, Hua S, Ding Z, Collins M, et al. FoxOs enforce a progression checkpoint to constrain mTORC1-activated renal tumorigenesis. Cancer Cell. 2010;18(5):472–84.

[133] Kress TR, Cannell IG, Brenkman AB, Samans B, Gaestel M, Roepman P, et al. The MK5/PRAK kinase and Myc form a negative feedback loop that is disrupted during colorectal tumorigenesis. Molecular Cell. 2011;41(4):445–57.

[134] Masui K, Tanaka K, Akhavan D, Babic I, Gini B, Matsutani T, et al. mTOR complex 2 controls glycolytic metabolism in glioblastoma through FoxO acetylation and upregulation of c-Myc. Cell Metabolism. 2013;18(5):726–39.

[135] Boyerinas B, Park SM, Shomron N, Hedegaard MM, Vinther J, Andersen JS, et al. Identification of let-7-regulated oncofetal genes. Cancer Research. 2008;68(8):2587–91.

[136] Kefas B, Comeau L, Erdle N, Montgomery E, Amos S, Purow B. Pyruvate kinase M2 is a target of the tumor-suppressive microRNA-326 and regulates the survival of glioma cells. Neuro-oncology. 2010;12(11):1102–12.

[137] Zhou J, Xu T, Yan Y, Qin R, Wang H, Zhang X, et al. MicroRNA-326 functions as a tumor suppressor in glioma by targeting the Nin one binding protein (NOB1). PloS One. 2013;8(7):e68469.

[138] de Visser KE, Eichten A, Coussens LM. Paradoxical roles of the immune system during cancer development. Nature Reviews Cancer. 2006;6(1):24–37.

[139] Mantovani A, Sozzani S, Locati M, Allavena P, Sica A. Macrophage polarization: tumor-associated macrophages as a paradigm for polarized M2 mononuclear phagocytes. Trends in Immunology. 2002;23(11):549–55.

[140] Graff JW, Dickson AM, Clay G, McCaffrey AP, Wilson ME. Identifying functional microRNAs in macrophages with polarized phenotypes. The Journal of Biological Chemistry. 2012;287(26):21816–25.

[141] Cai X, Yin Y, Li N, Zhu D, Zhang J, Zhang CY, et al. Re-polarization of tumor-associated macrophages to pro-inflammatory M1 macrophages by microRNA-155. Journal of Molecular Cell Biology. 2012;4(5):341–3.

[142] Tanikawa T, Wilke CM, Kryczek I, Chen GY, Kao J, Nunez G, et al. Interleukin-10 ablation promotes tumor development, growth, and metastasis. Cancer Research. 2012;72(2):420–9.

[143] Zhang C, Han L, Zhang A, Yang W, Zhou X, Pu P, et al. Global changes of mRNA expression reveals an increased activity of the interferon-induced signal transducer and activator of transcription (STAT) pathway by repression of miR-221/222 in glioblastoma U251 cells. International Journal of Oncology. 2010;36(6):1503–12.

[144] Raulet DH, Gasser S, Gowen BG, Deng W, Jung H. Regulation of ligands for the NKG2D activating receptor. Annual Review of Immunology. 2013;31:413–41.

[145] Friese MA, Platten M, Lutz SZ, Naumann U, Aulwurm S, Bischof F, et al. MICA/NKG2D-mediated immunogene therapy of experimental gliomas. Cancer Research. 2003;63(24):8996–9006.

[146] Codo P, Weller M, Meister G, Szabo E, Steinle A, Wolter M, et al. MicroRNA-mediated down-regulation of NKG2D ligands contributes to glioma immune escape. Oncotarget. 2014;5(17):7651–62.

[147] Wei J, Nduom EK, Kong LY, Hashimoto Y, Xu S, Gabrusiewicz K, et al. MiR-138 exerts anti-glioma efficacy by targeting immune checkpoints. Neuro-oncology. 2015.

[148] Ohno M, Natsume A, Kondo Y, Iwamizu H, Motomura K, Toda H, et al. The modulation of microRNAs by type I IFN through the activation of signal transducers and activators

of transcription 3 in human glioma. Molecular Cancer Research: MCR. 2009;7(12):2022–30.

[149] Aleckovic M, Kang Y. Regulation of cancer metastasis by cell-free miRNAs. Biochimica et Biophysica Acta. 2015;1855(1):24–42.

[150] Wang K, Yuan Y, Cho JH, McClarty S, Baxter D, Galas DJ. Comparing the MicroRNA spectrum between serum and plasma. PloS One. 2012;7(7):e41561.

[151] Cheng HH, Yi HS, Kim Y, Kroh EM, Chien JW, Eaton KD, et al. Plasma processing conditions substantially influence circulating microRNA biomarker levels. PloS One. 2013;8(6):e64795.

[152] Sasayama T, Nakamizo S, Nishihara M, Kawamura A, Tanaka H, Mizukawa K, et al. Cerebrospinal fluid interleukin-10 is a potentially useful biomarker in immunocompetent primary central nervous system lymphoma (PCNSL). Neuro-oncology. 2012;14(3):368–80.

[153] Skog J, Wurdinger T, van Rijn S, Meijer DH, Gainche L, Sena-Esteves M, et al. Glioblastoma microvesicles transport RNA and proteins that promote tumour growth and provide diagnostic biomarkers. Nature Cell Biology. 2008;10(12):1470–6.

[154] Roth P, Wischhusen J, Happold C, Chandran PA, Hofer S, Eisele G, et al. A specific miRNA signature in the peripheral blood of glioblastoma patients. Journal of Neurochemistry. 2011;118(3):449–57.

[155] Wang Q, Li P, Li A, Jiang W, Wang H, Wang J, et al. Plasma specific miRNAs as predictive biomarkers for diagnosis and prognosis of glioma. Journal of Experimental & Clinical Cancer Research: CR. 2012;31:97.

[156] Zhao Q, Yin T, Peng J, Zou Y, Yang J, Shen A, et al. Noninvasive metabolomic profiling of human embryo culture media using a simple spectroscopy adjunct to morphology for embryo assessment in in vitro fertilization (IVF). International Journal of Molecular Sciences. 2013;14(4):6556–70.

[157] Dong L, Li Y, Han C, Wang X, She L, Zhang H. miRNA microarray reveals specific expression in the peripheral blood of glioblastoma patients. International journal of oncology. 2014;45(2):746–56.

[158] Manterola L, Guruceaga E, Gallego Perez-Larraya J, Gonzalez-Huarriz M, Jauregui P, Tejada S, et al. A small noncoding RNA signature found in exosomes of GBM patient serum as a diagnostic tool. Neuro-oncology. 2014;16(4):520–7.

[159] Shao N, Wang L, Xue L, Wang R, Lan Q. Plasma miR-454-3p as a potential prognostic indicator in human glioma. Neurological Science. 2015;36(2):309–13.

[160] Wu J, Li L, Jiang C. Identification and Evaluation of Serum MicroRNA-29 Family for Glioma Screening. Molecular Neurobiology. 2015;52(3):1540–6.

[161] Liu Q, Liao F, Wu H, Cai T, Yang L, Fang J. Different expression of miR-29b and VEGFA in glioma. Artificial Cells, Nanomedicine, and Biotechnology. 2015:1–6.

[162] Wei X, Chen D, Lv T, Li G, Qu S. Serum microRNA-125b as a potential biomarker for glioma diagnosis. Molecular neurobiology. 2016;53(1):163–70.

[163] Lai NS, Wu DG, Fang XG, Lin YC, Chen SS, Li ZB, et al. Serum microRNA-210 as a potential noninvasive biomarker for the diagnosis and prognosis of glioma. British Journal of Cancer. 2015;112(7):1241–6.

[164] Ivan M, Huang X. miR-210: fine-tuning the hypoxic response. Advances in experimental medicine and biology. 2014;772:205–27.

[165] Zeng L, He X, Wang Y, Tang Y, Zheng C, Cai H, et al. MicroRNA-210 overexpression induces angiogenesis and neurogenesis in the normal adult mouse brain. Gene Therapy. 2014;21(1):37–43.

[166] Chio CC, Lin JW, Cheng HA, Chiu WT, Wang YH, Wang JJ, et al. MicroRNA-210 targets antiapoptotic Bcl-2 expression and mediates hypoxia-induced apoptosis of neuroblastoma cells. Archives of Toxicology. 2013;87(3):459–68.

[167] Cui H, Seubert B, Stahl E, Dietz H, Reuning U, Moreno-Leon L, et al. Tissue inhibitor of metalloproteinases-1 induces a pro-tumourigenic increase of miR-210 in lung adenocarcinoma cells and their exosomes. Oncogene. 2015;34(28):3640–50.

[168] Sun J, Liao K, Wu X, Huang J, Zhang S, Lu X. Serum microRNA-128 as a biomarker for diagnosis of glioma. International Journal of Clinical and Experimental Medicine. 2015;8(1):456–63.

[169] Yue X, Lan F, Hu M, Pan Q, Wang Q, Wang J. Downregulation of serum microRNA-205 as a potential diagnostic and prognostic biomarker for human glioma. Journal of Neurosurgery. 2016;124(1):122–8.

[170] Baraniskin A, Kuhnhenn J, Schlegel U, Maghnouj A, Zollner H, Schmiegel W, et al. Identification of microRNAs in the cerebrospinal fluid as biomarker for the diagnosis of glioma. Neuro-oncology. 2012;14(1):29–33.

[171] Teplyuk NM, Mollenhauer B, Gabriely G, Giese A, Kim E, Smolsky M, et al. MicroRNAs in cerebrospinal fluid identify glioblastoma and metastatic brain cancers and reflect disease activity. Neuro-oncology. 2012;14(6):689–700.

[172] Akers JC, Ramakrishnan V, Kim R, Skog J, Nakano I, Pingle S, et al. MiR-21 in the extracellular vesicles (EVs) of cerebrospinal fluid (CSF): a platform for glioblastoma biomarker development. PloS One. 2013;8(10):e78115.

[173] Shi R, Wang PY, Li XY, Chen JX, Li Y, Zhang XZ, et al. Exosomal levels of miRNA-21 from cerebrospinal fluids associated with poor prognosis and tumor recurrence of glioma patients. Oncotarget. 2015;6(29):26971–81.

7

Mechanisms of Glioma Cell Invasion

Scott G. Turner, Maleeha Ahmad and
Steven A. Toms

Abstract

Malignant gliomas are the most aggressive primary brain tumors. Although current treatment includes surgery and chemo/radiation therapy, life expectancy remains on the order of 2 years. One of the features, which make these tumors incurable, is their infiltration into normal brain tissue. This process is incompletely understood at a molecular level and appropriate targets need to be developed. This review discusses (1) the unique structure of the neural extracellular matrix (ECM), (2) the basis of the proliferation to migration transition that initiates the infiltrative process, (3) the remodeling of the ECM by degradation and synthesis of new components, and (4) trophic factors that act as chemoattractants and chemorepellents for migrating cells. Finally we briefly discuss the challenges facing the study of this complex process and future directions in attacking this important problem in neuro-oncology.

Keywords: glioma, migration, invasion, extracellular matrix, protease, signaling

1. Introduction

Malignant gliomas are the most common primary tumors of the central nervous system (CNS) accounting for over 22,000 new cases in the USA each year [1]. Glioblastoma multiforme (GBM) is the most aggressive (WHO grade IV) glioma and is characterized histologically by high mitotic activity leading to hypoxia and necrosis, nuclear atypia and cellular pleomorphism, and microvascular proliferation due to secretion of pro-angiogenic factors. These tumors are uniformly fatal with standard treatment consisting of maximal surgical resection followed by radiation and chemotherapy which targets cell proliferation (Temozolomide or other DNA modifying agents) [2] or angiogenesis (Bevacizumab) [3], as well as other newly developed methods of attacking dividing tumor cells (Optune-TTF) [4].

Gliomas differ from metastatic tumors in their ability to migrate into the surrounding brain parenchyma. While most recurrence occurs within 1–2 cm of the original tumor bed [5], seemingly multifocal disease or so-called "butterfly glioma" can develop at distant sites as a consequence of migration of cells along blood vessels and white matter tracts [6] (**Figure 1**). Although they are highly infiltrative, less than 2% of gliomas spread outside the CNS, suggesting that tumor cells are either not able to cross the basement membrane and enter the vasculature or that they require a specific neural environment containing specific molecules through which they can proliferate and migrate. Tumor cells switch from a proliferative to a migratory or mesenchymal phenotype, resorting to this more primitive state, which mimics the behavior of their migratory progenitors such as the radial glia that traversed white matter pathways and other structures during embryonic development [7]. The molecular mechanisms of this transition are currently poorly understood.

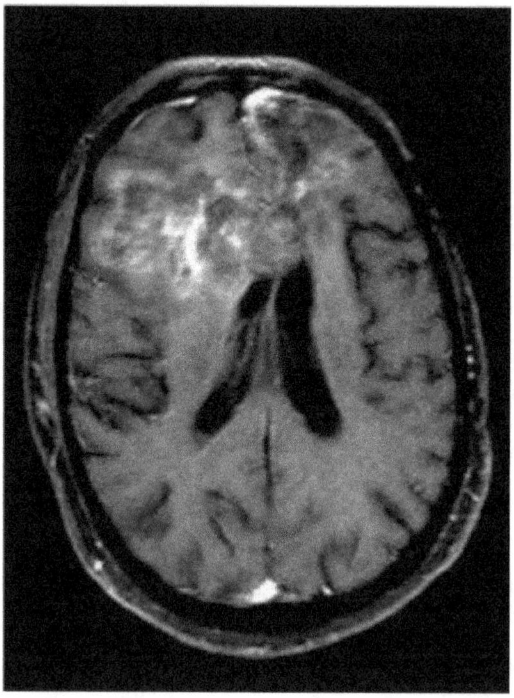

Figure 1. Butterfly glioma in a patient with bihemispheric spread due to involvement of the corpus callosum.

In this chapter, we discuss the composition of the brain's extracellular matrix, as well as the mechanisms by which tumor cells transition to a migratory phenotype and remodel the ECM through degradation by novel proteases and their inhibitors. We discuss the search for ECM molecules expressed by the tumor cells, which then respond to chemoattractants in the environment in order to direct growth. Finally, we discuss potential targets of anti-infiltrative therapy and the obstacles that must yet be overcome to address this important neuro-oncologic problem.

2. The Extracellular Matrix

The ECM consists of three components: (1) perineural nets (PN) which surround neural cells and their processes and provide support and regulate plasticity, (2) a complex interstitial matrix between cells, and (3) basement membranes that surround blood vessels made up primarily of laminin, fibronectin, and collagens. ECM components are secreted by resident cells and serve to provide structural cell support, regulate cell-cell connectivity and communication, and sequester growth factors and chemoattractants to regulate cell motility. The composition of the ECM varies from tissue to tissue and is comprised of proteoglycans such as chondroitin sulfate, heparin sulfate, keratin sulfate, and a lattice of interconnected fibrous proteins [8].

The neural extracellular matrix comprises 10–20% by volume of the brain and spinal cord and is structurally and functionally distinct from the ECM in other tissues [9] (**Figure 2**). The most abundant component of the neural ECM is hyaluronan (HA) and its associated glycoproteins. HA is a large hygroscopic glycosaminoglycan composed of alternating D-glucuronic acid and N-acetylglucosamine which is synthesized by hyaluronan synthase anchored to cell membranes [10]. In the developing brain, HA is organized into fiber-like structures along which neural precursors migrate. HA is anchored to astrocytes through its receptor, CD44, a transmembrane glycoprotein that couples the ECM to the actin cytoskeleton [11] and to hyaluronan synthase on neurons. Overexpression of CD44 was shown to increase the length of filopodia of neuroblastoma cells *in vitro* and promote invasion into a HA-rich matrix, demonstrating how overexpression of this single gene can affect the complex sequence of events for an invading cell to detach from its substrate, adhere to and degrade the surrounding matrix, and migrate through it [12].

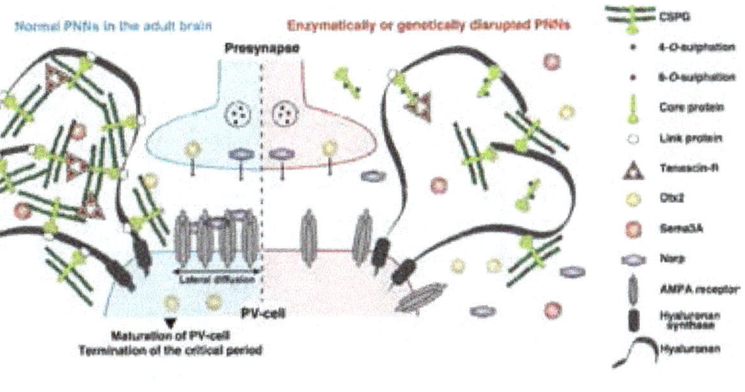

Figure 2. Structure of neural extracellular matrix (ECM). Reproduced with permission from Miyata et al. [14].

HA is associated with a number of proteins that are organized into a scaffold within the ECM. The major group is chondroitin sulfate proteoglycans (CSPGs) whose structure consists of a core protein covalently linked to chondroitin sulfate glycosaminoglycan (CS-GAG) through serine residues [13, 14]. Chondroitin sulfate is a disaccharide chain consisting of glucuronic acid and N-acetylgalactosamine linked via a β-glycosidic bond and is polymerized into chains through the activity of chondroitin synthase and polymerizing factor [15]. Variability within CSPG derives from variation within the core protein of CSPGs as well as the number and

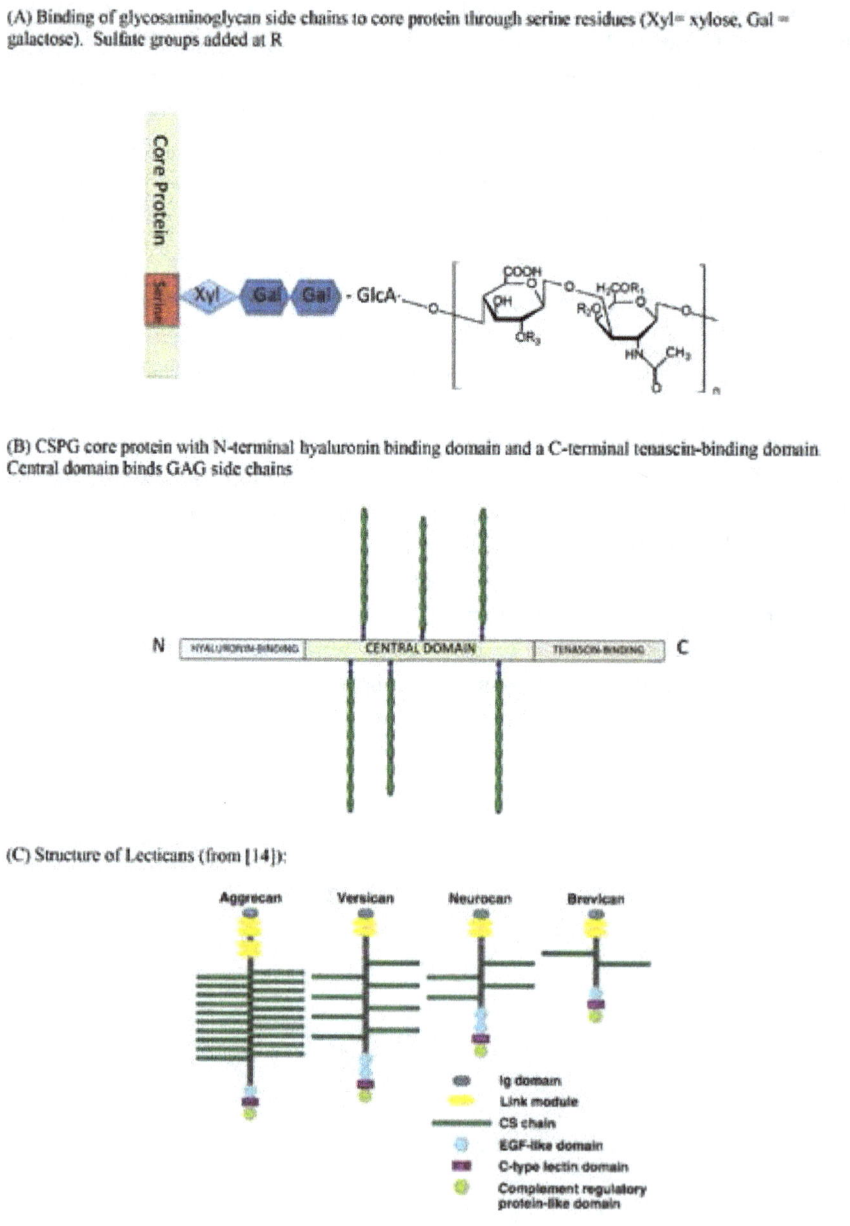

Figure 3. Chondroitin sulfate proteoglycan structure. (A) Binding of glycosaminoglycan side chains to core protein through serine residues (Xyl, xylose; Gal, galactose). Sulfate groups added at R. (B) CSPG core protein with N-terminal hyaluronan binding domain and a C-terminal tenascin-binding domain. Central domain binds GAG side chains. (C) Structure of Lecticans (Reproduced with permission from Miyata et al. [14]).

positions of sulfate groups, which are added via chondroitin sulfotransferases [16, 17]. This variability determines the CSPG binding properties and their function. Link proteins such as Bral-1 and 2, [18], Crtl1 [19], and HAPLN1 [20] stabilize the interaction between HA and CSPG within the PN. Mice lacking Crtl1 have attenuated PN and persistent plasticity in the visual cortex [21].

The classes of CSPG include (1) lecticans such as aggrecan, brevican, neurocan, and versican [22], (2) phosphacan (a tyrosine phosphatase) [23], and (3) small leucine-rich proteoglycans [24]. CSPG can be associated with the plasma membrane through a membrane-spanning domain [25] or a GPI-anchor [26], or can be secreted into the ECM (e.g., lecticans and phosphacan). In the CNS, the chondroitin sulfate side chains act as chemorepellents, and CPSGs are known to inhibit axon projection and cell motility and limit neural plasticity [27]. The lecticans are the principal CSPGs in the CNS, whose core proteins consist of an N-terminal HA-binding domain and a C-terminal domain that binds tenascin-R [28] and tenascin-C [29] (**Figure 3**).

The tenascin family of glycoproteins has four members, tenascin-R, -C, -X, and -W, which are encoded by four genes with a number of splice variants [30] and are believed to modulate cell adhesion and migration. Tenascin-R (formerly called restrictin) is found exclusively in the adult CNS and forms trimers which crosslink CSPGs. Tenascin-R inhibits adhesion of neural cells to fibronectin [31]. Tenascin-C is expressed during embryonic development by migrating neural crest cells, is re-expressed during wound healing and in gliomas, and is thought to be involved with increasing glioma cell proliferation and migration [32]. In tenascin-C knockout mice, CSPGs aggregate and fewer PN form [33]. Tenasacin-X is not found in the nervous system. Tenascin-W is expressed in blood vessels within gliomas and may be involved in angiogenesis [34].

The interstitial ECM forms a highly compressible network of HA and CSPG filaments that is resistant to cell migration by virtue of the inhibitory actions of CPSG, especially their CS components, paucity of anchorage points in the water-rich environment, and the presence of sequestered inhibitory molecules such as slits [35], semaphorins [36], and netrins [37].

In contrast to the hydrated PN that surrounds neurons and the loose interstitial matrix of the brain parenchyma, the ECM around the brain's vasculature and subpial surfaces forms a more rigid basal lamina that contains laminin, fibronectin, and type IV and VI collagens and is similar to the ECM in other tissues [35]. This substrate is more likely to allow adhesion of migrating cells and for this reason, gliomas tend to follow blood vessels and subpial surfaces as they invade into the surrounding tissue [36]. They do not, however, degrade the basal lamina and thus do not generally intravasate and spread hematogenously to distant sites.

3. Migration vs. proliferation

One of the characteristics of malignant gliomas that makes them universally fatal is their ability to infiltrate normal brain parenchyma. This diffuse spread makes surgical cure impossible and makes treatment with radiation and chemotherapy difficult and inefficient. The rapid proliferation of cells in malignant gliomas changes the tumor microenvironment, which becomes hypoxic, acidic, and devoid of glucose and other nutrients. Tumor cells must adapt to these changes to survive and thus change from a proliferative to a migratory phenotype in order to reach a more favorable environment. The mechanism by which tumor cells transition to this migratory state and the factors which trigger this process are therefore important to understand as it serves as an excellent target for therapy. This complex metabolic change, sometimes called the "epithelial-mesenchymal transition," is poorly understood, however, and involves multiple signal transduction pathways with many molecules needed to effect the changes in gene expression needed to bring about this transition.

One of the key molecules involved with sensing stress in a cell's microenvironment is the AMP-activated serine/threonine protein kinase (AMPK) [37]. AMPK is activated by a high AMP/ATP ratio and other conditions of metabolic stress and causes cells to conserve energy, thus regulating their cellular homeostasis in response to environmental cues. AMPK is activated in response to environmental stress through phosphorylation by three known protein kinases: liver kinase-B1 (LKB1) and the two calmodulin-dependent protein kinases, CaMKKα and CaMKKβ, that phosphorylate AMPK in response to high intracellular calcium levels [38]. Once activated, AMPK exerts its effects on cellular metabolism through many downstream molecules, one of which is cyclooxygenase-2 (COX2), whose inhibition by AMPK leads to more aggressive tumor growth and invasion [39]. Overexpression of COX2 has been seen in many types of cancer including colon, breast, and lung [40].

LKB1, a tumor suppressor gene, is constitutively active and is the primary AMPK kinase. Its phosphorylation of AMPK sets off a cascade that results in liberation of intracellular ATP and conservation of energy through regulation of biosynthetic pathways [41]. Mutations in LKB1 are found in Peutz-Jeghers syndrome [42] as well as melanoma [43], lung [44], and pancreatic cancers [45]. LKB1 signaling pathways also are involved in cell migration by virtue of their control of cytoskeletal proteins involved in cell polarization and migration. LKB1 deficiency leads to alterations in cell polarity and impaired migration of neural progenitor cells *in vivo* [46], while LKB1 activation is known to inhibit cell proliferation and can affect cellular polarity, which is essential for cell migration [47]. The latter effect is thought to be mediated, in part, through phosphorylation of MAP/microtubule affinity regulating kinase-3 (MARK-3), which regulates phosphorylation of microtubule-associated proteins [48] and phosphorylation of myosin light chain-2 directly by AMPK [49].

While the activation of AMPK leads to energy conservation in nutrient-poor environments, the mammalian target of rapamycin complex-1 (mTORC1) is a serine/threonine kinase, which promotes cell growth and proliferation. Inhibition of apoptosis [50] by mTOR overactivity has been observed in several types of cancers [51]. The balance between AMPK and mTOR is maintained in part by the tuberous sclerosis complex-2 gene (TSC-2), which is activated by AMPK and which, in turn, inactivates mTOR [50] (**Figure 4**). In addition, AMPK directly phosphorylates Raptor, a scaffold protein in the mTOR1 complex, resulting in direct inactivation of mTORC1 [52]. Mammalian target of rapamycin complex-2 (mTORC2) is considered resistant to rapamycin and is not sensitive to nutrients in the cellular microenvironment. It activates PKC-α and AKT to regulate the structure of the actin cytoskeleton [53].

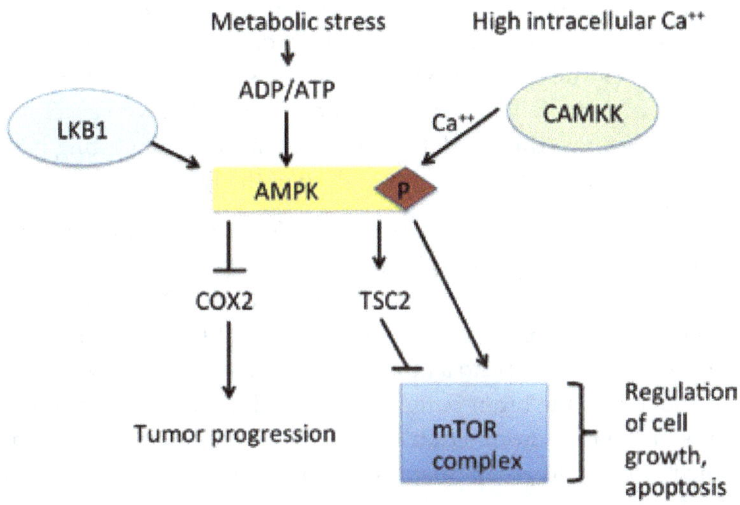

Figure 4. The AMPK/mTOR system. AMPK, AMP-activated serine/threonine protein kinase; CAMKK, Ca(2+)/calmodulin-dependent protein kinase kinase; COX2, cyclooxygenase-2; LKB1, liver kinase B1, mTOR, mammalian target of rapamycin; TSC2, tuberous sclerosis-2.

In addition to intracellular energy levels, hypoxia and acidity are triggers for cells to regulate their gene expression to adapt to a hostile environment. In tumors, hypoxia occurs due to rapid cell proliferation and inadequate blood supply from aberrant blood vessels. It leads to resistance to radiation and chemotherapy and is associated with a more aggressive disease and a poorer outcome. Oxygen homeostasis is mediated by the hypoxia-inducible factor (HIF) family of basic helix-loop-helix transcription factors, which consist of heterodimer of a constitutively expressed beta-subunit and an alpha-subunit which, when translated, is only stabilized under hypoxic conditions and is degraded once hypoxia has been corrected [54–56]. HIF-1 induces expression of dozens of target genes involved in the regulation of angiogenesis, cellular metabolism, and cell migration by binding to hypoxia-responsive elements (HREs) in their promoters. HIF-1α directly activates transcription of vascular endothelial growth factor (VEGF) [57, 58], which is the major regulator of angiogenesis and directs new blood vessel growth into hypoxic areas. HIF-2α knockdown leads to reduced levels of VEGF and poorly vascularized, highly necrotic tumors in neuroblastoma [59]. In order to adapt to hypoxia, cells switch from aerobic to anaerobic metabolism, and this shift is regulated, in part, by HIF-1. Glycolytic enzymes such as pyruvate kinase M2, phosphoglycerate kinase, and aldolase are induced by HIF-1 [60, 61] as are the glucose transporters, GLUT-1 and GLUT-3 [62]. Additionally, pyruvate dehydrogenase kinase-1 is activated, reducing mitochondrial oxygen consumption by preventing pyruvate from entering the citric acid cycle [63]. Finally,

HIF-1 is essential in the epithelial-mesenchymal transition by directly regulating the expression of Twist, which is essential for cancer metastasis [64]. Twist is a basic helix-loop-helix transcription factor whose expression is regulated through a number of signal transduction pathways including Akt, Ras, and Wnt and whose expression correlates with higher tumor grade [65]. It inhibits the E-cadherin-mediated adhesion between cells, which enables tumor cells to adopt a more motile phenotype [66]. Twist also serves as a survival factor by inhibiting p53-induced apoptosis by counteracting the effects of c-MYC in neuroblastoma [67]. HIF-1 regulates expression of a number of adhesion molecules, such as alpha- and beta-integrins and E-cadherin [68–70], matrix metalloproteinase-2 and -9 [71, 72] as well as a number of chemokines and their receptors including c-Met and CXCR4 [73–75], suggesting how hypoxia may play a role in triggering cell migration and digestion of the ECM.

Much remains to be elucidated regarding the molecular cascades through which cells transition to a migratory phenotype. Rapid proliferation creates a toxic microenvironment that, when sensed by the cell, sends a signal through the AMPK-mTORC axis or by HIF-1 and others to effect the changes in transcription needed to bring about the transformation to a migratory phenotype so the cell may escape to a more favorable environment. As they leave the main tumor mass and move into the brain parenchyma which limits and inhibits their migration, glioma cells remodel their environment by secreting degradative enzymes and novel ECM components which attempt to recapitulate the more permissive, primitive structure of the developing brain.

4. ECM Remodeling

4.1. Degradation

In 1946, Fisher [76] proposed that metastatic spread of tumors may be mediated by proteolytic degradation of the ECM. Since then, several classes of intracellular and extracellular proteases, both secreted and membrane-bound, have been identified which play roles in tumorigenesis including cell proliferation, adhesion, migration, angiogenesis, and apoptosis. The coordination between ECM degradation and subsequent cell adhesion to ECM components through integrin and other receptors followed by migration is the basis of glioma infiltration into brain parenchyma.

Lysosomal cathepsins are proteases, which are critical in removing other proteases which are in turn critical in removing unwanted cellular and extracellular components such as collagens, fibronectin, and laminin [77], and secreted cathepsins also mediate the activity of matrix metalloproteases (MMPs) by degrading their inhibitors TIMP-1 and TIMP-2 [78]. Cathepsin B promoter activity and protein levels are higher in high grade gliomas than in low-grade gliomas, and the protein is maximally expressed at the leading infiltrating edge of enlarging tumors [79]. Additionally, upregulation of cathepsins B and D has been shown to correlate with glioma tumor grade and invasiveness [80, 81], while inhibition inhibits glioma cell invasion *in vitro* [82]. Another class of intracellular proteases is the caspases, a family of intracellular cysteine proteases essential for apoptosis that are synthesized as inactive pro-caspases and activated by pro-apoptotic signals [83]. Malignant cells have the ability to escape apoptosis and, in neuroblastoma cells, the caspase 8 gene (CASP8) has been shown to be either deleted or silenced [84]. Loss of CASP8 correlates with increased risk of metastasis in patients with neuroblastoma. Other caspases, including CASP10, 3, 5, 6, and 7, have also found to be mutated in various tumor types [85–89].

Extracellular proteases are secreted by migrating tumor cells in order to degrade ECM components and to release chemoattractant and chemorepellent molecules to direct further tumor cell migration [90]. MMPs are a class of 28 zinc-dependent endopeptidases whose expression by tumor cells has been linked to increased invasion, proliferation, angiogenesis, and morbidity [91]. There are both membrane-bound MMPs and secreted forms which are released as inactive zymogens in response to growth factors such as platelet-derived growth factor (PDGF), epidermal growth factor (EGF), and transforming growth factor beta (TGF-β) [92], as well as in response to cell–cell and cell–ECM interactions and signaling [93]. These inactive proenzymes contain a pro-peptide residue at the N-terminus, which masks the zinc ion within the catalytic region. Proteolytic cleavage of this region exposes the catalytic domain and activates the enzyme [94]. MMP2 and MMP9 are both expressed in human glioma cells *in vitro* [95, 96] and overexpression in gliomas correlates with higher tumor grade and poorer prognosis [97]. The MMPs localize to the leading edges of migrating cells, and many components of the neural ECM have been identified as substrates for MMP2 and MMP9 including the lecticans-aggrecan [98], versican [99], brevican [100], and neurocan, as well as link protein and tenascin [101] and components of the vascular basement membrane such as laminin, fibronectin, and collagen [102]. Although these substrates have been demonstrated *in vitro*, the exact role of MMP *in vivo* is unclear. Versican, for example, appears not be a major MMP substrate *in vivo*, and glioma cells do not degrade the basal laminae of blood vessels to enter the bloodstream. MMP activity is tightly regulated at the level of transcription, activation of the zymogen, and by activity of tissue inhibitors of metalloproteases (TIMS) [103]; the degree of ECM digestion during migration is clearly a complex and carefully regulated process. MMPs are also involved in the "pro-angiogenic switch" that stimulates the production of new blood vessels into the growing tumor mass [104], a process mediated, in large part, by the VEGF signaling pathway [105]. The transmembrane metalloprotease, MT1-MMP, can directly degrade the ECM and also activate pro-MMP2 and upregulate VEGF expression [106], suggesting that this MMP may play a major role in tumor invasiveness and angiogenesis and may serve as a potential target for therapy.

Another class of zinc-dependent metalloproteases is the ADAMS (a disintegrin and metalloproteinase) and the related ADAMTS (a disintegrin and metalloproteinase with thrombospondin motifs). ADAMS are membrane-bound, zinc-dependent metalloproteases that contain a pro-domain which is cleaved to activate the metalloprotease, a disintegrin domain which can bind to integrin receptors, a cysteine-rich domain, an EGF-like domain, and a transmembrane domain at the C terminus [107] (**Figure 5**). ADAMTS are extracellular proteases similar in structure but lack the EGF and transmembrane domains and contain an additional thrombospondin type I motif at the C terminus which may bind them to the ECM [108]. ADAM-8 and ADAM-19 are expressed at high levels in gliomas, and its expression correlates with invasiveness [109]. ADAM-17 activates the EGF/phosphoinositide-3 kinase/serine/threonine kinase signal transduction pathway under hypoxic conditions and leads to increased tumor cell invasion [110]. ADAM-22 normally inhibits astrocyte proliferation in normal brain via interactions between its disintegrin domain and cell surface integrins. It is downregulated in high-grade gliomas leading to elimination of this growth inhibition [111]. ADAMTS-4 and ADAMTS-5 degrade the lectican and small leucine-rich repeat families of proteoglycans, and their expression also correlates with glioma invasiveness [112].

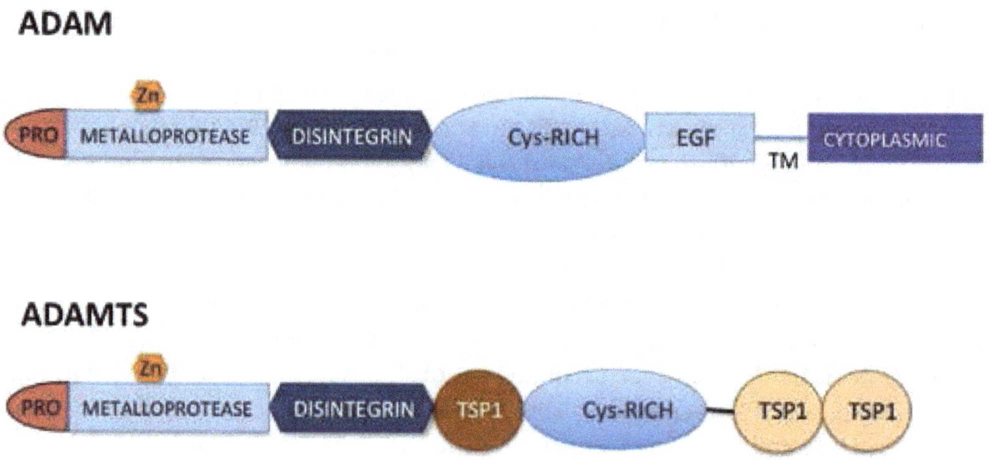

Figure 5. ADAM/ADAMT structure. ADAM and ADAMT members contain a propeptide domain (Pro) followed by the enzymatic metalloprotease domain containing the Zn-binding site followed by the disintegrin- and cystein-rich domains. ADAM members contain an EGF-like domain and ADAMTS contain additional thrombospondin type 1 motifs (TSP1) transmembrane (TM).

Finally, plasmin degrades ECM components and activates several MMPs, and the plasminogen activators, urokinase-type PA (uPA), expressed by glioma cells, and tissue-type PA (tPA) transmembrane (TM) expressed in the endothelium of blood vessels, both play an important role in tumor cell invasion and angiogenesis [113, 114]. There is a higher level of expression of uPA in higher-grade gliomas than in lower-grade gliomas [115] and its binding to its receptor (uPAR) causes it to form a heteromeric complex with integrin receptors, which are also highly expressed on glioma cells. These then initiate signal transduction cascades that result in the upregulation of uPA, MMP, and other molecules that promote cell migration through the ECM [116].

4.2. Synthesis

It is evident that intracellular and extracellular proteases play important roles in the complex process of glioma cell-cell adhesion and attachment and detachment to ECM components during migration. This process is mediated by a well-regulated cascade of signal transduction pathways that also lead to the production of novel ECM components to create a new scaffold on which tumor cells can migrate. As migrating cells degrade the ECM, they further change their microenvironment by secreting novel proteins and liberating peptides on which to migrate and generating chemoattractants and chemorepellents for guidance. In many ways, this new environment is reminiscent of that of the primitive CNS in which cell migration was abundant in setting up the organization of the brain.

One of the earliest events in glioma formation is the loss of the p53 tumor suppressor gene and upregulation of secreted protein acidic and rich in cysteine (SPARC), an ECM-associated glycoprotein that has an anti-adhesive role and leads to cell rounding and detachment from the ECM [117]. This is thought to be accomplished through the activation of P38 mitogen-activated protein kinase (MAPK)-heat shock protein (HSP)-27, Akt, and Shc-Raf-extracellular signal-regulated kinase (ERK) signaling pathways [118]. SPARC is secreted at the leading edge of the invading cells [119] and has been shown to increase invasion *in vitro* [120] and *in vivo* [121]. Additionally, the combination of SPARC overexpression and loss of p53 may play a role in promoting cell survival by escaping immune surveillance [122]. SPARC is highly expressed in gliomas, and increased levels are associated with poorer prognosis [123]. Interestingly, SPARC levels are higher in developing brain, where cell migration is necessary for setting up the architecture of the developing brain, so it is not surprising that invading glioma cells try to recapitulate this more permissive environment.

The Receptor-type protein tyrosine phosphatase mu (PTPμ) is a cell adhesion molecule normally found in neurons and glia but is absent in higher-grade, infiltrative gliomas. It is hypothesized to be involved with cell-cell adhesion and contact inhibition and that its loss allows for cell migration [124]. PTPμ is cleaved in human GBM tumor tissue and cell lines by a number of proteases including ADAMS, calpain, and serine proteases to generate protein fragments with unique biologic functions affecting cell adhesion and migration [125]. In addition to the degradation of the protein component of the ECM, glioma cells secrete hyaluronidases, which break down HA in the ECM, generating soluble HA, which activates MMP and promotes invasion [126]. Increased levels of HA and hyaluronectin are found in peripherally invasive regions of certain tumors [127] creating a more disorganized matrix through which cells can migrate. Receptor-type protein tyrosine phosphatase zeta (RPTP-ζ) is a membrane-bound proteoglycan expressed in developing and adult brains as well as in migrating glioma cells [128]. The soluble factor pleiotrophin is overexpressed in gliomas and, through binding to RPTP-ζ, promotes cytoskeletal changes through modification of beta-catenin, beta-adducin, and Fyn [129]. RPTP-ζ undergoes differential splicing and one splice variant, phosphacan, is a soluble factor lacking the cytoplasmic phosphatase domain. Phosphacan is also highly expressed during embryogenesis and in migrating glioma cells and may regulate glioma migration through interactions with tenascin in the ECM [130] and axonin [131].

Two members of the lectican family, which are normally inhibitory to cell migration, versican and brevican, have unique isoforms that are present at different times of development, and these tumor-specific isoforms have been shown to promote invasion. Versican undergoes differential splicing to generate four different isoforms (V0, V1, V2, and V3), which vary in their GAG-binding domains. The V2 isoform is predominant in the adult CNS and is a potent inhibitor of axonal growth into the ECM [132]. The V0/V1 isoform, however, is found in the primitive developing brain and is upregulated by TGF-β in malignant glioma [133], where it acts as a pro-migratory factor by upregulating membrane type 1 matrix metalloprotease (MT1-MMP) through the activation of microglial Toll-like receptor 2 (TLR2) [134]. Brevican, on the other hand, undergoes differential glycosylation and there are novel glycoforms in gliomas in developing and mature brain [135]. It is overexpressed in malignant gliomas, and its brevican knockdown inhibits proliferation, invasion, and spread of brevican-expressing glioma cells *in vitro* [136]. Not only is brevican overexpressed in gliomas, it is also proteolytically cleaved by metalloproteases of the ADAMTS family including ADAMTS-4 and -5, which are also overexpressed in gliomas [137]. If this posttranslational cleavage is blocked, brevican does not enhance glioma cell invasion *in vitro* or tumor progression *in vivo* [138].

Because the basal lamina of blood vessels presents a more favorable substrate for migration, it is not surprising that migrating glioma cells secrete basal lamina components to travel on. For example, certain laminin isoforms are secreted by glioma cells, and these cells interact with these isoforms and others on the tumor vasculature through the alpha3beta1 integrin during migration [139]. As tumor cells proliferate, the tumor mass becomes denser, and this mechanical stress induces secretion of collagens, their crosslinker LOX, and the angiogenic factor VEGF [140]. Collagens bind to integrins via integrin-binding domains at the cell surface and can thus activate signal transduction pathways that control proliferation, angiogenesis, and migration [141]. Integrins are associated with the actin cytoskeleton through the interaction with talin and with the microtubule network via paxillin and binding to components of the cytoskeleton modulates the affinity of integrins for the ECM [142]. Glioma cells can migrate along fibronectin in the vascular ECM, and both versican and brevican can increase synthesis of fibronectin through an EGFR-dependent mechanism by binding to β-1 integrin and β-3 integrin, respectively [143–145]. These newly synthesized fibronectin fibrils accumulate at the migrating cell surface and serve to reorganize the ECM and promote cell attachment [146, 147].

4.3. Transcriptional control

The regulation of the expression of novel proteins in gliomas is poorly understood but is surely a complex process involving many signal transduction pathways and transcription factors, and some candidates have emerged that may regulate cell migration. The Oct-3/4 transcription factor is involved in regulating self-renewal in stem cells and was recently found to be overexpressed in malignant gliomas. Oct-3/4 expressing-glioblastoma cells exhibited increased migration and invasion *in vitro* and resulted in upregulated FAK and c-Src expression, which mediate integrin signals as well as increased MMP-13 expression [148]. ATF2, another transcription factor expressed in malignant glioma, is thought to be involved in the regulation of cell invasion as its level of expression is correlated with cell invasion *in vitro* [149]. Finally, suppressor of fused (Sufu) is a tumor suppressor which downregulates hedgehog, WNT, and other signaling pathways to prevent tumorigenesis [150, 151]. Overexpression suppresses glioma cell proliferation and invasiveness, angiogenesis, and *in vivo* tumor growth, while knockdown of Sufu promoted these effects, possibly by directly affecting Gli1, a transcription factor in the hedgehog signaling pathway [152].

4.4. Chemotaxis

Once glial cells switch to a migratory phenotype, they degrade the ECM surrounding them, detach from the matrix and extend "invadopodia", actin-rich protrusions with ECM proteolytic activity that bind to and digest ECM components as a result of complex signal transduction pathways linking the extracellular microenvironment to the actin cytoskeleton [153]. Cells respond to soluble molecules in this environment and use these cues to direct migration through various signal transduction pathways. These include growth factors, soluble peptides generated by proteolysis of cell surface adhesion molecules [118], and small chemotactic cytokines.

The EGF family of growth factors is known to stimulate cell proliferation and migration [154], and overexpression of EGF receptor (EGFR) is an important feature distinguishing high-grade from low-grade gliomas [155], and the highest level of expression is found at the invasive border of the expanding tumor [156]. EGFR is amplified in 40% of GBM and of these, half have a mutant form of the receptor (EGFRvIII) lacking the ligand-binding domain leading to constitutive activation [157]. Ligand binding induces dimerization and activation of EGFR, a receptor tyrosine kinase (RTK), whose signaling results in cell proliferation, angiogenesis as well as metastatic spread through the activation of PI3K-AKT-GSK3b-Rac1 and Ras-Raf-MEK-ERK signal transduction pathways [158]. However, the activation of wild-type EGFR promotes invasion independent of angiogenesis, whereas loss of its activity results in angiogenic tumor growth. EGFRvIII might only be involved in stimulating angiogenic tumor growth when wild-type EGFR expression is lost [159,160]. Formylpeptide receptor (FPR) is a G-protein-coupled receptor that has been shown to be expressed in highly malignant gliomas [161]. Necrotic GBM cells release a number of potential ligands for FPR, and the activation of this pathway promotes chemotaxis as well as the production of VEGF [162, 163]. In addition, FPR has been shown to transactivate EGFR leading to increased chemotaxis and proliferation [164].

Scatter factor/hepatocyte growth factor (SF/HGF) as well as its receptor which is encoded by the c-MET proto-oncogene are both are upregulated in malignant gliomas. MET is a transmembrane RTK whose signal transduction cascade leads to increased gliomas motility *in vitro* as well as survival and angiogenesis [165]. Fibroblast growth factor (FGF) may act synergistically with upregulated VEGF and SF/HGF in GBM cells to enhance malignancy [166].

Serine-threonine kinases also play a role in tumorigenesis. TGF-β is an important growth factor whose signaling is involved in invasion as well as proliferation and survival of glioma cells [167]. Its receptor is a serine-threonine kinase that, on ligand binding, oligomerizes and activates a signal transduction cascade that results in the translocation of activated Smads to the nucleus where they interact with other transcription factors to regulate expression of genes involved in cell motility and proliferation [168]. TGF-β signaling upregulates MMP expression and suppresses tissue inhibitors of metalloproteinase (TIMP), thus promoting invasion [169] and inhibition of TGF-β1 or knockdown of its receptor reduces invasiveness *in vitro* [170].

Chemotactic cytokines are a group of small molecules that have been found to regulate the migration of leukocytes in the immune system and have been found to be involved in metastatic behavior of certain cancers [171]. Chemokine receptors are G-protein-coupled transmembrane receptors whose signaling pathways regulate many cellular activities including motility. Chemokines and their receptors are expressed throughout the CNS by neurons and glia and are overexpressed in high-grade gliomas [172]. Stromal-derived factor 1 (SDF-1) also called CXCL2 is a chemotactic cytokine, which, along with its receptor CXCR4, is overexpressed in gliomas as well as within the vascular endothelium along the hypoxic rim of the tumor [173, 174]. SDF-1 has been shown to promote the migration of glioma cells *in vitro* [175] by upregulating the expression of membrane type-2 matrix metalloproteinase (MT2-MMP) [176]. CXCL1 is another small chemokine known to be involved in the metastatic spread in melanoma [177] and has been shown to be highly expressed in glioma samples and promotes migration *in vitro* by upregulating MMP-2 and β1-integrin [178]. TGF-β signaling promotes invasion by reducing expression of neurotactin, a chemokine also known as CX3CL1 whose pro-adhesive properties must be overcome to allow cells to detach and migrate. The treatment of glioma cells with recombinant TGF-β1 reduced CX3CL1, expression and facilitated glioma cell detachment and dispersion [179].

Both positive and negative signals exist within the microenvironment of glioma cells, and hypoxia is an important chemorepellent as described previously which induces cell migration away from the tumor mass. HIF-1α is stabilized at the leading tumor edge and mediates cell invasion and angiogenesis through integrin and RTK signaling pathways [180]. Slit glycoproteins are secreted into the ECM and normally serve as chemorepulsive factors but whose expression is diminished in invasive gliomas through promoter methylation. They normally bind to members of the Roundabout (Robo) family of transmembrane receptors and lead to depolymerization of the actin cytoskeleton within the invadopodia to promote cell adhesion [181, 182]. This may be accomplished through the inactivation of Cdc42, a Rho GTPase known to be involved in cell motility [183].

Semaphorins and their receptors (plexins and neuropilins) have been found to be involved in cell migration and metastasis as well as proliferation and angiogenesis in several types of cancers [184–188], and different members of the family have different functions depending on the type of tumor involved. For example, Sema 3A inhibits migration in GBM and has anti-angiogenic properties in meningioma [189, 190]. Secreted semaphorins contain an N-terminal sema domain followed by variable numbers of PSI (plexins, semaphorins, and integrins) and immunoglobulin-like domains in their extracellular regions [191]. Sema 3A binds to the Neuropilin-1 receptor that recruits the PlexinA1 receptor to transduce a chemorepulsive signal. Sema3A also binds Neuropilin-2 but at a lower affinity than Neuropilin-1, and the binding of Neuropilin-2 acts to modulate cell signaling and converts the repulsive signal into an attractive one. Blocking Neuropilin-1 or Plexin A1 switches the Sema3A response from repulsion to attraction, while blockade of Neuropilin-2 suppresses Sema3A's typical chemorepulsive effect [192]. Similarly, Sema 4D which binds to PlexinB1 and acts through Rho [193], and Sema5A which binds to PlexinB3 and acts through Rac1, both act as chemorepellents by ultimately affecting the actin cytoskeleton and altering cell morphology [194].

Finally, Netrins are secreted laminin-associated chemotactic molecules that regulate embryonic axon migration [195] which have also been shown to be involved in glioma cell migration, mediated by binding to their receptors, deleted in colorectal cancer (DCC), neogenin, and uncoordinated-5 (UNC5) [196–198]. Netrins have been shown to localize to cell surfaces and interact with laminins in the basement membrane of blood vessels. Netrin-1 binding to DCC receptors on migrating glia promotes the formation of focal adhesions, limiting migration. GBMs have been shown to downregulate Netrins, thus releasing the inhibition and promoting loss of cell-cell interaction, promoting migration along basement membranes [199]. Though Netrin-1 binding to the DCC receptor tends to promote adhesion, limiting migration, UNC5 binding transforms this to repulsion [200]. This switch from attachment to motility is reminiscent of that described earlier with the semaphorins.

5. Future Directions

Current therapy for malignant gliomas is aimed at reducing tumor burden and targeting dividing cells with cytotoxic chemotherapy, anti-angiogenic agents, or tumor-treating fields. New agents targeting new pathways are desperately needed as survival still remains extremely poor and glioma cells become resistant over time to current therapies. Delivering therapy to normal brain parenchyma containing infiltrating tumor cells is also difficult as the blood-brain barrier remains largely intact, though several strategies have been attempted to overcome this [201]. Limiting the invasiveness of these aggressive tumors is desirable; however, the molecular pathways involved in this complex process remain incompletely understood and new targets and therapies are lacking. Additionally, because tumor cells seem to adopt either a proliferative or migratory phenotype, preventing migration may impose a selective advantage for cells to proliferate rather than migrate leading to more rapid local recurrences. There is also no way to visualize invading cells until they stop migrating and proliferate to create a radiographically evident tumor mass. Two-dimensional *in vitro* assays have been used to study this process using glass or plastic substrates and more recently, assays using hydrogels or nanofiber scaffolds have been developed to better simulate the three-dimensional microenvironment encountered by migrating tumor cells [202–204].

Identifying molecular targets has been a priority in developing new therapies for GBM, and the complex process of cell migration offers many potential targets including ECM components, proteases, and members of signal transduction pathways. The neural ECM has many unique components that are potential targets for therapy. Because tenascin is upregulated in malignant gliomas and may be a stem cell marker [205], it is an attractive target and phase I trials are underway exploring the use of radiolabeled monoclonal antibodies to tenascin-C or tenascin-R to deliver a radiation boost to the resection cavity. Since many signal transduction pathways involved in glioma invasion often involve RTKs, and since various RTKs are mutated or overexpressed in GBM, RTK inhibitors are an obvious choice of targeted therapy. The results, however, have been disappointing, and no clear RTK inhibitor or combination has demonstrated a significant survival benefit [206]. Similarly, several inhibitors of MMPs have been investigated and, though some have shown efficacy *in vitro*, no clear clinical benefit has yet been demonstrated [207–209]. Cilengitide is an arginine-glycine-aspartic acid containing peptide that targets integrins and, though it was promising in preclinical studies, it failed to show improvement in progression-free survival or overall survival in both the CENTRIC [210] and CORE [211] trials investigating the addition of cilengitide to standard therapy in patients with newly diagnosed GBM with or without MGMT promoter methylation.

Many molecules involved in regulating cell migration in malignant gliomas are also involved in angiogenesis, cell proliferation, and avoidance of apoptosis; so agents targeting these molecules would be expected to have multiple antitumor effects. However, results have been mixed and, though *in vitro* data are encouraging for many agents, none has proven successful in showing clinical improvement in survival. There is apparently much redundancy in these signaling pathways, requiring a more complete understanding of these molecular events as well as more accurate modeling with which to study the complex processes involved in tumor spread. The earliest events leading to a migratory phenotype would be ideal candidates for therapy, though inhibiting migration could select for a proliferating phenotype leading to faster local recurrence. Hopefully, as we achieve a better understanding of the genetics and molecular alterations leading to glioma invasion, new therapies will arise to limit this aggressive, deadly disease.

Author details

Scott G. Turner*, Maleeha Ahmad and Steven A. Toms

*Address all correspondence to: sgturner@geisinger.edu

Departments of Neurology and Neurosurgery, Geisinger Medical Center, Danville, PA, USA

References

[1] Dolecek TA, Propp JM, Stroup NE, Kruchko C. CBTRUS statistical report: primary brain and central nervous system tumors diagnosed in the United States in 2005–2009. Neuro Oncol. 2012; 14 Suppl 5:v1-49.

[2] Stupp R, Mason WP, van den Bent MJ, et al. Radiotherapy plus Concomitant and Adjuvant Temozolomide for Glioblastoma. N Engl J Med. 2005; 352:987–996.

[3] Vredenburgh JJ, Desjardins A, Herndon JE, Marcello J, Reardon DA, Quinn JA, Rich JN, Sathornsumetee S, Gururangan S, Sampson J, Wagner M, Bailey L, Bigner DD, Friedman AH, Friedman HS. Bevacizumab plus irinotecan in recurrent glioblastoma multiforme. J Clin Oncol. 2007; 25(30):4722–9.

[4] Stupp R, Taillibert S, Kanner AA, et al. Maintenance Therapy With Tumor-Treating Fields Plus Temozolomide vs Temozolomide Alone for Glioblastoma: A Randomized Clinical Trial. JAMA. 2015; 314(23):2535–2543.

[5] Hou LC, Veeravagu A, Hsu AR, Tse VCK. Recurrent Glioblastoma Multiforme: A Review of Natural History and Management Options. Neurosurg Focus. 2006; 20(4):E5.

[6] Giese A, Westphal M. Glioma invasion in the central nervous system. Neurosurgery. 1996;39(2):235–250.

[7] Wolf K, Mazo I, Leung H, Engelke K , von Andrian UH., Deryugina EI, Strongin AY, Bröcker EB, Friedl P. Compensation mechanism in tumor cell migration/mesenchymal–amoeboid transition after blocking of pericellular proteolysis. JCB. 2003; 160(2): 267–277.

[8] Lau LW, Cua R, Keough MB, Haylock-Jacobs S, Yong VW. Pathophysiology of the Brian Extracellular Matrix: a new target of remyelination. Natire Reviews. 2013; 14:722–729.

[9] Bignami A, Hosley M, Dahl D. Hyaluronic Acid and Hyaluronic Acid-Binding Proteins in Brain Extracellular Matrix. Anat. Embryol. 1993; 188:419–433.

[10] Delpech B, Maingonnat C, Girard N, Chauzy C, Maunoury R, Olivier A, Tayot J, Creissard P. Hyaluronan and hyaluronectin in the extracellular matrix of human brain tumour stroma. Eur J Cancer. 1993; 29A(7):1012–7.

[11] Misra S, Heldin P, Hascall VC, Karamanos NK, Skandalis SS, Markwald RR, Ghatak S. Hyaluronan-CD44 interactions as potential targets for cancer therapy. FEBS J. 2011; 278(9):1429–43.

[12] Pusch A, Boeckenhoff A, Glaser T, Kaminski T, Kirfel G, Hans M, Steinfarz B, Swandulla D, Kubitscheck U, Gieselmann V, Brüstle O, Kappler J. CD44 and hyaluronan promote invasive growth of B35 neuroblastoma cells into the brain. Biochimica et Biophysica Acta (BBA) - Molecular Cell Research. 2010; 1803(2): 261–274.

[13] Mikami T, Kitagawa H. Biosynthesis and function of chondroitin sulfate. Biochim. Biophys Acta. 2013; 1830: 4719–4733.

[14] Sugahara K, Mikami T. Chondroitin/der- matan sulfate in the central nervous system. Curr. Opin. Struct. Biol. 2007; 17:536–545.

[15] Mikami T, Kitagawa H. Biosynthesis and function of chondroitin sulfate. Biochim. Biophys. Acta. 2013; 1830:4719–4733.

[16] Ohtake S, Ito Y, Fukuta M, Habuchi O. Human N-acetylgalactosamine 4-sulfate 6-O-sulfotrans- ferase cDNA is related to human B cell recombination activating gene-associated gene. J. Biol. Chem. 2001; 276: 43894–43900.

[17] Kobayashi M, Sugumaran G, Liu J, Shworak NW, Silbert JE, Rosenberg RD. Molecular cloning and characterization of a human uronyl 2-sulfo- transferase that sulfates iduronyl and glucuronyl residues in dermatan/chondroitin sulfate. J. Biol. Chem. 1999; 274:10474–10480.

[18] Oohashi T, Hirakawa S, Bekku Y, Rauch U, Zimmermann DR, Su WD, Ohtsuka A, Murakami T, Ninomiya Y. Bral1, a brain-specific link protein, colocalizing with the

versican V2 isoform at the nodes of Ranvier in developing and adult mouse central nervous systems. Mol. Cell. Neurosci. 2002; 19:43–57.

[19] Carulli D, Pizzorusso T, Kwok JCF, Putignano E, Poli A, Forostyak S, Andrews MR, Deepa SS, Glant TT, Fawcett JW. Animals lacking link protein have attenuated perineuronal nets and persistent plasticity. Brain 2010; 133:2331–2347.

[20] Sim H, Hu B, Viapiano MS. Reduced Expression of the Hyaluronan and Proteoglycan Link Proteins in Malignant Gliomas. J Biol Chem. 2009; 284(39):26547–26556.

[21] Carulli D, Pizzorusso T, Kwok JCF, Putignano E, Poli A, Forostyak S, Andrews MR, Deepa SS, Glant TT, Fawcett JW. Animals lacking link protein have attenuated perineuronal nets and persistent plasticity. Brain 2010; 133:2331–2347.

[22] Yamaguchi Y. Lecticans: organizers of the brain extracellular matrix. Cell. Mol. Life Sci. 2000; 57:276–289.

[23] Levy JB, Canoll PD, Silvennoinen O, Barnea G, Morse B, Honegger AM, Huang JT, Cannizzaro LA, Park SH, Druck T. The cloning of a receptor-type protein tyrosine phosphatase expressed in the central nervous system. J Biol Chem. 1993; 268(14):10573–10581.

[24] Dellett M, Hu W, Papadaki V, Ohnuma S. Small leucine rich proteoglycan family regulates multiple signalling pathways in neural development and maintenance. Dev Growth Differ. 2012; 54(3):327–340.

[25] Kinugasa Y, Ishiguro H, Tokita Y, Oohira A, Ohmoto H, Higashiyama S. Neuroglycan C, a novel member of the neuregulin family. Biochem Biophys Res Commun. 2004; 321(4):1045–9.

[26] Seidenbecher CI, Smalla KH, Fischer N, Gundelfinger ED, Kreutz MR. Brevican isoforms associate with neural membranes. Journal of Neurochemistry. 2002; 83(3):738–746.

[27] Niederost BP, Zimmermann DR, Schwab ME, Bandtlow CE. Bovine CNS myelin contains neurite growth-inhibitory activity associated with chondroitin sulfate proteoglycans. J. Neurosci. 1999; 19:8979–8989.

[28] Yamaguchi Y. Lecticans: organizers of the brain extracellular matrix. Cell. Mol. Life Sci. 2000; 57:276–289.

[29] Day JM, Olin AI, Murdoch AD, Canfield A, Sasaki T, Timpl R, Hardingham TE, Aspberg A. Alternative splicing in the aggrecan G3 domain influences binding interactions with Tenascin-C and other extracellular matrix proteins. J. Biol. Chem. 2004; 279:12511–12518.

[30] Hsia H, Schwarzbauer J. Meet the tenascins: multifunctional and mysterious. J Biol Chem. 2005; 280 (29): 26641–26644.

[31] Pesheva P, Probstmeier R, Skubitz AP, McCarthy JB, Furcht LT, Schachner M. Tenascin-R (J1 160/180) inhibits fibronectin-mediated cell adhesion–functional relatedness to tenascin-C. J Cell Sci. 1994; 107: 2323–2333.

[32] Herold-Mende C, Mueller MM, Bonsanto MM, Schmitt HP, Kunze S, Steiner HH. Clinical impact and functional aspects of tenascin-C expression during glioma progression. Int. J. Cancer. March 2002; 98(3): 362–369.

[33] Garcion E, Faissner A, Ffrench-Constant C. Knockout mice reveal a contribution of the extracellular matrix molecule tenascin-C to neural precursor proliferation and migration. Development. 2001; 128(13):2485–2496.

[34] Martina E, Degen M, Rüegg C, Merlo A, Lino MM, Chiquet-Ehrismann R, Brellier F. Tenascin-W is a specific marker of glioma-associated blood vessels and stimulates angiogenesis in vitro. FASEB J. 2010; 24(3):778–787.

[35] Gladson CL. The extracellular matrix of gliomas: modulation of cell function. J Neuropathol Exp Neurol. 1999; 58(10):1029–1040.

[36] Cuddapah VA, Robel S, Watkins S, Sontheimer HA. Neurocentric perspective on glioma invasion. Nature Reviews. 2014; 15: 455–465.

[37] Hue L, Rider MH. The AMP-activated protein kinase: more than an energy sensor. Essays Biochem. 2007; 43:121–137.

[38] Woods A, Dickerson K, Heath R, Hong SP, Momcilovic M, Johnstone SR, Carlson M, Carling D. Ca2+/calmodulin-dependent protein kinase kinase-beta acts upstream of AMP-activated protein kinase in mammalian cells. Cell Metab. 2005; 2(1):21–33.

[39] Lee YK, Park SY, Kim YM, Lee WS, Park OJ. AMP kinase/cyclooxygenase-2 pathway regulates proliferation and apoptosis of cancer cells treated with quercetin. Experimental & Molecular Medicine. 2009; 41:201–207.

[40] Sobolewski C, Cerella C, Dicato M, Ghibelli L, Diederich M. The Role of Cyclooxygenase-2 in Cell Proliferation and Cell Death in Human Malignancies. International Journal of Cell Biology. 2009; 2010:1–21.

[41] Woods A, Johnstone SR, Dickerson K, Leiper FC, Fryer LG, Neumann D, Schlattner U, Wallimann T, Carlson M, Carling D. LKB1 is the upstream kinase in the AMP-activated protein kinase cascade. Curr Biol. 2003; 13(22):2004–2008.

[42] Hemminki A, Avizienyte E, Roth S, Loukola A, Aaltonen LA, Jarvinen H, de la Chapelle A. A serine/ threonine kinase gene defective in Peutz–Jeghers syndrome. Duodecim 1998; 114:667–668.

[43] Guldberg P, thor Straten P, Ahrenkiel V, Seremet T, Kirkin AF, Zeuthen J. Somatic mutation of the Peutz–Jeghers syndrome gene, LKB1/STK11, in malignant melanoma. Oncogene 1999; 18:1777–1780.

[44] Hearle N, Schumacher V, Menko FH, Olschwang S, Boardman LA, Gille JJ, Keller JJ, Westerman AM, Scott RJ, Lim W, et al. Frequency and spectrum of cancers in the Peutz–Jeghers syndrome. Clin Cancer Res. 2006; 12:3209–3215.

[45] Su GH, Hruban RH, Bansal RK, Bova GS, Tang DJ, Shekher MC, Westerman AM, Entius MM, Goggins M, Yeo CJ, Kern SE. Germline and somatic mutations of the STK11/LKB1 Peutz–Jeghers gene in pancreatic and biliary cancers. Am J Pathol 1999; 154:1835–1840.

[46] Asada N, Sanada K, Fukada Y. LKB1 regulates neuronal migration and neuronal differentiation in the developing neocortex through centrosomal positioning. J Neurosci. 2007; 27(43):11769–11775.

[47] Alessi DR, Sakamoto K, Bayascas JR. LKB1-dependent signaling pathways. Annu Rev Biochem. 2006; 75:137–163.

[48] Sapir T, Sapoznik S, Levy T, Finkelshtein D, Shmueli A, Timm T, Mandelkow EM, Reiner O. Accurate balance of the polarity kinase MARK2/Par-1 is required for proper cortical neuronal migration. J Neurosci. 2008; 28(22):5710–5720.

[49] Lee JH, Koh H, Kim M, Kim Y, Lee SY, Karess RE, Lee SH, Shong M, Kim JM, Kim J, Chung J. Energy-dependent regulation of cell structure by AMP-activated protein kinase. Nature. 2007; 447(7147):1017–1020.

[50] Shaw RJ. LKB1 and AMPK control of mTOR signalling and growth Acta Physiol (Oxf). 2009; 196(1): 65–80.

[51] Hardt M, Chantaravisoot N, Tamanoi F. Activating mutations of TOR (target of rapamycin). Genes Cells. 2011; 16(2):141–151.

[52] Gwinn DM, Shackelford DB, Egan DF, Mihaylova MM, Mery A, Vasquez DS, Turk BE, Shaw RJ. AMPK phosphorylation of raptor mediates a metabolic checkpoint. Mol Cell. 2008; 30(2):214–26.

[53] Jacinto E, Loewith R, Schmidt A, Lin S, Rüegg MA, Hall A, Hall MN. Mammalian TOR complex 2 controls the actin cytoskeleton and is rapamycin insensitive. Nat Cell Biol. 2004 ;6(11):1122–1128.

[54] Wang GL, Jiang B, Rue EA, Semenza GL. Hypoxia-inducible factor 1 is a basic-helix-loop-helix-PAS heterodimer regulated by cel- lular O2 tension. Proc Natl Acad Sci USA. 1995; 92:5510–5514.

[55] Yang J, Zhang L, Erbel PJ, Gardner KH, Ding K, Garcia JA, Bruick RK. Functions of the Per/ARNT/Sim domains of the hypoxia-in- ducible factor. J Biol Chem. 2005; 280:36047–36054 .

[56] Chapman-Smith A, Lutwyche JK, Whitelaw ML. Contribution of the Per/Arnt/Sim (PAS) domains to DNA binding by the basic helix-loop-helix PAS transcriptional regulators. J Biol Chem. 2004; 279:5353- 5362.

[57] Dery MA, Michaud MD, Richard DE. Hypoxia-inducible factor 1: regulation by hypoxic and non-hypoxic activators. Int J Biochem Cell Bio. 2004; 37:535–540.

[58] Vaupel P. The Role of Hypoxia-Induced Factors in Tumor Progression. Oncologist. 2004; 9:10–17.

[59] Pietras A, Johnsson AS, Påhlman S. The HIF-2α-driven pseudo-hypoxic phenotype in tumor aggressiveness, differentiation, and vascularization. Curr Top Microbiol Immunol. 2010; 345:1–20.

[60] Luo W, Hu H, Chang R, Zhong J, Knabel M, O'Meally R, Cole RN, Pandey A, Semenza GL. Pyruvate kinase M2 is a PHD3-stimulated coactivator for hypoxia-inducible factor 1. Cell. 2011; 145(5):732–744.

[61] Kress S, Stein A, Maurer P, Weber B, Reichert J, Buchmann A, Huppert P, Schwarz M. Expression of hypoxia-inducible genes in tumor cells. J Cancer Res Clin Oncol. 1998; 124(6):315–320.

[62] Mobasheri A, Richardson S, Mobasheri R, Shakibaei M, Hoyland JA. Hypoxia inducible factor-1 and facilitative glucose transporters GLUT1 and GLUT3: putative molecular components of the oxygen and glucose sensing apparatus in articular chondrocytes. Histol Histopathol. 2005; 20(4):1327–1338.

[63] Papandreou I, Cairns RA, Fontana L, Lim AL, Denko NC. HIF-1 mediates adaptation to hypoxia by actively downregulating mito- chondrial oxygen consumption. Cell Metab. 2006; 3:150–151.

[64] Yang MH, Wu MZ, Chiou SH, Chen PM, Chang SY, Liu CJ, Teng SC, Wu KJ. Direct regulation of TWIST by HIF-1alpha promotes metastasis. Nat Cell Biol. 2008; 10(3):295–305.

[65] Je EC, Lca BS, Ga GA. The Role of Transcription Factor TWIST in Cancer Cells. Je et al. J Genet Syndr Gene Ther 2013; 4:1.

[66] Martin A, Cano A. Tumorigenesis: Twist1 links EMT to self-renewal. Nat Cell Biol. 2010; 12(10):924–925.

[67] Valsesia-Wittmann S, Magdeleine M, Dupasquier S, Garin E, Jallas AC, Combaret V, Krause A, Leissner P, Puisieux A. Oncogenic cooperation between H-Twist and N-Myc overrides failsafe programs in cancer cells. Cancer Cell. 2004; 6(6):625–630.

[68] Lee SH, Lee YJ, Han HJ. Role of hypoxia- induced fibronectin-integrin beta1 expression in embryonic stem cell proliferation and migra- tion: Involvement of PI3K/Akt and FAK. J Cell Physiol 2011; 226:484–493.

[69] Ryu MH, Park HM, Chung J, Lee CH and Park HR. Hypoxia-inducible factor-1alpha mediates oral squamous cell carcinoma invasion via upregulation of alpha5 integrin and fibronectin. Biochem Biophys Res Commun 2010; 393:11–15.

[70] Krishnamachary B, Zagzag D, Nagasawa H, Rainey K, Okuyama H, Baek JH, Semenza GL. Hypoxia-inducible factor-1-dependent re- pression of E-cadherin in von Hippel-

Lindau tumor suppressor-null renal cell carcinoma mediated by TCF3, ZFHX1A, and ZFHX1B. Can- cer Res. 2006; 66:2725–2731.

[71] LuoY, He DL, Ning L, Shen SL, Li L, Li X, Zhau HE, Chung LW. Over-expression of hypoxia- inducible factor-1alpha increases the invasive potency of LNCaP cells in vitro. BJU Int. 2006; 98:1315–1319.

[72] O'Toole EA, van Koningsveld R, Chen M, Woodley DT. Hypoxia induces epidermal kerati- nocyte matrix metalloproteinase-9 secretion via the protein kinase C pathway. J Cell Physiol. 2008; 214:47–55.

[73] Pennacchietti S, Michieli P, Galluzzo M, Mazzone M, Giordano S, Comoglio PM. Hypoxia promotes invasive growth by transcriptional activation of the met protooncogene. Cancer Cell. 2003; 3:347–361.

[74] Ishikawa T, Nakashiro K, Klosek SK, Goda H, Hara S, Uchida D, Hamakawa H. Hypoxia enhances CXCR4 expression by activating HIF-1 in oral squamous cell carcinoma. Oncol Rep. 2009; 21:707–712.

[75] Li Y, Qiu X, Zhang S, Zhang Q, Wang E. Hypoxia induced CCR7 expression via HIF-1alpha and HIF-2alpha correlates with migration and invasion in lung cancer cells. Cancer Biol Ther. 2009; 8:322–330.

[76] Fisher, A. Mechanism of the proteolytic activity of malignant tissue cells. Nature 1946;157:442.

[77] Buck MR, Karustis DG, Day NA, Honn KV, and Sloane BF. Degradation of extracellular-matrix proteins by human cathepsin B from normal and tumour tissues. Biochem J. 1992; 282(Pt 1):273–278.

[78] Kostoulas G, Lang A, Nagase H, Baici A. Stimulation of angiogenesis through cathepsin B inactivation of the tissue inhibitors of matrix metalloproteinases. FEBS Lett. 1999; 455:286–290.

[79] Mikkelsen T, et al. Immunolocalization of cathepsin B in human glioma: implications for tumor invasion and angiogenesis. J. Neurosurg. 1995; 83:285–290.

[80] Demchik LL, Sameni M, Nelson K, Mikkelsen T, Sloane BF. Cathepsin B and glioma invasion. Int J Dev Neurosci. 1999;17(5–6):483–94.

[81] Rempel SA, Rosenblum ML, Mikkelsen T, Yan PS, Ellis KD, Golembieski WA, Sameni M, Rozhin J, Ziegler G, Sloane BF. Cathepsin B expression and localization in glioma progression and invasion. Cancer Res. 1994; 54:6027–6031.

[82] Liu Y, Zhou Y, Zhu K. Inhibition of glioma cell lysosome exocytosis inhibits glioma invasion. PLoS One. 2012;7(9):e45910.

[83] López-Otín C, Lynn M. Matrisian Emerging roles of proteases in tumour suppression. Nature Reviews Cancer. 2007; 7:800–808.

[84] Teitz T, Wei T, Valentine MB, Vanin EF, Grenet J, Valentine VA, Behm FG, Look AT, Lahti JM, Kidd VJ. Caspase 8 is deleted or silenced preferentially in childhood neuroblastomas with amplification of MYCN. Nature Med. 2000; 6:529–535.

[85] Harada K, Toyooka S, et al. Deregulation of caspase 8 and 10 expression in pediatric tumors and cell lines. Cancer Res. 2002; 62:5897–5901.

[86] Soung YH, Lee JW, Kim SY, Park WS, Nam SW, Lee JY, Yoo NJ, Lee SH. Somatic mutations of CASP3 gene in human cancers. Hum. Genet. 2004; 115:112–115.

[87] Offman J, Gascolgne K, et al. Repeated sequences in CASPASE-5 and FANCD2 but not NF1 are targets for mutation in microsatellite-unstable acute leukemia/ myelodysplastic syndrome. Mol. Cancer Res. 2005; 3: 251–260.

[88] Lee JW, Kim MR, Soung YH, Nam SW, Kim SH, Lee JY, Yoo NJ, Lee SH. Mutational analysis of the CASP6 gene in colorectal and gastric carcinomas. APMIS. 2006; 114:646–650.

[89] Soung YH, Lee JW, et al. Inactivating mutations of CASPASE-7 gene in human cancers. Oncogene. 2003; 22:8048–8052.

[90] McCawley LJ , and Matrisian LM. Matrix metalloproteinases: they're not just for matrix anymore! Curr. Opin. Cell Biol. 2001; 13:534–540.

[91] Hagemann C, Anacker J, Ernestus R, Vince GH. A complete compilation of matrix metalloproteinase expression in human malignant gliomas. World J Clin Oncol. 2012; 3(5):67–79.

[92] Borden P, Heller RA. Transcriptional control of matrix me- talloproteinases and the tissue inhibitors of matrix metallo- proteinases. Crit Rev Eukaryot Gene Expr. 1997; 7:159–178.

[93] Nagase H, Woessner JF. Matrix metalloproteinases. J Biol Chem 1999; 274:21491–21494.

[94] Van Wart HE, Birkedal-Hansen H. The cysteine switch: a principle of regulation of metalloproteinase activity with potential applicability to the entire matrix metalloproteinase gene family. Proc Natl Acad Sci USA 1990; 87:5578–5582.

[95] Rao JS, Go Y, Kyritisis AP, Uhm J, Venkaiah B, Mohanam S, Gokaslan ZL, Rao JS. Elevated levels of Mr 92,000 type IV collagenase in human brain tumors. Cancer Res. 1993; 53:2208–2211.

[96] Forsyth PA, Wong H, Laing TD, Rewcastle NB, Morris DG, Muzik H, Leco KJ, Johnston RN, Brasher PM, Sutherland G, Edwards DR. Gelatinase-A (MMP-2), gelatinase-B (MMP-9) and membrane type matrix metalloproteinase-1 (MT1-MMP) are involved in different aspects of the pathophysiology of malignant gliomas. Br. J. Cancer 1999; 79:1828–1835.

[97] Rao JS. Molecular mechanisms of glioma invasiveness: the role of proteases. Nat Rev Cancer. 2003; 3(7):489–501.

[98] Struglics A, Hansson M. MMP proteolysis of the human extracellular matrix protein aggrecan is mainly a process of normal turnover. Biochem J. 2012; 446(2):213–223.

[99] Barascuk NF, Genovese F, et al. A MMP derived versican neo-epitope is elevated in plasma from patients with atherosclerotic heart disease. Int. J. Clin. Exp. Med (2013); 6:174–184.

[100] Nakamura H, Fujii Y, et al. Brevican Is Degraded by Matrix Metalloproteinases and Aggrecanase-1 (ADAMTS4) at Different Sites. The Journal of Biological Chemistry. 2000; 275(49):38885–38890.

[101] Hagemann C, Anacker J, Ernestus RI, Vince GH. A complete compilation of matrix metalloproteinase expression in human malignant gliomas. World J Clin Oncol. 2012; 3(5):67–79.

[102] Wang M, Wang T, Liu S, Yoshida D, Teramoto A.The expression of matrix metalloproteinase-2 and -9 in human gliomas of different pathological grades. Brain Tumor Pathol. 2003;20(2):65–72.

[103] Bergers G, Brekken R, McMahon G, Vu TH, Itoh T, Tamaki K, Tanzawa K, Thorpe P, Itohara S, Werb Z, Hanahan D. Matrix metalloproteinase-9 triggers the angiogenic switch during carcinogenesis. Nat Cell Biol. 2000; 2(10):737–744.

[104] Plate KH, Breier G, Weich HA, Risau W. Vascular endothelial growth factor is a potential tumour angiogenesis factor in human gliomas in vivo. Nature 1992; 359:845–848.

[105] Sounni NE, Devy L, Hajitou A, Frankenne F, Munaut C, Gilles C, Deroanne C, Thompson EW, Foidart JM, Noel A. MT1-MMP expression promotes tumor growth and angiogenesis through an up-regulation of vascular endothelial growth factor expression. FASEB J. 2002; 16(6):555–64.

[106] Viapiano MS, Hockfield S, Matthews RT. BEHAB/brevican requires ADAMTS-mediated proteolytic cleavage to promote glioma invasion. J Neurooncol. 2008; 88(3): 261–272.

[107] Wolfsberg TG, Straight PD, Gerena RL, et al. ADAM, a widely distributed and developmentally regulated gene family encoding membrane proteins with a disintegrin and metalloprotease domain. Dev. Biol. 1995; 169(1):378–383.

[108] Porter S, Clark IM, Kevorkian L, Edwards DR. The ADAMTS metalloproteinases. Biochemical Journal 2005; 386 (1): 15–27.

[109] Wildeboer D, Naus S, Amy Sang QX, Bartsch JW, Pagenstecher A. Metalloproteinase disintegrins ADAM8 and ADAM19 are highly regulated in human primary brain tumors and their expression levels and activities are associated with invasiveness. J Neuropathol Exp Neurol. 2006; 65(5):516–527.

[110] Zheng X, Jiang F, Katakowski M, Kalkanis SN, Hong X, Zhang X, Zhang ZG, Yang H, Chopp M. Inhibition of ADAM17 reduces hypoxia-induced brain tumor cell invasiveness. Cancer Sci. 2007; 98(5):674–684.

[111] D'Abaco GM, Ng K, Paradiso L, Godde NJ, Kaye A, Novak U. ADAM22, expressed in normal brain but not in high-grade gliomas, inhibits cellular proliferation via the disintegrin domain. Neurosurgery. 2006; 58(1):179–186.

[112] Stanton H, Melrose J, Little CB, Fosang AF. Proteoglycan degradation by the ADAMTS family of proteinases. Biochimica et Biophysica Acta (BBA) - Molecular Basis of Disease. 2011; 1812(12):1616–1629.

[113] Akai T, Niiya K, Sakuragawa N, Iizuka H, Endo S. Modulation of tissue-type plasminogen activator expression by platelet activating factor in human glioma cells. J Neurooncol. 2002; 59(3):193–198.

[114] Rustamzadeh E, Li C, Doumbia S, Hall WA, Vallera DA. Targeting the over-expressed urokinase-type plasminogen activator receptor on glioblastoma multiforme. J Neurooncol. 2003; 65(1):63–75.

[115] Yamamoto M, Sawaya R, Mohanam S, Rao VH, Bruner JM, Nicolson GL, et al. Expression and localization of urokinase-type plasminogen activator receptor in human gliomas. Cancer Res. 1994; 54:5016–5020.

[116] Lakka SS, Gondi CS, Yanamandra N, Dinh DH, Olivero WC, Gujrati M, Rao JS. Synergistic down-regulation of urokinase plasminogen activator receptor and matrix metalloproteinase-9 in SNB19 glioblastoma cells efficiently inhibits glioma cell invasion, angiogenesis, and tumor growth. Cancer Res. 2003; 63(10):2454–24561.

[117] Sage EH, Bornstein P. Extracellular proteins that modulate cell-matrix interactions. SPARC, tenascin and thrombospondin. J Biol Chem. 1991; 266:14831–14834.

[118] Alam R, Schultz CR, Golembieski WA, Poisson LM, Rempel SA. PTEN suppresses SPARC-induced pMAPKAPK2 and inhibits SPARC-induced Ser78 HSP27 phosphorylation in glioma. Neuro Oncol. 2013; 15(4):451–461.

[119] Rempel SA, Golembieski WA, Ge S, Lemke N, Elisevich K, Mikkelsen T, Gutiérrez JA: SPARC: a signal of astrocytic neoplastic transformation and reactive response in human primary and xenograft gliomas. J Neuropathol Exp Neurol. 1998; 57:1112–1121.

[120] Rempel SA, Golembieski WA, Fisher JL, Maile M, Nakeff A. SPARC modulates cell growth, attachment and migration of U87 glioma cells on brain extracellular matrix proteins. J Neurooncol. 2001; 53:149–160.

[121] Schultz C, Lemke N, Ge S, Golembieski WA, Rempel SA. Secreted protein acidic and rich in cysteine promotes glioma invasion and delays tumor growth in vivo. Cancer Res 2002; 62:6270–6277.

[122] Rich JN, Hans C, Jones B, et al. Gene expression profiling and genetic markers in glioblastoma survival. Cancer Res. 2005; 65:4051–4058.

[123] Thomas SL, Schultz CR, Mouzon E, Golembieski WA, El Naili R, Radakrishnan A, Lemke N, Poisson LM, Gutiérrez JA, Cottingham S, Rempel SA. Loss of Sparc in p53-null Astrocytes Promotes Macrophage Activation and Phagocytosis Resulting in Decreased Tumor Size and Tumor Cell Survival . Brain Pathology. 2015; 25:391–400.

[124] Burgoyne AM, Palomo JM, Phillips-Mason PJ, Burden-Gulley SM, Major DL, Zaremba A, Robinson S, Sloan AE, Vogelbaum MA, Miller RH, Brady-Kalnay SM. PTPμ suppresses glioma cell migration and dispersal. Neuro Oncol. 2009; 11(6):767–778.

[125] Phillips-Mason PJ, Craig SE, Brady-Kalnay SM. A protease storm cleaves a cell-cell adhesion molecule in cancer: multiple proteases converge to regulate PTPmu in glioma cells. J Cell Biochem. 2014; 115(9):1609–1623.

[126] Isnard N, Legeais JM, Renard G, Robert L. Effect of hyaluronan on MMP expression and activation. Cell Biol Int. 2001; 25(8):735–739.

[127] Bertrand P, Girard N, Delpech B, Duval C, d'Anjou J, Dauce JP. Hyaluronan (hyaluronic acid) and hyaluronectin in the extracellular matrix of human breast carcinomas: comparison between invasive and non-invasive areas. Int J Cancer. 1992; 52(1):1–6.

[128] Sakurai T, Friedlander DR, Grumet M. Expression of polypeptide variants of receptor- type protein tyrosine phosphatase beta: the secreted form, phosphacan, increases dramatically during embryonic development and modulates glial cell behavior in vitro. J Neurosci Res. 1996; 43(6):694–706.

[129] Pariser H, Ezquerra L, Herradon G, Perez-Pinera P, Deuel TF. Fyn is a downstream target of the pleiotrophin/receptor protein tyrosine phosphatase beta/zeta-signaling pathway: regulation of tyrosine phosphorylation of Fyn by pleiotrophin. Biochem Biophys Res Commun. 2005; 332:664–669.

[130] Grumet M, Milev P, Sakurai T, Karthikeyan L, Bourdon M, Margolis RK, Margolis RU. Interactions with tenascin and differential effects on cell adhesion of neurocan and phosphacan, two major chondroitin sulfate proteoglycans of nervous tissue. The Journal of Biological Chemistry. 1994; 269:12142–12146.

[131] Milev P, Maurel P, Häring M, Margolis RK, Margolis RU. TAG-1/Axonin-1 Is a High-affinity Ligand of Neurocan, Phosphacan/Protein-tyrosine Phosphatase-ζ/β, and N-CAM. The Journal of Biological Chemistry.1996; 27:15716–15723.

[132] Schmalfeldt M, Bandtlow CE, Dours-Zimmermann MT, Winterhalter KH, Zimmermann DR. Brain derived versican V2 is a potent inhibitor of axonal growth. J Cell Sci. 2000; 113(Pt 5):807–816.

[133] Arslan F, Bosserhoff AK, Nickl-Jockschat T, Doerfelt A, Bogdahn U, Hau P. The role of versican isoforms V0/V1 in glioma migration mediated by transforming growth factor-β2. British Journal of Cancer. 2007; 96, 1560–1568.

[134] Hu F, a Dzaye OD, Hahn A, Yu Y, Scavetta RJ, Dittmar G, Kaczmarek AK1, Dunning KR, Ricciardelli C, Rinnenthal JL, Heppner FL, Lehnardt S, Synowitz M, Wolf SA, Kettenmann H. Glioma-derived versican promotes tumor expansion via glioma-associated microglial/macrophages Toll-like receptor 2 signaling. Neuro-Oncology. 2015; 17(2), 200–210.

[135] Viapiano MS, Bi WL, Piepmeier J, Hockfield S, Matthews RT. Novel tumor-specific isoforms of BEHAB/brevican identified in human malignant gliomas. Cancer Res. 2005; 65(15):6726–6733.

[136] Lu R, Wu C, et al. The role of brevican in glioma: promoting tumor cell motility in vitro and in vivo. BMC Cancer. 2012; 12:607–616.

[137] Held-Feindt J, Paredes EB, Blömer U, Seidenbecher C, Stark AM, Mehdorn HM, Mentlein R. Matrix-degrading proteases ADAMTS4 and ADAMTS5 (disintegrins and metalloproteinases with thrombospondin motifs 4 and 5) are expressed in human glioblastomas. Int J Cancer. 2006; 118(1):55–61.

[138] Viapiano MS, Hockfield S, Matthews RT. BEHAB/brevican requires ADAMTS-mediated proteolytic cleavage to promote glioma invasion. J Neurooncol. 2008; 88(3): 261–272.

[139] Kawataki T, Yamane T, Naganuma H, Rousselle P, Andurén I, Tryggvason K, Patarroyo M. Laminin isoforms and their integrin receptors in glioma cell migration and invasiveness: Evidence for a role of alpha5-laminin(s) and alpha3beta1 integrin. Exp Cell Res. 2007; 313(18):3819–3831.

[140] Mammoto T, Jiang A, Jiang E, Panigrahy D, Kieran M W, Mammoto A. Role of Collagen Matrix in Tumor Angiogenesis and Glioblastoma Multiforme Progression. Am J Pathol. 2013; 183(4):1293–1305.

[141] Leitinger B. Transmembrane collagen receptors. Annu Rev Cell Dev Biol. 2011; 27:265–290.

[142] Tanentzapf G, Brown NH. An interaction between integrin and the talin FERM domain mediates integrin activation but not linkage to the cytoskeleton. Nat Cell Biol. 2006; 8:601–606.

[143] Xiang YY, Dong H, Wan Y, Li J, Yee A, Yang BB, Lu WY. Versican G3 domain regulates neurite growth and synaptic transmission of hippocampal neurons by activation of epidermal growth factor receptor. J Biol Chem. 2006; 281(28):19358–19368.

[144] Wu Y, Sheng W, Chen L, Dong H, Lee V, Lu F, Wong CS, Lu WY, Yang BB. Versican V1 isoform induces neuronal differentiation and promotes neurite outgrowth. Mol Biol Cell. 2004; 15(5):2093–2104.

[145] Hu B, Kong LL, Matthews RT, Viapiano M S. The Proteoglycan Brevican Binds to Fibronectin after Proteolytic Cleavage and Promotes Glioma Cell Motility. J Biol Chem. 2008; 283(36): 24848–24859.

[146] Schwarzbauer JE, Sechler JL. Fibronectin fibrillogenesis: a paradigm for extracellular matrix assembly. Curr Opin Cell Biol. 1999; 11(5):622–627.

[147] Larsen M, Artym VV, Green JA, Yamada KM. The matrix reorganized: extracellular matrix remodeling and integrin signaling. Curr Opin Cell Biol. 2006; 18(5):463–471.

[148] Kobayashi K, Takahashi H, Inoue A, Harada H, Toshimori S, Kobayashi Y, Goto K, Sugimoto K, Yano H, Ohnishi T, Tanaka J. Oct-3/4 promotes migration and invasion of glioblastoma cells. J Cell Biochem. 2012; 113(2):508–517.

[149] Zhang R, Luo H, Wang S, Chen Z, Hua L, Wang HW, Chen W, Yuan Y, Zhou X, Li D, Shen S, Jiang T, You Y, Liu N, Wang H. MiR-622 suppresses proliferation, invasion and migration by directly targeting activating transcription factor 2 in glioma cells. J Neurooncol. 2015; 121(1):63–72.

[150] Lee Y, Kawagoe R, Sasai K, Li Y, Russell HR, Curran T, McKinnon PJ. Loss of suppressor-of-fused function promotes tumorigenesis. Oncogene. 2007; 26:6442–6447.

[151] Jenkins D. Hedgehog signalling: emerging evidence for non-canonical pathways. Cellular signalling. 2009; 21:1023–1034.

[152] Liu X, Wang X, et al. Suppressor of fused (Sufu) represses Gli1 transcription and nuclear accumulation, inhibits glioma cell proliferation, invasion and vasculogenic mimicry, improving glioma chemo-sensitivity and prognosis. Oncotarget. 2014; 5(22):11681–11694.

[153] Stylli SS, Kaye AH, Lock P. Invadopodia: at the cutting edge of tumour invasion. J Clin Neurosci. 2008; 15(7):725–737.

[154] Herbst RS. Review of epidermal growth factor receptor biology. International Journal of Radiation Oncology, Biology, Physics. 2004; 59(2 Suppl):21–26.

[155] Huang PH, Xu AM, White FM. Oncogenic EGFR signaling networks in glioma. Sci Signal. 2009; 2(87):re6.

[156] Okada Y, Hurwitz EE, Esposito JM, Brower MA, Nutt CL, Louis DN. Selection pressures of TP53 mutation and microenvironmental location influence epidermal growth factor receptor gene amplification in human glioblastomas. Cancer Res. 2003; 63(2):413–416.

[157] Ekstrand AJ, James CD, Cavenee WK, Seliger B, Pettersson RF, Collins VP. Genes for epidermal growth factor receptor, transforming growth factor α, and epidermal growth factor and their expression in human gliomas in vivo. Cancer Res. 1991; 51, 2164–2172.

[158] Guillamo JS, de Bouard S, Valable S, Marteau L, Leuraud P, Marie Y, Poupon MF, Parienti JJ, Raymond E, Peschanski M. Molecular mechanisms underlying effects of epidermal growth factor receptor inhibition on invasion, proliferation, and angiogenesis in experimental glioma. Clin Cancer Res. 2009; 15:3697–3704.

[159] Talasila KM, Soentgerath A, et al. EGFR wild-type amplification and activation promote invasion and development of glioblastoma independent of angiogenesis. Acta Neuropathol. 2013; 125(5):683–698.

[160] Huang J, Hu J, et al. Transactivation of the Epidermal Growth Factor Receptor by Formylpeptide Receptor Exacerbates the Malignant Behavior of Human Glioblastoma Cells. Cancer Res. 2007; 67(12):5906–5913.

[161] Zhou Y, Bian X, Le Y, et al. Formylpeptide receptor FPR and the rapid growth of malignant human gliomas. J Natl Cancer Inst. 2005; 97:823–835.

[162] Le Y, Gong W, Li B, et al. Utilization of two seven-transmembrane, G protein-coupled receptors, formyl peptide receptor-like 1 and formyl peptide receptor, by the synthetic hexapeptide WKYMVm for human phagocyte activation. J Immunol. 1999; 163:6777–6784.

[163] Zhou Y, Bian X, Le Y, et al. Formylpeptide receptor FPR and the rapid growth of malignant human gliomas. J Natl Cancer Inst. 2005; 97:823–835.

[164] Huang J, et al. Receptor "hijacking" by malignant glioma cells: a tactic for tumor progression. Cancer Lett. 2008; 267(2):254–261.

[165] Brockmann MA, Papadimitriou A, Brandt M, Fillbrandt R, Westphal M, Lamszus K. Inhibition of intracerebral glioblastoma growth by local treatment with the scatter factor/hepatocyte growth factor-antagonist NK4. Clin Cancer Res. 2003; 9(12):4578–4585.

[166] Lamszus K, Laterra J, Westphal M, Rosen EM. Scatter factor/hepatocyte growth factor (SF/HGF) content and function in human gliomas. Int J Dev Neurosci. 1999; 17(5–6):517–530.

[167] Kaminska B, Kocyk M, Kijewska M. TGF beta signaling and its role in glioma pathogenesis. Adv Exp Med Biol. 2013; 986:171–87.

[168] Derynck R, Zhang Y, Feng XH. SMADS: transcriptional activators of TGF beta responses. Cell. 1998; 95 (6): 737–40.

[169] Wick W, Platten M, Weller M. Glioma cell invasion: regulation of metalloproteinase activity by TGF-beta. J Neurooncol. 2001; 53:177–185.

[170] Ye XZ, Xu SL, Xin YH, Yu SC, Ping YF, Chen L, Xiao HL, Wang B, Yi L, Wang QL, Jiang XF, Yang L, Zhang P, Qian C, Cui YH, Zhang X, Bian XW. Tumor-associated microglia/macrophages enhance the invasion of glioma stem-like cells via TGF-beta1 signaling pathway. J Immunol. 2012; 189:444–453.

[171] Balkwill F. Cancer and the chemokine network. Nature Reviews Cancer. 2004; 4:540–550.

[172] Ambrosini E, Aloisi F. Chemokines and glial cells: a complex network in the central nervous system. Neurochem Res. 2004; 29(5):1017–1038.

[173] Rempel SA, Dudas S, Ge S, Gutiérrez JA. Identification and localization of the cytokine SDF1 and its receptor, CXC chemokine receptor 4, to regions of necrosis and angiogenesis in human glioblastoma. Clin Cancer Res. 2000; 6(1):102–111.

[174] Ehtesham M, Winston JA, Kabos P, Thompson RC.. CXCR4 expression mediates glioma cell invasiveness. Oncogene. 2006; 25(19):2801–2806.

[175] Barbieri F, Bajetto A, Porcile C, Pattarozzi A, Massa A, Lunardi G, Zona G, Dorcaratto A, Ravetti JL, Spaziante R, Schettini G, Florio T. CXC receptor and chemokine expression in human meningioma: SDF1/CXCR4 signaling activates ERK1/2 and stimulates meningioma cell proliferation. Ann N Y Acad Sci. 2006; 1090:332–343.

[176] Zhang J, Sarkar S, Yong VW. The chemokine stromal cell derived factor-1 (CXCL12) promotes glioma invasiveness through MT2-matrix metalloproteinase. Carcinogenesis. 2005; 26(12):2069–2077.

[177] Zhou Y, Zhang J, Liu Q, Bell R, Muruve DA, Forsyth P, Arcellana-Panlilio M, Robbins S, Yong VW. The chemokine GRO-alpha (CXCL1) confers increased tumorigenicity to glioma cells. Carcinogenesis. 2005; 26(12):2058–2068.

[178] Richmond A, Thomas HG. Melanoma growth stimulatory activity: isolation from human melanoma tumors and characterization of tissue distribution. J. Cell. Biochem. 2008; 36(2):185–198.

[179] Sciumé G, Soriani A, Piccoli M, Frati L, Santoni A, Bernardini G. CX3CR1/CX3CL1 axis negatively controls glioma cell invasion and is modulated by transforming growth factor-beta. Neuro-Oncology. 2010; (7)701–710.

[180] Kaur B, Khwaja FW, Severson EA, Matheny SL, Brat DJ, Van Meir EG. Hypoxia and the hypoxia-inducible-factor pathway in glioma growth and angiogenesis. Neuro Oncol. 2005; 7(2):134–153.

[181] Spitzweck B, Brankatschk M, Dickson BJ. Distinct protein domains and expression patterns confer divergent axon guidance functions for Drosophila Robo receptors. Cell. 2010; 140(3):409–420.

[182] Evans TA, Bashaw GJ. Functional diversity of Robo receptor immunoglobulin domains promotes distinct axon guidance decisions. Curr. Biol. 2010; 20(6):567–572.

[183] Wong K, Ren XR, Huang YZ, Xie Y, Liu G, Saito H, Tang H, Wen L, Brady-Kalnay SM, Mei L, Wu JY, Xiong WC, Rao Y. Signal transduction in neuronal migration: roles of GTPase activating proteins and the small GTPase Cdc42 in the Slit-Robo pathway. Cell. 2001; 107(2):209–221.

[184] Xiang RH, Hensel CH, Garciaeta DK. Isolationofthe human semaphorin III/F Gene (SEM A3F) at chromosome 3p21, a region deleted in lung cancer. Genomics. 1996; 32(1): 39–48.

[185] Tomizawa Y, Sekido Y, and Kondo Y, et al., Inhibition of lung cancer cell growth and induction of apoptosis after reexpres- sion of 3p21.3 candidate tumor suppressor gene

SEMA3B, Proceedings of the National Academy of Sciences of the United States of America. 2001; 98(24):13954–13959.

[186] Castro-Rivera E, Ran S, Thorpe P, Minna JD. Semaphorin 3B (SEMA3B) induces apoptosis in lung and breast cancer, whereas VEGF165 antagonizes this effect. Proceedings of the National Academy of Sciences of the United States of America. 2004; 101(31):11432–11437.

[187] De Ponnat C, Buffard V, Leroy K, et al. Antiproliferative effect of semaphorin 3F on human melanoma cell lines. Journal of Investigative Dermatology. 2006; 126(10):2343–2345.

[188] Wu F, Zhou Q, Yang J, et al. Endogenous axon guiding chemorepulsant semaphorin-3F inhibits the growth and metastasis of colorectal carcinoma. Clinical Cancer Research 2011; 17(9):2702–2711.

[189] Tamagnone L, Artigiani S, Chen H, et al. Plexins are a large family of receptors for transmembrane, secreted, and GPI- anchored semaphorins in vertebrates. Cell. 1999; 99(1):71–80.

[190] Bagci T, Wu JK, Pfannl R, Ilag LL, Jay DG. Autocrine semaphorin 3A signaling promotes glioblastoma dispersal. Oncogene. 2009; 28(40):3537–3550.

[191] Barresi V, Vitarelli E, Cerasoli S. Semaphorin3A immunohistochemical expression in human meningiomas: cor- relation with the microvessel density. Virchows Archiv. 2009; 454(5):563–571.

[192] Nasarre C, Concina E, et al. Neuropilin-2 acts as a modulator of Sema3A-dependent glioma cell migration. Cell Adh Migr. 2009; 3(4):383–389.

[193] Swiercz JM, Kuner R, Behrens K, and Offermanns S. Plexin-B1 directly interacts with PDZ-RhoGEF/LARG to regulate RhoA and growth cone morphology. Neuron. 2002; 35(1):51–63.

[194] Li X, Lee, AYW. Semaphorin 5A and plexin-B3 inhibit human glioma cell motility through RhoGDIα-mediated inactivation of Rac1 GTPase. The Journal of Biological Chemistry. 2010; 285(42):32436–32445.

[195] Rajasekharan S, Kennedy TE. The netrin protein family. Genome Biol. 2009; 10:239.1–239.8.

[196] Meyerhardt JA, Look AT, Bigner SH, Fearon ER. Identification and characterization of neogenin, a DCC-related gene. Oncogene1997; 14:1129–1136.

[197] Meyerhardt JA, Caca K, et al. Netrin- 1: interaction with deleted in colorectal cancer (DCC) and alterations in brain tumors and neuroblastomas. Cell Growth Differ. 1999; 10:35–42.

[198] Thiebault K, Mazelin L, et al. The netrin-1 receptors UNC5H are putative tumor suppressors controlling cell death commitment. Proceedings of the National Academy of Sciences of the United States of America. 2003; 100:4173–4178.

[199] Jarjour AA, Durko M, Luk TL, Marçal N, Shekarabi M, Kennedy TE. Autocrine netrin function inhibits glioma cell motility and promotes focal adhesion formation. PLoS One. 2011; 6(9):e25408.

[200] Hong K, Hinck L, Nishiyama M, Poo MM, Tessier-Lavigne M, Stein E. A Ligand-Gated Association between Cytoplasmic Domains of UNC5 and DCC Family Receptors Converts Netrin-Induced Growth Cone Attraction to Repulsion. Cell. 1999; 97(7):927–941.

[201] van Tellingen O, Yetkin-Arik B, de Gooijer MC, Wesseling P, Wurdinger T, de Vries HE. Overcoming the blood-brain tumor barrier for effective glioblastoma treatment. Drug Resist Updat. 2015; 19:1–12.

[202] Agudelo-Garcia PA, De Jesus JK, et al. Glioma Cell Migration on Three-dimensional Nanofiber Scaffolds Is Regulated by Substrate Topography and Abolished by Inhibition of STAT3 Signaling. Neoplasia. 2011; 13(9):831–840.

[203] Viapiano MS, Lawler SE. Glioma invasion: mechanisms and therapeutic challenges. In: Van Meir, E.G., ed. CNS Cancer: Models, Markers, Prognostic Factors, Targets, and Therapeutic Approaches. 1st ed. New York: Humana Press (Springer), 2009. pp. 1219.

[204] Valster A, Tran NL, Nakada M, Berens ME, Chan AY, Symons M. Cell migration and invasion assays. Methods. 2005; 37(2):208–15.

[205] Nie S, Gurrea M, Zhu J, Thakolwiboon S, Heth JA, Muraszko KM, Fan X, Lubman DM. Tenascin-C: a novel candidate marker for cancer stem cells in glioblastoma identified by tissue microarrays. J Proteome Res. 2015; 14(2):814–822.

[206] Joshi AD, Loilome W, Siu IM, Tyler B, Gallia GL, Riggins GJ. Evaluation of tyrosine kinase inhibitor combinations for glioblastoma therapy. PLoS One. 2012; 7(10):e44372.

[207] Wang M, Yoshida D, Liu S, Teramoto A. Inhibition of cell invasion by indomethacin on glioma cell lines: in vitro study. J Neurooncol. 2005; 72(1):1–9.

[208] Blázquez C, Salazar M, Carracedo A, Lorente M, Egia A, González-Feria L, Haro A, Velasco G, Guzmán M. Cannabinoids Inhibit Glioma Cell Invasion by Down-regulating Matrix Metalloproteinase-2 Expression. Cancer Res. 2008; 68:1945–1952.

[209] Gabelloni P, Da Pozzo E, Bendinelli S, Costa B, Nuti E, Casalini F, Orlandini E, Da Settimo F, Rossello A, Martini C. Inhibition of metalloproteinases derived from tumours: new insights in the treatment of human glioblastoma. Neuroscience. 2010; 168(2):514–522.

[210] Stupp R, Hegi ME, et al. Cilengitide combined with standard treatment for patients with newly diagnosed glioblastoma with methylated MGMT promoter (CENTRIC

EORTC 26071–22072 study): a multicentre, randomised, open-label, phase 3 trial. Lancet Oncol. 2014; 15(10):1100–108.

[211] Nabors LB, Fink KL, et al. Two cilengitide regimens in combination with standard treatment for patients with newly diagnosed glioblastoma and unmethylated MGMT gene promoter: results of the open-label, controlled, randomized phase II CORE study. Neuro Oncol. 2015; 17(5):708–717.

8

Intraoperative Neurophysiological Monitoring in Neuro-oncology

Lorena Vega-Zelaya, Rafael G. Sola and Jesús Pastor

Abstract

Neurosurgery can be considered a radical method to treat some illnesses and can seriously damage the nervous system. To avoid deleterious effects, such injuries must be detected during their initial development by means of intraoperative neurophysiological techniques (including intraoperative neurophysiological monitoring (IONM) and functional mapping).

In this chapter, we review the most relevant and frequently performed IONM/mapping techniques. Some insight about the electrophysiological basis of stimulation and recording of the nervous system are provided. Intraoperative neurophysiological techniques can be divided into free running or evoked elicited. Among the first we discuss EMG, EEG and ECoG. Evoked potentials discussed include somato-sensory (SSEPs), auditory (BAEPs), visual (VEPs), motor (MEPs) and stimulated EMG. We are especially interested in the clear and concise exposition of the methodological peculiarities, the fields of application and the flaws associated with the different techniques discussed, with a focus on practical applications. Therefore, we show examples of real operations performed at our institution.

We conclude that IONM and mapping are some of the techniques with more relevance during recent decades for oncological neurosurgery. The widespread use and improvement of these techniques have allowed a safer removal of a radical tumour, reducing the risk of permanent postoperative deficits and better functional postsurgical outcomes during neuro-oncological surgery.

Keywords: anaesthetized craniotomy, awake craniotomy, intraoperative neurophysiology, motor evoked potentials, multimodal evoked potentials

1. Introduction

Neuro-oncology is a great challenge for neurosurgeons from two perspectives: first, in some types of tumours, gross total resection (GTR) is the best predictor of outcome in terms of life expectancy [1,2]; second, a main goal of every surgery is to avoid introducing new iatrogenic lesions. The relative weight of every one of these principles can be changed based on individual considerations of the type of tumour, the structures affected, the life expectancy and even the social considerations of each patient. These features are particularly relevant to patients suffering from high-grade gliomas, for whom survival is directly related to the degree of tumour removal. Therefore, to maintain an adequate quality of life, the primary goal of surgery is to achieve GTR without compromising neurological function.

Central nervous system tumours are relatively common in adults; they are the second most common form of cancer and the most common type of solid tumour in children. Although more than half of these tumours are benign, they can cause substantial morbidity. The most common tumours in adolescents and adults aged 15–34 years are gliomas and meningiomas [3]. Glioblastoma multiforme (GBM) is the most common type of glioma. Meningiomas derive from meningothelial cells and comprise approximately 20 percent of primary brain tumours. GBM are more commonly located in the supratentorial region, with the frontal lobe being the most common site [3].

Advances in surgical techniques, such as intraoperative neurophysiological monitoring (IONM), intraoperative magnetic resonance imaging (MRI), diffusion tensor imaging (DTI), stereotactic guidance and fluorescent-guided resection (FGR), have facilitated the delineation of tumour borders and can aid in optimizing safe surgical resection [4–6].

Neurosurgery can be considered a radical method to treat some illnesses and can seriously damage the nervous system (NS). These injuries may not be apparent by visual inspection by the surgeon in the operating room but subsequently evolve into a definite lesion [7]. To avoid deleterious effects, such injuries can be detected during their initial development by IONM. Therefore, IONM is a powerful set of techniques that provide increased functional knowledge during a surgical operation, resulting in the safer removal of a radical tumour [8,9].

The operating room is an aggressive environment to perform recordings due to the presence of several sources of noise. Therefore, it is very important to identify the source of electromagnetic noise and to determine how to manage it. Unfortunately, this subject is beyond the scope of this chapter, but we refer the reader to Pastor J, 2014, [10] for a detailed discussion of these topics.

In this chapter, we review the most relevant and frequently performed IONM techniques. We are especially interested in the clear and concise exposition of the methodological peculiarities, the fields of application and the flaws associated with the different techniques discussed, with a focus on practical applications. Therefore, we show examples of real operations performed at our institution.

2. Neurophysiological techniques

The possibility of using neurophysiological techniques to study the physiology of the NS is based on the way of function of the NS. Therefore, before introducing the techniques, we must understand, at least in a general manner, the function of this system for recording signals because all of the information that can be obtained and used clinically ultimately depends on both features.

2.1. Some insight regarding the function and recordings of the nervous system

The basic functional unit of the NS is the action potential (AP), which is the stereotypical change in the transmembrane voltage of a neuron [11–13]. In general, the AP originates in the neural soma or axon hillock and is transmitted by the axon to the synapse. All potentials originate from closed circuits of current [14], and the extracellular component can be recorded using the appropriate electrodes. In general, small metal electrodes are used to detect these currents.

Bioelectrical signals coming from the brain originate from synaptic currents in the cortex [13,14], or in deep nuclei of the thalamus or brainstem. These currents (clearly together with their intracellular components) form closed circuits that spread via volume conduction. The relationship between the current density (mA/cm^2) and the electric field ($\vec{E}$, in V/cm) is given by the generalized Ohm's law:

$$\vec{J} = \sigma \vec{E} \tag{1}$$

where σ is the tensor of conductivity (mS/cm). Considering that conductivity is the inverse of resistivity, ϱ (kΩ cm). In the electrostatic approach, the electric field can be expressed in terms of the electrostatic potential ($\varnothing$, in V) by the following expression:

$$\vec{E} = -\nabla \varnothing \tag{2}$$

where ∇ is the symbol for the gradient operator.[1] Substituting this expression into the first equation, we obtain the following:

$$\vec{J} = -\sigma \nabla \varnothing \tag{3}$$

which provides the current in terms of the potential. We want to highlight the presence of symbol σ. In the real head, conductivity depends on position (inhomogeneity) and direction (anisotropy). Therefore, it is not possible avoid the vectorial approach in Eq. (3) that can be written in the three spatial dimensions (x, y, z) as follows:

---

[1] The gradient operator is the partial derivative for the space and is given by $\nabla = \frac{\partial}{\partial x}\vec{i} + \frac{\partial}{\partial y}\vec{j} + \frac{\partial}{\partial z}\vec{k}$

$$\begin{pmatrix} J_x \\ J_y \\ J_z \end{pmatrix} = -\begin{bmatrix} \sigma_{xx} & \sigma_{xy} & \sigma_{xz} \\ \sigma_{yx} & \sigma_{yy} & \sigma_{yz} \\ \sigma_{zx} & \sigma_{zy} & \sigma_{zz} \end{bmatrix} \begin{pmatrix} \frac{\partial \varnothing}{\partial x} \\ \frac{\partial \varnothing}{\partial y} \\ \frac{\partial \varnothing}{\partial z} \end{pmatrix} \tag{4}$$

This tensorial equation can be represented for every spatial dimension *x, y, z* as follows:

$$\vec{J}_i = -\sigma_{ix}\frac{\partial \varnothing}{\partial x}\vec{i} - \sigma_{iy}\frac{\partial \varnothing}{\partial y}\vec{j} - \sigma_{iz}\frac{\partial \varnothing}{\partial z}\vec{k}; i = x, y, z \tag{5}$$

Hence, for the same voltage source, the current obtained depends on the conductivity of the different structures. Consequently, structures with higher resistivity, such as the skull and the skin, will only allow a lower current [14]. Similarly, if we recall that higher frequency oscillations of the cortex imply smaller synchronized regions, we can understand why frequencies above the beta band (13–30 Hz) are extremely difficult to record from the scalp. The necessity to record very small currents is the main reason why a low impedance is needed at the patient–electrode interface.

In general, two types of recordings can be distinguished in neurophysiology [15]: near-field and far-field potentials. These concepts are completely different from the same words used in electromagnetic theory. The generators of near-field potentials are located in the cerebral cortex with limited spreading on the scalp. That is, we assume that the neurons responsible for the potential are in the immediate proximity of the region in which this potential is observed. However, far-field potentials originate from the deepest structures (white matter, basal ganglia or brainstem nuclei), and their distribution throughout the scalp is more extensive.

We can divide the neural response recorded by electrodes into three types according to the type of stimuli that induces the response in the neural tissue [13]: (i) electrically induced responses. We apply a controlled stimulation to activate different structures. Among these, we have all the types of evoked potentials or the response of a muscle after electrical stimulation of its innervating nerve (stimulated electromyography or sEMG); (ii) neural response by involuntary stimulation. Those responses appearing in the neural tissue after surgical aggression, e.g., mechanical compression or torsion, ischemia or heating induced by electrocoagulation, must be included in this group. A typical example of this is the neurotonic discharge of a muscle (free electromyography or fEMG) induced by stretching or overheating of a cranial nerve (CN); (iii) physiological response of the NS. These are spontaneously induced responses that are intrinsically generated by the neural activity, either as a physiological or pathological expression of the activity, and can include electrocorticography (ECoG) or electrocardiography (EKG).

Neurophysiological techniques can be classified according to the manner by which the signals can be obtained, by means of a previous stimulation (a) or without that stimulus (b and c).

2.2. Free-running techniques

The recordings obtained using these techniques can be acquired continuously and do not require a command from the neurophysiologist to be released.

2.2.1. Electromyography (EMG)

Free EMG (or fEMG) is the recording of the bioelectrical activity from muscles. Usually, fEMG is recorded by a pair of intramuscular stainless steel electrodes that are inserted into the muscle separated by a distance of 2 cm.

Although we may be interested in the state of the muscle, the most common use of the fEMG signal is to identify changes in the CN or peripheral nerves. In fact, we used nerve-induced electrical activity of the muscle as a measure of the state of that nerve. In this way, we could be aware of irritative activity originating in the nerve as a consequence of traction, torsion, compression, or heat injury, among others. In addition, the patient should not be curarized during most of the surgery. It is important to distinguish between mechanical activity induced by surgical activity, which is usually transient, and neurotonic discharges, which are continuous and persist after the surgeon leaves the surgical field.

Settings that are used to record fEMG depend on the muscle being recorded, the size of the electrodes and the objective. However, it is quite common to use a 10–3000 Hz bandwidth, with either the notch on or off (in this case, the high pass filter should be increased up to 50 Hz), a gain always greater than 30 μV/div (the most common is 50 μV/div), and a time base between 100 ms/div (for small periods) and 750 ms/div (for longer periods). In the last case, we are aware that the shape of the muscle activity can be distorted (depending on the screen resolution) and could be misinterpreted as an artefact.

2.2.2. Electroencephalography (EEG) and electrocorticography (ECoG)

The difference between EEG and ECoG resides in the location of the recording electrodes. However, this difference is sufficient great to warrant separate discussion of the methods. As a result of the analysis of volume conduction, among other dissimilarities that are not discussed herein, EEG and ECoG will be differentiated based on the magnitude of the current and the frequency composition.

2.2.2.1. EEG

Recording electrodes are placed onto the skin of the scalp. The most common types are subdermal stainless steel needles that are placed inside the skin or cork-screw electrodes, which are more easily fixed to the patient but are clearly also more aggressive. Subdermal electrodes allow low impedance (less than 5 kΩ is fine), which is important for acquiring a good recording. We can use the International System 10–20 [16] to position the electrodes, but it is more common to use a reduced version of this system.

EEG can be used to monitor the state of the cerebral cortex, and the main indications in IONM are blood flow alterations and epileptic activity. Bioelectrical activity directly depends on blood flow, and a reduction of this variable will be observed as a slowing of the brain activity denoted by the appearance of theta/delta activity [17]. Epileptic activity can appear after a perfusion alteration or as a consequence of an insult to the cortex (mechanical, chemical or electrical). Considering that high-voltage electrical stimulation is common during IONM, EEG should be used in all patients with an increased risk of epileptic seizure. Similarly, we must be aware that general anaesthetics can increase the likelihood of seizures [18]. Customarily, some degree of quantification should be useful.

The bandwidth filter should be at least 0.5–30 Hz, with the notch on. For this type of recording, higher frequencies are uncommon in the presence of anaesthesia. The gain must be set between 7 and 15 μV/div and the time base at approximately 15–30 mm/s.

2.2.2.2. ECoG

ECoG is used to record the bioelectrical activity directly from the cortical surface. Several types of tumours that are located in the cortex can induce epilepsy or irritative activity, which are defined by the presence of a spike or sharp waves and its combinations. Hence, it is very relevant to assess the presence of these activities. In this sense, ECoG can discriminate between different functional regions in the cortex, namely [9,19] (i) the spiking area, where the irritative activity can be observed; (ii) the lesional area, where abnormal slowing or loss of activity is observed; and (iii) the non-pathological area, which is defined by the absence of the above-mentioned activities. The identification of these regions helps the surgeon to select the cortical region through which to approach the tumour [6,20].

As we have stated previously, it is very important to monitor the presence of epileptic activity during electrical stimulation of the cerebral cortex.

The settings for ECoG should consist of a bandwidth filter of 0.5–100 Hz, with the notch on, a gain of 750–1500 μV/div and a time base of 15–30 mm/s. As stated previously, some type of mathematical analysis can be helpful for the assessment of ECoG [5,6].

2.3. Evoked potentials

The signals recorded using these techniques have the common feature that a previous stimulation must be elicited. Some of these, due to a very small amplitude, must be averaged. Before each technique is discussed in detail, we shall briefly explain why an average is needed [21,22]. Averaging is an extraordinarily powerful tool to separate the signal from its noisy environment.

A neurophysiological measurement (m) consists of the signal to be acquired (s) and the noise (n) [23]. Consider $m(t)=s(t)+n(t)$. In many cases, the noise amplitude is greater than the signal ($n > s$). Therefore, to reduce the noise and enhance the signal we perform several rounds of stimulation (say M), such that, for each kth stimulus, the expression of the measure will be as follows:

$$m_k(t) = s_k(t) + n_k(t); k = 1,2,\ldots M \tag{6}$$

We can see that the average of M leads to $m(t)$, $s(t)$ and $n(t)$, denoted by, $\bar{m}$, $\bar{s}$, $\bar{n}$, and can be written as follows:

$$\bar{m} = \frac{1}{M}\sum_{i=1}^{M} m_i(t) = \frac{1}{M}\sum_{i=1}^{M} s_i(t) + \frac{1}{M}\sum_{i=1}^{M} n_i(t) = \bar{s} + \bar{n} \tag{7}$$

This expression embodies the justification of the method. However, to be truly useful, it is necessary that two conditions are met: (i) there is no causal relationship between the signal and the noise and (ii) the noise varies randomly from one stimulus to the next. The mean for any variable that varies randomly is $\bar{n}=0$; therefore, the greater the stimulus number, then the greater will be the similarity between $\bar{m}$ and $\bar{s}$. Furthermore, it is easy to prove (see Van Drongelen), but omitted here, the signal estimated from the measurement, improves by a factor of $^1/_{\sqrt{M}}$.

2.3.1. *Somato-sensory evoked potentials (SSEPs)*

These are potentials that are generated at several points of the somato-sensory pathway.

Electrical stimulation is performed along the path of a peripheral nerve. In the upper limb, the median nerve or ulnar nerve (at wrist or elbow) is commonly used. In the lower limb, the posterior tibial nerve is commonly used. In general terms, nerve stimulation is achieved in the region closest to the cathode (i.e., negative electrode), where it produces a cationic output current [24] that depolarizes the membrane. To avoid anodic block, it is very important to place the anode distally and the cathode proximally.

Stimulation can be performed through the use of auto-adherence electrodes or subdermal needles [23].

It is customary to name the recorded waves (potentials) according to two criteria: polarity; the downward deflection of the wave is considered to be positive (P) and upward deflection negative (N) and latency; the time (measured in milliseconds) during which the potential appears with greater frequency.

Different points will be used throughout the path that reflect the activity of various nerve structures [15]. Recording is performed by placing and properly fixing subdermal electrodes (other types, such as cork-screws or discs, can clearly also be used) according to the 10–20 IS.

2.3.1.1. *Upper limb SSEP*

- Erb's point. The active electrode is located on the midclavicular line, 2 cm above the clavicle. The reference electrode can be placed several centimetres away. A wave called N9 is recorded. It represents the near-field generated by the afferent arrival of CNAP in the brachial plexus.
- Cervical. The active electrode is located on the second spinose apophysis (C2) or fifth (C5) cervical vertebra, with the reference electrode in the Fz. At this location, we can identify several potentials as follows: (a) N11. This potential is likely a presynaptic travelling wave arising near the root entry zone of C6 and C7 and action potentials ascending in the dorsal columns. It is also known as the dorsal column volley. (b) N13. This potential is generated by the synapse of neurons spanning from dorsal columns onto the nucleus cuneatus. (c) P/N14. This is a distant potential generated by the caudal part of the medial lemniscus at the location of the brainstem. Latency and morphology can vary between individuals (i.e., they can be positive or negative) and may have one or more phases.
- Scalp. The active electrode is placed 5 cm in the lateral direction and 2 cm caudally in relation to the vertex (C4′/C3′ for right/left). The reference electrode is located on Fz. Typically, several potentials are registered as follows: (a) N18. Reflecting the postsynaptic potential activity of the ventrocaudal nucleus of the thalamus. (b) N20. This is a near-field potential that is generated by postsynaptic potentials at the hand cortical region. (c) P25 may be an average of the independent posterior frontal and parietal generators. (d) The N35 peak is attributed to the sense of pain and temperature (conveyed by small myelinated fibres).

2.3.1.2. *Lower limb SSEP*

- Popliteal fossa. Labelled N8.
- Lumbar point. The reference electrode is located in the spinous process of L1 with the reference electrode on the iliac crest. It is called LP (lumbar point) or N22.
- Cervical. It is known as N30.
- Scalp. The active electrode is located in the midline, 2 cm caudal to the vertex (Cz′), with the reference electrode located at Fz. The waves are called P37 and originate from the cortical area of the foot. A potential can also be registered in the fronto-central region with a latency of 38 ms (N38). Because the orientation of the dipole inside the longitudinal fissure is variable, P38 is sometimes maximal over the ipsilateral scalp (paradoxical localization).

The most common parameters employed for stimulation are trains between 4.18 and 7.1 Hz, with a 200–300 μs pulse width and an amplitude that is double the threshold of the motor response. In general, the amplitudes are approximately 15–30 mA, and 200–300 pulses/train is recommended. The recording will have a bandwidth of 10–1500 Hz, with the notch off, a gain of 0.1–2 μV/div and a base time of 5–10 ms/div for the upper and the lower limbs, respectively. It is very important to recall that impedances must be below 5 kΩ.

Warning criteria include increase the latency greater than 10% and/or a decrease in amplitude to less than 50% with respect to baseline.

2.3.1.3. Cortical SSEP

During surgery of the cortex, it is very common to use phase reversal of SSEP to identify the transition between motor and somato-sensory areas, which usually occurs at the central sulcus (CS).

Thalamo-cortical projections from the ventrocaudal nucleus synapse in layer IV of the primary somato-sensory area. However, the rostral part of area 3 is located in the anterior wall of the central sulcus, and thus the current sources generated by these afferents can be modelled by a dipole oriented parieto-frontally rather than in a normal position relative to the surface.

We always use cortical SSEP when we need to identify the primary somato-sensory region and/or the motor area (Brodmann area 4). It is very important to keep in mind that in the case of tumours, a significant distortion of the anatomy can be observed [25,26].

The somato-sensory region corresponding to the forearm can be easily identified by the greater amplitude of the complex N1/P1/N2 waves [25].

The recording will have a bandwidth of 10–1500 Hz, with the notch off, a gain of 10–30 μV/div and a base time of 5–10 ms/div for the upper and the lower limbs, respectively. A 20-electrode grid placed at the lateral region of the fronto-parietal transition can be very helpful. By contrast, for the lower limb SSEP, a 4-8-electrode strip is placed at the medial region. The reference electrode should be placed as far as possible, i.e., at the contralateral earlobe, whereas the ground electrode should be as close as possible, e.g., at the ipsilateral earlobe [13,20].

2.3.2. Auditory evoked potentials (AEPs)

Brainstem AEPs (BAEP) are generated by different relay nuclei along the auditory pathway. They are far-field potentials that originate from very deep structures.

2.3.2.1. Brainstem auditory evoked potentials (BAEPs)

BAEPs are the set of waveforms that are recorded at the scalp after auditory stimulation of the middle ear. They are formed by the following potentials [26]: (a) wave I. Originates at the distal action potential of cranial nerve (CN) VIII, typically has a latency of 1.5 ms; (b) wave II. This potential is generated at the entry of CN VIII into the brainstem; (c) wave III. Synapse at the ipsilateral superior olivary nucleus. Latency of 3.5 ms; (d) wave IV is produced by activation of the nucleus or axons of the lateral lemniscus; (e) wave V appears to result from activation of the inferior colliculus; (f) waves VI and VII are presumed to be generated by the medial geniculate body and the thalamo-cortical pathways, respectively.

BAEPs are indicated when tumours affect the auditory system (mainly schwannomas of CN VIII) and tumours affecting the brainstem.

A high intensity (greater than 80 dB) is usually used during IONM. The frequency is 21.14 Hz, and a bandwidth of 10/30–1500 Hz is optimal (a broader bandwidth can allow too much noise), with the notch on. A minimum of 1000 stimuli/train are needed to obtain reproducible and stable waveforms.

2.3.2.2. Cortical auditory evoked potentials (cAEPs)

These potentials were initially thought to be generated in the primary auditory cortex (PAC), located deeply in the white matter of the lateral fissure of the transverse gyrus of Heschl. However, other different areas, including the second auditory cortex (SAC) and the insula are capable of eliciting cAEPs. There is considerable inter-subject and inter-hemispheric variability [27], and the whole structure remains to be elucidated.

cAEPs are characterized by a series of waves, which can be systematized as follows: (a) short latency waves: N13/P17/N30. These waves are typically recorded from the PAC. This complex is absent in the SAC and (b) intermediate latency waves: peak between 60 and 100 ms. These waves, which are always present in the SAC, can also be present in the PAC.

A stimulation frequency of 2.18 would be adequate. The bandwidth filter is 0.5–1500 Hz, with the notch filter off, and a minimum intensity of 70 dB (sensation level) is applied to the contralateral ear.

2.3.3. Visual evoked potentials (VEPs)

These waves exhibit the characteristics of near-field potentials generated from the primary visual cortex. In the surgery room, the most widely (and probably the only) technique used for stimulation is the application of flashes of light. A normal VEP in response to a pattern-reversal checkerboard is a positive midoccipital peak that occurs at a mean latency of 100 ms with three separate phases: an initial negative deflection (Nl or N75), a prominent positive deflection (P1 or P100) and a later negative deflection (N2 or N145).

Although we think that VEP has undeniable utility, there have been some questions about its efficacy. However, more recent results have demonstrated stable recordings and a strong correlation with the postoperative visual function [28,29]. Therefore, intraoperative VEP monitoring will be mandatory for surgeries harbouring a risk of visual impairment [30].

Stimulation is performed by flashing light-emitting diodes at 2.18 Hz, with 10 μs pulse width, and a bandwidth of 10–1000 Hz. We considered an increase in latency of 10% or a reduction in amplitude greater than 50% amplitude compared with baseline as alarm criteria [6].

In some cases, VEP can be directly recorded from the cortical surface. In these cases, potentials are much more stable, require fewer stimuli (in fact, a very small number of stimuli can induce the response) and are 2–3 orders of magnitude higher than the scalp recording [31].

2.3.4. Motor evoked potentials (MEPs)

Motor evoked potentials are the recordings that are obtained from muscles in response to stimulation of the motor system at different levels (cortex, inner capsule, corticospinal/corticobulbar tracts or spinal cord) [22]. Considering the amplitude of the response, these types of evoked potentials do not need to be averaged.

2.3.4.1. Transcranial electrical stimulation (TES)

This technique consists of the stimulation of the motor pathway by an electrical current delivered through electrodes placed outside the cranium, usually in the scalp [32]. The introduction of TES revolutionized the field of IONM [33].

It is commonly believed that TES excites the white matter of the inner capsule (IC) rather than cortical neurons. In fact, an increase in the magnitude of the current provides stimulation at the level of the brainstem [34]. This possibility must be recognized and kept in mind by the neurophysiologist, especially in the case of surgery at the supratentorial level.

Electrodes can be subdermal needles or cork-screws and are placed at different sites, depending on the region to be stimulated. The most common sites are as follows [35].

- C3/C4, positioned 6 cm from the vertex and in the same plane. These are adequate to elicit responses from the contralateral body, especially from the upper member.
- C1/C2, positioned in the same plane but separated 3 cm from the vertex. This configuration is suitable to elicit response from the lower limbs. However, it has the inconvenience of eliciting too much movement in the patient.
- Fz–Cz′: this configuration is adequate to elicit responses from the lower limbs simultaneously. Unfortunately, the response is more variable than the above configurations.
- M1/M2: the electrodes are located 9 cm from the vertex and usually 1 cm in the rostral direction. This configuration is suitable to elicit responses from facial and cranial nerves starting from the brainstem.
- C3/C4–Cz: in this montage, a hemispheric stimulation is elicited with an anode located 6 cm lateral from the vertex and a cathode at Cz. We have modified this configuration with a cathode located 2 cm from the vertex in the contralateral hemisphere [36]. This modification allowed a response not only from the face and contralateral upper limb but also from the lower member.

The parameters used to elicit MEP through TES are variable, but we use trains of 4–6 pulses, with a 50–75 μs pulse width, an inter-stimulus interval (ISI) of 2 ms (i.e., 500 Hz) and a voltage ranging from 120 to 450 V. It is extremely unusual to use a higher voltage. The recording should be performed with at least 50 μV/div, although it is quite common to use up to 500 μV/div for some muscles.

In some tumours located in the brainstem, cervical or upper thoracic cord, it can be useful to use a D wave recording rather than MEP. This wave reflects the travel wave of CNAP from the lateral cortico-spinal tract and must be recorded through electrodes placed in the immediacy of the spinal cord [32]. This technique is very useful because it can be performed under total neuromuscular relaxation and elicited by only one pulse. However, it cannot be used for vascular pathology of the spinal cord and must be cautiously considered when tumours are located near the anterior horns.

There is a false dispute, in our opinion, regarding the superiority of constant-current over constant-voltage stimulation. Of course, there are benefits and flaws of both techniques, but safe and reliable monitoring can be performed using voltage stimulation. Moreover, using a current of 61 mA with a pulse width of 500 μs [35], the total charge applied is 30.5 μC. However, a current of 340 mA over 50 μs [36] supplies a charge of 17 μC, which is approximately half of the total charge supplied with longer pulses.

2.3.4.2. Direct cortical stimulation (DCS)

For this technique, electrodes are applied directly to the cortical/subcortical surface. Direct cortical stimulation (DCS) to identify the primary motor cortex (PMC) is accomplished using paired electrodes. Stimulation is performed using 4–6 pulse trains at 500 Hz (the reason we denote this paradigm high frequency; this technique is also known as multipulse, which is misleading), with biphasic pulses of 150–200 μs in the duration/phase. Motor evoked potentials are assessed using pairs of subdermal needles spaced approximately 2 cm apart that are inserted into the contralateral muscles, but surface electrodes attached to the skin can also be used. Depending on the location of the tumour, it is customary to use the following muscles: the orbicularis oculi, orbicularis oris, deltoid, brachial biceps, extensor digitorum carpal flexor, abductor pollicis brevis, abductor digiti minimi, quadriceps, tibialis anterior and abductor hallucis.

Stimulation is initiated at 4 mA and increased continuously in increments of 1–2 mA until a stable compound muscle action potential (CMAP) is recorded, at a minimum amplitude of 30 μV or until an upper limit of 30 mA is achieved without eliciting a CMAP [5,6].

An alternative strategy entails the use of Ojemann's stimulation or low-frequency stimulation, which consists of a 50–60 Hz train that is 3–5 seconds in length and has a pulse width as high as 0.5 ms [37,38].

Although a systematic comparison between both strategies remains to be performed, it is important to be aware that neither electrical thresholds nor muscle response or electrical safety are equivalent.

In this sense, it is important at this point to consider some electrophysiological variables concerning patient safety. The effect of any type of electrical stimulation over the neural tissue is mediated by the total amount of charge applied to the system and the duration of application [39]. The electric current (*i*, in mA) is defined as follows:

$$i(t) = \frac{dq}{dt} \tag{8}$$

where q is the charge (in μC) and t is time (in ms). Thus, the total charge applied during time t_{pw} (time of pulse width) can be calculated from Eq. (8) as $q(t) = \int_0^{t_{pw}} i(t)dt$. For square pulses (which are the most common), the integral equals the amplitude × duration, e.g.:

$$q(t) = i \times t_{pw} \tag{9}$$

However, this expression only provides information about the charge/pulse. Therefore, to elucidate the total charge administered to the tissue (q_{total}), we must multiply by the number of pulses (N) as follows:

$$q_{total} = i \times t_{pw} \times N \tag{10}$$

Another relevant feature concerning safety is the maximum charge density (ρ_{max}), which is defined as q_{max}/A (μC/cm²/phase), where A is the area (usually in cm²). This parameter directly depends on the size and shape of the stimulation electrode.

A comparison of these magnitudes is provided in **Table 1** for three different stimulation paradigms.

Technique	i_{max} (mA)	Pulse width (μs)	Number of pulses	Surface (cm²)	q_{max}/pulse (μC)	q_{total}/train (μC)	ρ_{max} (μC/cm²)
HF	25	300	6	0.0133*	7.5	45	563.9
Awake craniotomy	10	1000	1	0.0079**	10.0	10	1265.8
Ojemann	10	500	240	0.0079	5.0	120	632.9

HF, high frequency.
*The surface is calculated from a 1.3 mm diameter disk electrode.
**The surface is calculated from a 1 mm diameter spherical electrode, assuming that only 1/4th of the surface is in contact with the cortex.

Table 1. Comparison of magnitudes.

Although there are no well-defined limits for the above-mentioned magnitudes, from the table we can observe that Ojemann's technique is the paradigm with the highest q_{total}/train, and the stimulation for awake craniotomy has the highest ρ_{max}.

2.3.5. Stimulated electromyography (sEMG)

For this technique, EMG is induced by an electrical shock that is delivered consciously, in contrast to the application described for fEMG. The pulses are usually delivered through bipolar (either concentric or parallel) or monopolar probes. In the latter case, it is important to use a cathodal current to stimulate the nerve and place the anode at a non-stimulated tissue.

The parameters must include pulses of a short length to avoid diffusion of the current. Normally, 50–100 μs should be adequate. The current must be maintained as low as possible to avoid injury to the neural tissue and diffusion. The latter effect must be considered in particular when a functional block is apparent because a high current or a long pulse (or both) can stimulate a region of the nerve distal in the damaged or blocked area and result in misleading information.

It is common to use sEMG in the next situation: (i) to explore a region to identify the proximity of nerves that are not easily visible (e.g., when the CN runs inside a schwannoma); (ii) to determine the identity of a nerve; (iii) to evaluate the functionality of the nerve. We usually measure the threshold to elicit a muscular response at two different points (proximal and distal to the region at risk or more damaged by the surgery) and calculate the ratio of $i_{distal}/i_{proximal}$. The closer this ratio is to 1, the better the function of the nerve.

The settings used to record sEMG depend on the muscle being recorded, but it is quite common to use a 50–3000 Hz bandwidth, with the notch off, a gain consistently greater than 30 μV/div (typically 50 μV/div), and a time base between 1.5 and 4.5 ms/div.

2.4. Cortical and subcortical surgery in awake patients

In recent years, there has been a renewed interest in surgery in awake patients [38,40,41]. This procedure uses the asleep–awake–sleep anaesthetic technique, which consists of induction with propofol + sevoflurane and topical blocking with svedocain + lidocaine around the skin incision. During exploration, the patient must be awaken slowly by removing the sedation. In recent years, a new anaesthetic, dexmedetomidine, has been introduced for this type of surgery and is considered the most effective [18].

Cortical stimulation is usually performed through a bipolar probe with ball-tips that are separated by 0.5 cm. It is common to use 60 Hz trains over 1–4 s. The pulse width is usually 1 ms, with a current intensity of 2.5–10 mA [42,43].

A low rate of intraoperative seizures has been reported (approximately 3–3.4%) [44], and some authors have concluded that control by ECoG is not mandatory [42]. However, this conclusion has been debated and remains to be validated.

In addition to this prevention, some authors have focussed on possible secondary effects derived from this technique. A normal human response to such an exceptional situation as awake craniotomy can, for instance, result in the delayed appearance of unintentional distressing recollections of the event or some type of post-traumatic stress disorder (as yet undescribed), despite the satisfaction of the patient concerning the procedure [45].

The limitations of awake surgery must be considered seriously. During such surgeries, the patient is awake with the head fixed and covered with cloth; and the patient may be kept awake for up to 2 h. Hence, patients must have both adequate cognitive function and the emotional maturity necessary to withstand such an environment. In fact, the Japan Society for Awake Surgery Guidelines limits the target patient population to those ranging from 15 to 65 years of age. Although with some limitations, awake craniotomy can be used in the paediatric population [50]. Nevertheless, use in mentally handicapped patients remains problematic or impossible.

However, no differences in the immediate postoperative motor status, extent of resection, or threshold intensity were found between IONM in anaesthetized patients and stimulation during awake craniotomy [46], although a detailed evaluation has not been performed for the different techniques or surgeries.

For selected patients, an awake craniotomy presents an option to reduce the risk of surgery-related neurological deficits, especially for language mapping. However, the benefits and risks of this type of procedure should be carefully considered, and the decision should serve the interests of the patient.

3. Different features of intraoperative neurophysiology

From a conceptual perspective, intraoperative clinical neurophysiology can be divided into two features: mapping and monitoring [47,48]. The characteristics of these features will be briefly described because neither their requirements nor the expectations associated with each are equivalent. The main differences between the features are the duration of study, the objectives and the modifications introduced to the surgery. However, in clinical practice, both features very often largely overlap or are used at different epochs of the same surgery.

3.1. Functional mapping

Functional mapping generally consists of the topographic assessment (although sometimes it is merely qualitative) of various structures to determine the functions that lead to or sit on the structures [9].

From the perspective of duration, it is usually short so that mapping ceases as soon as the function is positively identified. The objectives, as mentioned previously, are purely descriptive.

The changes during surgery are usually minor, especially because the surgery has a limited duration.

A typical example of mapping is the identification of eloquent areas in cortical surgery. In this case, the issue is to identify the eloquent regions. Thus, the surgeon knows the function of each region so he/she can decide where to position the incision or how far it can be moved prior to the detection of eloquent structures.

3.2. Intraoperative monitoring

Monitoring consists of the surveillance of the functional state(s)/structure(s) that is(are) being monitored for all or most of the surgical action, given the risk of iatrogenic injury [9].

Therefore, the duration of monitoring is considerably greater than in the case of mapping, and it usually lasts as long as the surgery itself. This condition naturally requires more dramatic changes than those used for mapping, beyond the modification of anaesthesia.

The objectives in this case are not just the functional identification but also the preservation of functional integrity, which can be compromised by many medical/surgical procedures, ranging from problems related to tissue perfusion (for example, by actively inducing hypotension or bleeding) to inadvertent surgical injuries such as the placement of spatulas.

In general, neurophysiological monitoring is widely employed in oncological or vascular neurosurgery.

4. Topographical approach to IONM

4.1. Cortical surgery

4.1.1. Anatomical and surgical considerations

IONM of cortical tumours is indicated when the lesion is in or near an eloquent area (areas responsible for carrying out basic neurological functions) such as the sensorimotor cortex or the language cortex. IONM enables clinicians to access the function of the motor and sensory systems of the patient during surgery to preserve neurological function, and it increases the success of radical tumour resection [6].

Functional mapping is initially performed to identify functional areas and their relationship with the tumour. This procedure might help the surgeon to determine the site at which to initiate resection of the tumour. Mapping is then followed by monitoring of the structures requiring continuous vigilance.

4.1.2. Particularities of IONM

As mentioned previously, ECoG is used to define functional areas. Moreover, electrical stimulation can elicit epileptiform discharges before, after and during mapping and IONM, considering that seizures in brain tumour patients are a common phenomenon accounting for 20–40 percent of cases [49].

Following the identification of functional areas via ECoG (**Figure 1B**), the location of the CS is determined by cSSEP phase reversal (**Figure 1C**). Accurate identification of the CS is extremely important because it permits identification of the PMC (**Figure 1C**) [5,6]. There is evidence that cSSEP phase reversal increases both the efficiency and the safety of PMC identification

[50]. Thereafter, DCS for the identification of PMC is performed. Of course, the motor map reference is always the Penfield homunculus [51]. However, when performing motor mapping, we must not forget that it does not conform strictly to reality [52]. It is a scheme upon which there are local movements in different directions [53].

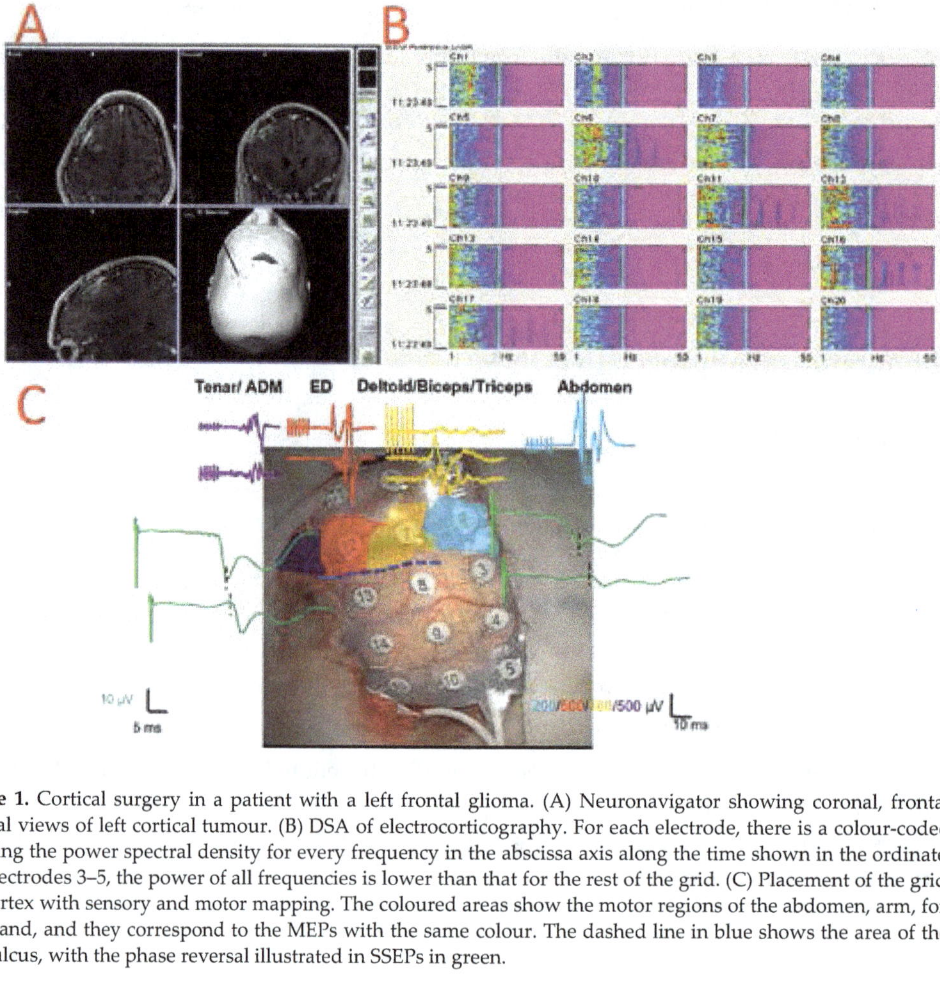

Figure 1. Cortical surgery in a patient with a left frontal glioma. (A) Neuronavigator showing coronal, frontal and sagittal views of left cortical tumour. (B) DSA of electrocorticography. For each electrode, there is a colour-coded plot showing the power spectral density for every frequency in the abscissa axis along the time shown in the ordinate axis. For electrodes 3–5, the power of all frequencies is lower than that for the rest of the grid. (C) Placement of the grid over the cortex with sensory and motor mapping. The coloured areas show the motor regions of the abdomen, arm, forearm and hand, and they correspond to the MEPs with the same colour. The dashed line in blue shows the area of the central sulcus, with the phase reversal illustrated in SSEPs in green.

4.1.3. Cortical language mapping

Locating the functional cortical regions related to language is the goal of intraoperative language mapping stimulation, which is performed during awake surgery. DCS is the technique of choice, as has been widely discussed in the previous section. Concerning this area of the cortex, we have provided additional information about the procedure employed for this type of surgery. The cortex is mapped every 5–10 mm, and positive stimulation sites responsible for language impairment are marked; the same technique is utilized during resection of the tumour via subcortical stimulation. A series of language tasks is conducted by a trained neuropsychologist throughout the duration of the tumour resection.

Although the risk of intraoperative seizures related to DCS is low, it is a real possibility. Additionally, considering that the patients are awake, this complication seems to be a particularly undesirable effect, not only from the perspective of patient discomfort but also because it would interfere with mapping by post-ictal hyperpolarisation. Using ECoG in this type of surgery could prevent, by monitoring and identifying discharges, the occurrence of seizures (**Figure 2**).

The identification of language areas and their fibres is not as successful as the localization of the cortical white matter in the PMC. Sanai and Berger [54] successfully identified the language areas in 145 (58%) of 250 patients with gliomas. Regarding neurological outcome, temporary language deficits were observed in 22% of patients, whereas permanent language deficits were observed in only 1.6% of patients.

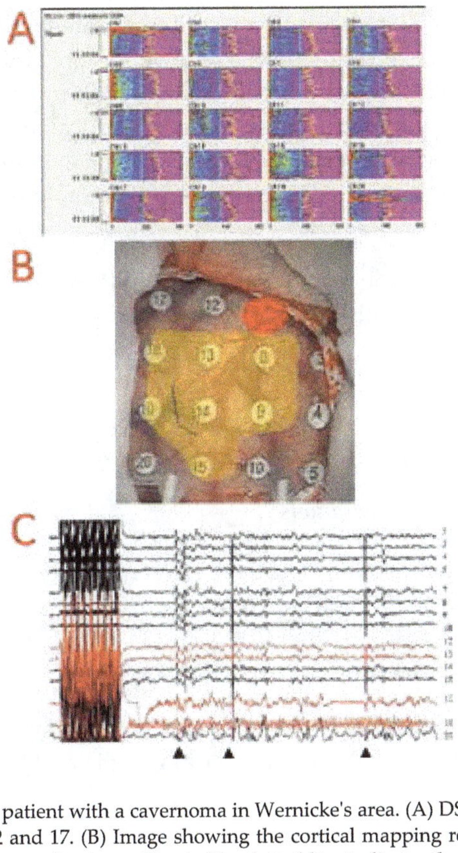

Figure 2. Mapping language in a patient with a cavernoma in Wernicke's area. (A) DSA showing a relative loss of cortical fast rhythms in electrodes 12 and 17. (B) Image showing the cortical mapping results. Red: Wernicke's area to 13 mA. Orange: region with negative results above 12 mA. The dotted line indicates the cortical incision for approaching. (C) Recording showing long-term after-discharges following stimulation by electrodes 18/1 –9 mA. The widespread artefact (arrowhead) corresponds to the moment at which cool serum was administered. The channels affected by after-discharges are shown in red.

4.1.4. *Continuous IONM techniques*

Following the determination of the relationship between the tumour and the PMC, continuous monitoring is performed via DCS using pairs of grid electrodes and employing high-frequency stimulation (**Figure 2B**).

It is accepted that the primary criterion for monitoring MEP in the setting of supratentorial surgery is an amplitude reduction of >50%. Temporary motor deficits have been linked to reversible declines in MEP amplitude of >50%, whereas irreversible declines and losses in MEP are predictors of permanent motor deficits [5]. Pastor et al. [5] described a study involving 34 patients who underwent surgical resection of glioma that was guided using 5-aminolevulinic acid (5-ALA) with no false-negative results. Nevertheless, postoperative neurological deficits without alterations in MEP are possible. This scenario, may be explained by secondary events such as postoperative oedema, haemorrhage and tumour resection from the supplementary motor area (SMA) [55].

An interesting issue for discussion is whether patients who harbour tumours in a region of the eloquent cortex other than the language area must be operated under general anaesthesia. As we have highlighted, there has recently been a renewed use of awake craniotomies [40,41]. In our experience, no new neurological deficits are observed in anaesthetized patients [5,20]. Accordingly, surgery near motor and somato-sensory cortical areas can be performed safely with the concomitant use of intensive neurophysiological mapping and monitoring [5]. Moreover, this combined approach is much more comfortable for both the patient and the surgical team.

When sensory function monitoring is also required, cSSEP are directly recorded from the grid. Monitoring the electrode entails the selection of higher amplitude responses for N1/P1/N2 potentials.

4.2. Semi-oval centre surgery

4.2.1. *Anatomical and surgical considerations*

The white matter in each hemisphere located between the cerebral cortex and deep nuclei together has a semi-oval shape. It consists of an association, a commissural and projecting cortical fibres. It contains, among others, the corticospinal, thalamo-cortical (containing somato-sensory and visual projections) or corticobulbar tracts.

In these patients, surgical removal of the tumour is performed far away from the motor cortex but near the subcortical structures such as the basal ganglia and the IC.

4.2.2. *Particularities of IONM*

As stated, DCS in these cases is usually precluded, and TES is the technique of choice. Because there is a risk of stimulation beneath the lesion, hemispheric TES must be performed. The somato-sensory pathway should also be monitored through the SSEP and, in a number of cases, even the VEP.

An interesting point is that warning criteria for the motor response may occur segmentally in isolated muscles. As previously described, these segmented changes are the most commonly observed changes [5] (**Figure 3**).

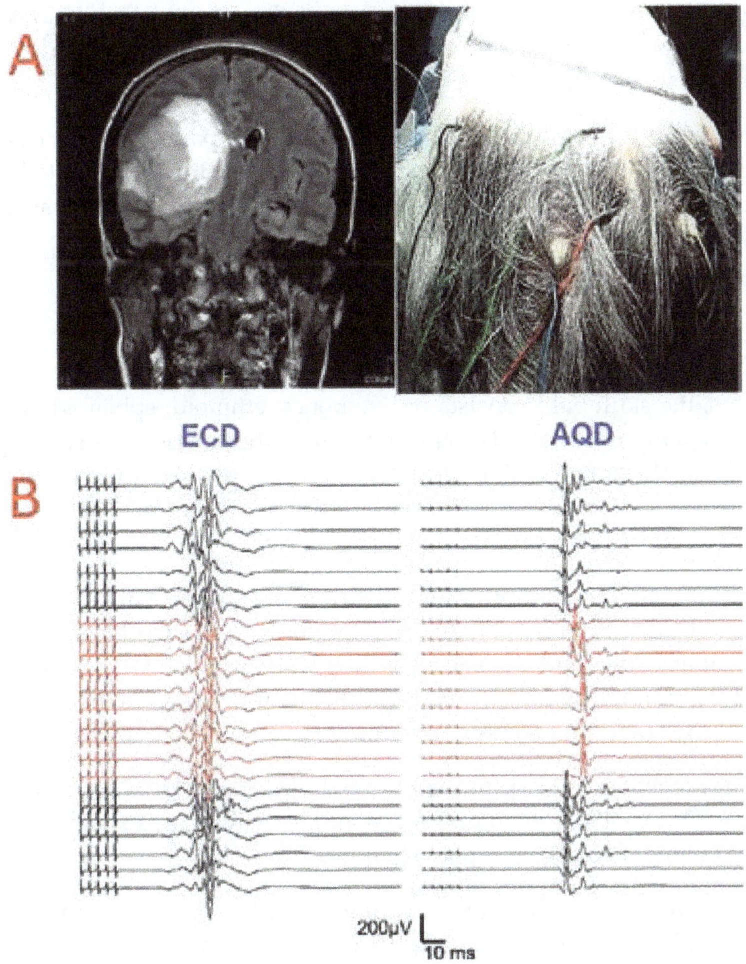

Figure 3. Monitoring of a patient with a tumour in the right semi-oval centre. (A) Frontal MRI before surgery, and an image indicating the placement of the electrodes for TES (B) MEPs monitoring of the upper limb at the moment a reversible segmental alteration occurred in the MEPs of the hand is shown in red.

Subcortical electrical stimulation is an important technique for the identification of the corticospinal tract [35]. The most accepted technique to date, in terms of effectiveness with respect to subcortical activation with a lower motor threshold (MT), is monopolar cathodal stimulation [39].

In general, a linear relationship is considered to be present among the five monopolar 0.2–0.5 ms pulses and the 3–4 ms ISI, as well as a threshold of 1 mA of stimulation, which is equivalent to approximately 1 mm of distance from the CST [56]. Some studies have attempted to determine the lowest intensity of stimulation allowed before resection should be terminated to prevent injury to the CST. This safety margin has not been standardized and has been defined as 6 mA in some studies, whereas other studies have suggested that both significant signal changes in MEP and permanent motor deficits do not occur below a threshold of 1–3 mA [57]. Regardless, it seems reasonable to follow these motor threshold safety margins provided that no alterations in MEP are observed during continuous motor monitoring; otherwise, the resection must be stopped immediately.

VEP are needed when the tumour is located in the occipito-parietal region due to the risk of injury to the thalamo-cortical projections to the visual cortex. In fact, we noted that up to 50% of patients monitored by VEP during semi-oval centre surgery displayed warning criteria [5].

4.3. Cranial base and anterior fossa surgery

4.3.1. Anatomical and surgical considerations

In general terms, the skull base consists of five bones: ethmoid, sphenoid, occipital, paired frontal and paired temporal bones. The anterior limit of the anterior fossa is the posterior wall of the frontal sinus. The anterior clinoid processes and the planum sphenoidale, which forms the roof of the sphenoid sinus, mark the posterior limit. The frontal bone forms the lateral boundaries.

The posterior aspect includes the optic canal, the superior orbital fissure (SOF), and the inferior orbital fissure (IOF). The SOF conveys the oculomotor (CN III), trochlear (CN IV), abducens (CN VI), ophthalmic nerves and V1, as well as the ophthalmic veins. An understanding of the relationship of the tumour to vital structures is essential to preserve these structures and to minimize morbidity associated with treatment.

The greater wing of the sphenoid forms the anterior limit of the middle skull base. The posterior limit is the clivus. The SOF, foramen rotundum, foramen ovale, and foramen spinosum lie in an anteroposterior and medio-lateral plane [58].

A significant structure that can be found lateral to the sphenoid sinus is the cavernous sinus. Along it lateral wall runs the internal carotid artery (ICA), CNs III, IV, V, and VI and the maxillary nerve (CN V2).The facial nerve (CN VII) and vestibule cochlear nerve (CN VIII) originate from the caudal pons. They course through the subarachnoid space and enter the porus acusticus and IAC.

With a suitable understanding of skull base anatomy and surgical access, diverse IONM techniques has been steadily improving the outcome of surgery, both in terms of disease-free survival and morbidity associated with treatment.

4.3.2. Particularities of IONM

According to the anatomy of the anterior and middle fosses, the main structures to monitor are the CNs. Therefore, the standard technique is recording fEMG to identify different discharge patterns related to either irritative or injury activity. Several criteria have been advanced to identify patterns that predict transitory or permanent nerve injury, but these criteria lack uniformity, and the correlation with the postoperative outcome is often unsatisfactory [59]. sEMG is a functional technique that is also essential during these types of surgeries.

Various techniques have been used for the placement and recording of the superior rectus muscle for CN III and the lateral rectus muscle for CN VI. These include the manual placement of bipolar needles, or single-shafted bipolar needles using an orbital ultrasound [60] or image guidance [61].

Corticobulbar tract (CBT) MEP monitoring is a neurophysiological technique that has improved greatly over time and is increasingly used in brainstem tumour surgery. Although the correlation between the intraoperative corticobulbar response and the postoperative outcome may not be completely accurate due to the possibility of false-positive and false-negative responses [62], experience seems to indicate that the complete disappearance of a corticobulbar MEP usually correlates with a severe, mostly irreversible, postoperative deficit. Conversely, when the corticobulbar MEP remains unchanged at the end of surgery, a transient deficit may not be prevented, but the great majority of these patients have recovered their preoperative status at the time of follow-up [59].

The vestibulocochlear nerve (CN VIII) and, to a greater extent, the auditory pathways as they pass through the brainstem are especially at risk during cerebellopontine angle (CPA), posterior/middle fossa or brainstem surgery. CN VIII can be damaged by several mechanisms, from vascular compromise to mechanical injury by stretch, compression, dissection and heat injury. Additionally, the cochlea itself can be significantly damaged during temporal bone drilling, by noise, mechanical destruction, or infarction, and due to rupture, occlusion or vasospasm of the internal auditory artery. CN VIII monitoring can be successfully achieved by live recording of the function of one of its parts, the cochlear or auditory nerve (AN), using the BAEPs [63].

The necessity to protect the optic tract is not uncommon in this setting, and thus intraoperative monitoring of the VEP is mandatory. Although such monitoring techniques were previously not well-established, high rates of feasibility have recently been reported in a number of publications, and stable VEPs have been associated with good postoperative visual function [30].

From a neurophysiological perspective the ICA emits at the supraclinoid segment, an important collateral branch: the posterior communicating. This artery is of paramount importance because in addition to providing branches to the optic chiasm and oculomotor nerve, it is also responsible for irrigating the thalamus. Therefore, in this type of surgery, the MEP and SSEP must be monitored.

4.4. Posterior fossa surgery

4.4.1. Anatomical and surgical considerations

The posterior cranial fossa is the deepest and most capacious fossa of the skull base. It contains the cerebellum, pons and medulla oblongata. Recent advances in diagnostic and surgical techniques have increased the accessibility of this region to surgery, providing new and neurologically safer treatments for these patients [64].

Tumours of the skull base show a tendency to be large in size, they are critical brain lesions because they extend inside and around the brainstem, placing not only the CNs and/or their motor nuclei at risk of injury but also the motor and somato-sensory pathways.

The particular approach is determined not simply by the location of the lesion but largely by the path that allows access to the lesion while minimally disturbing critical structures. The surgeon must select a cranial approach that provides line-of-sight access to the lesion while avoiding excessive manipulation; however, this achievement is not simple due to the high density of critical structures in the brainstem, and even a mild manoeuvre can result in the injury to the delicate nuclei, tracts, or nerves.

4.4.2. Particularities of IONM

There is a critically high potential risk of damage to neural structures during the resection of these tumours, and therefore IONM is an indispensable tool for posterior fossa surgery. The decision to monitor certain structures depends on both the anatomical location of the tumour and the surgical approach selected by the surgeon.

In general, IONM consists of three procedures (**Figure 4**): (i) brainstem mapping (BSM), (ii) CBT-MEP monitoring and (iii) monitoring of ascending and descending long pathways and transverse auditory radiations. BSM is a neurophysiological technique that is used to locate cranial nerves and their motor nuclei on the floor of the fourth ventricle [65] through sEMG. During resection of brainstem tumours involving incision of the fourth ventricle, the facial colliculus (intramedullary roots of the CN VII around the abducens nucleus) and motor nuclei of the lower CNs nucleus are especially prone to injury because the tumour often grossly distorts the brainstem anatomy, and the normal landmarks on the floor of the fourth ventricle are missing. If the neurosurgeon cannot identify these landmarks, he will not be able to make a safe incision. Hence, the mapping assists surgeons in locating these important structures.

The recording technique used for targeted muscles is the same as discussed previously, and the standard set of muscles used to record muscle activity are as follows: the orbicularis oris, orbicularis oculi, and mentalis for the VII cranial motor nucleus (CMN), the posterior pharyngeal wall for CMN IX, the cricothyroid or vocalis muscle for X and the intrinsic tongue muscles for CMN XII. Electrical stimulation of the floor of the fourth ventricle is delivered through a monopolar hand-held probe using the same parameters described above for the stimulated EMG technique. It is important to stress that during this procedure, the threshold intensity is essential for proper localization of the CMN.

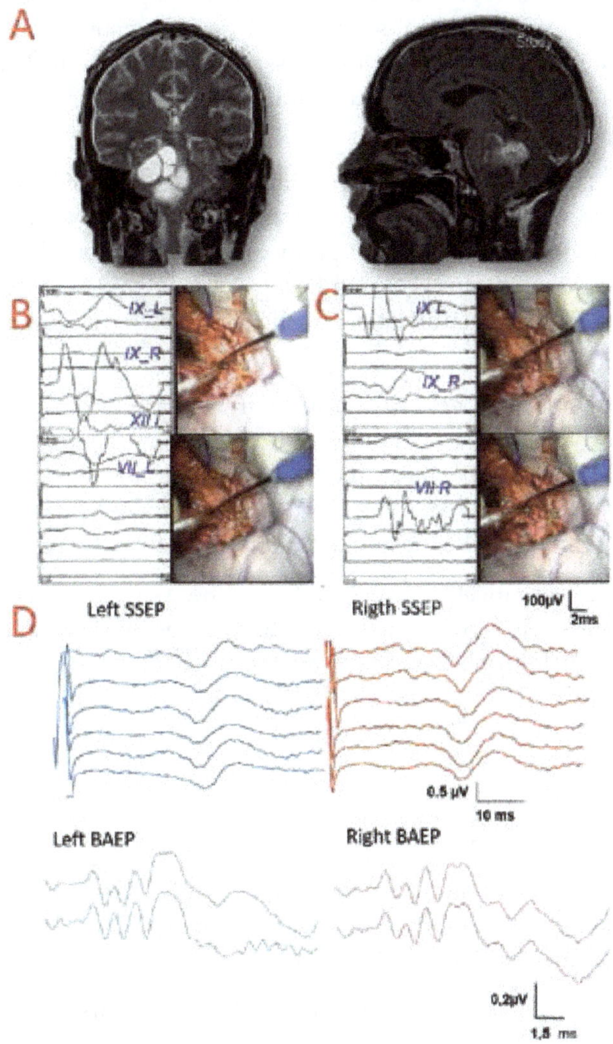

Figure 4. Brain stem mapping in a patient with a tumour locate on the floor of the fourth ventricle. (A) Frontal and sagittal MRI before surgery. (B) Stimulated EMG during identification of the right CN IX (above) and the left CN VII (below). (C) Identification of the left CN IX (above) and the right CN VII (below). (D) Brain stem monitoring comprising SSEPs (top) and BAEPs (bottom).

This technique is very valuable because although there has been a recent advancement of neuroimaging techniques, BSM remains the only way to reveal the surgical anatomy in the operative field [65,66]. We must not forget that it is a functional localization technique and can be performed only intermittently. Moreover, discrepancies between the final intraoperative recordings and postoperative function may occur. This situation can be explained by an injury to the afferent fibres during resection, in which the lower motoneuron is still intact or a nuclear injury results from a stimulation-elicited response activating the intramedullary root. Both instances can produce false-negative results [59,65]. A similar situation may occur during monitoring of the IX and X cranial nerve, difficulties in coughing or swallowing can occur postoperatively despite positive and normal CMAP recordings at the end of surgery. This phenomenon may be explained by BSM responses reflecting only the functional preservation of the efferent arc of these reflexes, but no information has been provided regarding the integrity of the sensory afferents.

For lesions that compress the brainstem ventrally or laterally, BSM provides a minimal contribution. In these cases, CBT-MEP monitoring is the neurophysiological technique indicated to monitor the entire CMN motor pathway from the cerebral cortex to the targeted muscle [59]. Likewise, when motor CN monitoring is considered, as mentioned previously, recording of fEMG with the identification of different discharge patterns will allow the identification of injury activity.

Electrical stimulation must be performed with extreme care due to the presence of vital structures within a very small space. Therefore, the frequency should be approximately 2.45 Hz, and the pulse width should be maintained as low as possible to provide specific stimulation and avoid current spreading. However, a compromise between current intensity and pulse width is essential, and therefore 100 μs and a current lower than 2 mA should be desirable.

Regarding the remaining critical neural structures, the ascending sensory pathways are monitored by BAEPs as well as SSEP, which together can be used to monitor approximately 20% of the brainstem [59]. Information concerning the descending motor pathways is provided by the use of MEP.

4.5. Spinal cord surgery

4.5.1. Anatomical and surgical considerations

Intramedullary spinal cord tumours (ISCTs) comprise 15% of intradural spinal tumours in adults [67]. Tumours of glial origin represent approximately 68% of ISCTs, most of which are ependymomas or astrocytomas [68].

Microsurgery plays a central role in the treatment of these tumours, and the main goal is the complete surgical removal. This aim is limited because preservation of spinal cord function with minimum neurological morbidity it is also desired, representing another challenge of these surgeries.

Microsurgical resection and the surgical strategy may vary, depending on the histological type of each tumour. However overall, there are well-defined steps during the surgical approach to ISCTs: opening of the posterior median sulcus, exposure and initial tumour debulking with separation between the sidewall of the tumour and spinal cord tissue and complete removal of the tumour, which requires the dissection and coagulation of the vascular afferences from the anterior spinal artery.

4.5.2. Particularities of IONM

During the resection of ISCT, lesions in neural structures can inadvertently occur, potentially creating severe neurological deficits. IONM of the spinal cord plays an important role in facilitating the resection of these tumours [69].

As previously described, an effective strategy could be to adapt IONM to the steps of the surgery to protect the somato-sensory and motor pathways [70]. Therefore, monitoring with SSEP and MEP is indicated.

Additionally, for spinal cord surgery, D wave recording is widely used and recommended. In well-documented studies of more than 100 ISCT surgeries, a preserved D wave up to 50% of the original amplitude, with a complete loss of muscle MEPs, has been shown to result in only transient paraplegia [71].

Although it also has disadvantages, we generally consider that under those circumstances in which the mechanism of injury to the spinal cord is purely ischemic, D wave monitoring does not add a significantly value to muscle MEP monitoring. Grey matter is more sensitive than white matter to cord ischemia, and both clinical and experimental data suggest that both peripheral and myogenic MEP disappear earlier than the D wave when spinal cord vascularisation is acutely compromised [72]. Regarding this issue, it seems logical to postulate that the nerve structures most likely to be affected during an ischemic alteration in ISCT surgery are the anterior horns (AH).

It is important to note that previous observations of EMG may improve the reliability of IONM during spinal cord surgery [73, 74]. Skinner and Transfeldt [75] have reported experience with EMG for monitoring ISCT in 14 patients. They described segmental and suprasegmental elicitation of neurotonic discharges that could anticipate the loss of MEP and predict a postoperative motor deficit. Moreover, some studies have associated spinal cord mechanical and thermal injury with EMG activity and motor conduction block (MEP loss) in animals [75, 76].

In our experience, we can define three different phases of the surgical approach to ISCTs that must be followed by the neurophysiological techniques used (**Figure 5**).(i) Phase A: during posterior median sulcus opening, it is important to protect the dorsal columns by monitoring the somato-sensory evoked potentials (SSEPs). (ii) Phase B: working at the cleavage plane, monitoring of motor evoked potentials (MEPs) is mandatory, mainly to protect the corticospinal tract in the lateral cords during the separation between the sidewall of the tumour and the spinal cord tissue. (iii) Phase C: the final phase of complete tumour removal during which, as previously mentioned, the anterior vascular supply is threatened and consequently there is a certain risk of injuring the AH. Thus, fEMG is critical during this phase.

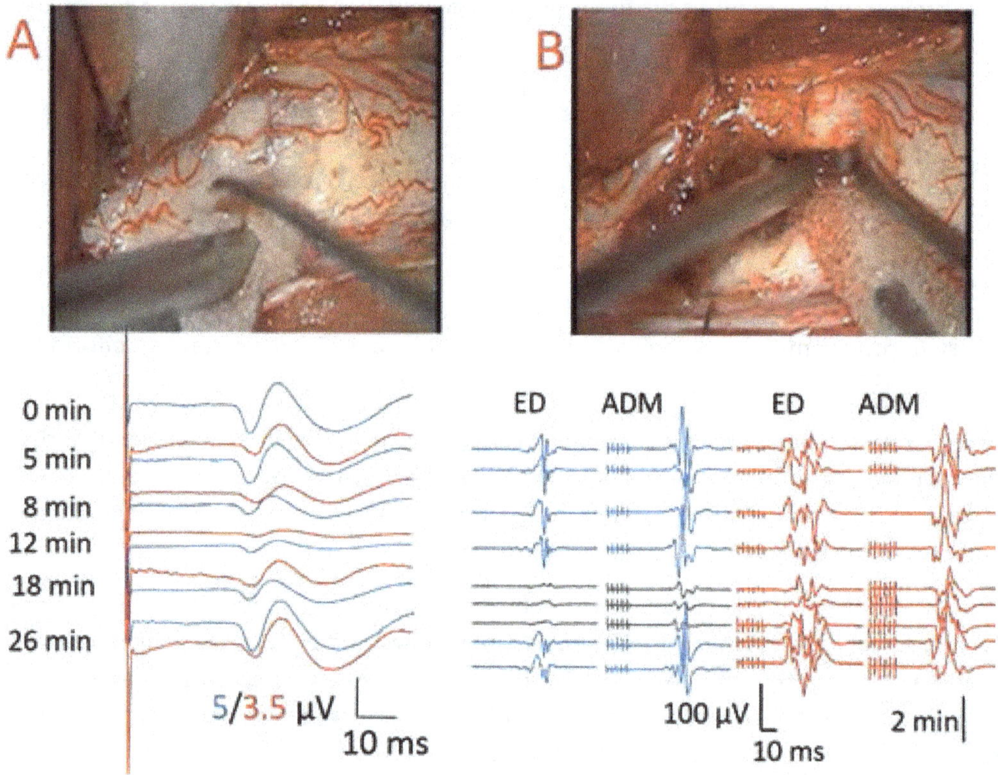

Figure 5. Two different times during monitoring of ISCT surgery. (A) (Top) Microphotograph during incision of the dorsal median raphe. (Bottom) SSEPs for the left (blue) and right (red) sides. Times are shown on the left. Zero min indicates opening of the dura. Between 8 and 18 min, both SSEPs, displayed a decrease in amplitude and an increase in latency (right SSEPs at 8 min). (B) (Top) Microphotograph during tumour removal from the lateral walls. (Bottom) MEPs for the left (blue) and right (red) sides. Grey lines indicate significant changes in MEPs. Times are shown on the left.

5. Conclusion

IONM is a cheap and effective method for reducing the risk of permanent postoperative deficits in many different operations in which NS is undergoing manipulation. It provides real-time monitoring of function to an extent that makes it superior to imaging methods that provide information about structures but not about the physiological state of the patient.

Intraoperative neurophysiology must be conducted by teams of experts that include a clinical neurophysiologist with a thorough understanding of neuroscience and the pathophysiology of the disorders that are to be treated.

Therefore, we can conclude without exaggerating that IONM and mapping are some of the techniques with more relevance during recent decades for oncological neurosurgery. The widespread use and improvement of these techniques have allowed better functional post-surgical outcomes, increasing life expectancy together with better functionality.

However, different topics have been debated that must be clarified. Among these are parameters for stimulation, indications regarding awake versus anaesthetized craniotomy, different types of DCS, and a better definition of the warning criteria or the prognostic utility of some surgeries. Future investigations will clarify most of these features and will undoubtedly contribute to improve outcomes in neuro-oncology.

Acknowledgements

This work was supported by a grant from the Plan Nacional de Investigación Científica, Desarrollo e Innovación Tecnológica (I+D+I), Instituto de Salud Carlos III, Subdirección General de Evaluación y Fomento de la Investigación PI12/02839 and partially supported by F.E.D.E.R.

Author details

Lorena Vega-Zelaya[1,3], Rafael G. Sola[2] and Jesús Pastor[1,3*]

*Address all correspondence to: jesus.pastor@salud.madrid.org

1 Clinical Neurophysiology, Hospital Universitario de la Princesa, Madrid, Spain

2 Neurosurgery, Hospital Universitario de la Princesa, Madrid, Spain

3 Biomedical Research Institute, Hospital Universitario de la Princesa, Madrid, Spain

References

[1] Stummer W, Reulen HJ, Novotny A, Stepp H, Tonn JC. Fluorescence-guided resections of malignant gliomas–an overview. Acta Neurochir Suppl. 2003; 88: 9–12.

[2] Stummer W, Pichlmeier U, Meinel T, Wiestler OD, Zanella F, Reulen HJ. Fluorescence-guided surgery with 5-aminolevulinic acid for resection of malignant glioma: a randomized controlled multicenter phase III trial. Lancet Oncol. 2006; 7: 392–401.

[3] Thakkar JP, Dolecek TA, Horbinski C, Ostrom QT, Lightner DD, Barnholtz-Sloan JS, et al. Epidemiologic and molecular prognostic review of glioblastoma. Cancer Epidemiol Biomarkers Prev. 2014 Oct; 23(10): 1985–1996. doi: 10.1158/1055-9965.

[4] Perry J, Okamoto M, Guiou M, Shirai K, Errett A, Chakravarti A. Novel therapies in glioblastoma. Neurol Res Int. 2012; 428565. http://dx.doi.org/10.1155/2012/428565.

[5] Pastor J, Vega-Zelaya L, Pulido P, Garnés-Camarena O, Abreu A, Sola RG. Role of intraoperative neurophysiological monitoring during fluorescence-guided resection surgery. Acta Neurochir (Wien). 2013; 155(12): 2201–2213.

[6] Vega-Zelaya L, Pastor J. Intraoperative neurophysiological monitoring techniques for the resection of malignant brain tumors located in eloquent cortical areas. Austin J Neurosurg. 2015; 2(4): 1038.

[7] Møller AR. Introduction. Intraoperative Neurophysiological Monitoring. 2nd edition. Humana Press, Totowa, 2006; pp: 1–8.

[8] Krieg SM, Shiban E, Droese D, Gempt J, Buchmann N, Pape H, et al. Predictive value and safety of intraoperative neurophysiological monitoring with motor evoked potentials in glioma surgery. Neurosurgery. 2012; 70(5): 1060–1071.

[9] Pastor J. Conceptos de Neurofisiología en Neurocirugía Funcional, in Navarrete EG y Sola RG (ed): Neurocirugía Funcional y Estereotáxica. Barcelona: Viguera Editores, 2011, pp. 17–27.

[10] Pastor J. Quirófano: Neurofisiología intraoperatoria. En: Cirugía raquimedular. Eds. C Botella, RG Sola, A Isla. Viguera Editores, Barcelona, 2014; pp. 157–170 ISBN 978-84-92931-26-2

[11] Koester J, Siegelbaum SA. Propagated signalling: the action potential. In: Principles of Neural Sciences, 5th edition, Eds: Kandel ER, Schwartz JH, Jessell TM, Siegelbaum SA, Hudspeth AJ. Elsevier, New York, 2013; pp. 148–176.

[12] Pastor J. Biophysical foundations of neural activity. Rev Neurol. 2000; 30(8): 741–755.

[13] Pastor J: Neurofisiología Intraoperatoria, in Navarrete EG y Sola RG (ed): Neurocirugía Funcional y Estereotáxica. Barcelona: Viguera Editores, 2011, pp. 589–604

[14] Nunez P, Srinivasan R. The physics-EEG interface. In: Electric Fields of the Brain, 2nd Edition. Oxford University Press, New York, 2006; pp. 3–55.

[15] Stevens JC. Somatosensory evoked potentials. In: Clinical Neurophysiology, 2nd ed., Ed: Daube JR. Oxford University Press; 2002. pp. 181–203.

[16] Nuwer MR, Comi C, Emerson R, Fuglsang-Frederiksen A, Guérit J-M, Hinrichs H, et al. IFCN standards for digital recording of clinical EEG. Electroencephalogr Clin Neurophysiol. 1998; 106: 259–261.

[17] Finnigan S, Wong A, Read S. Defining abnormal slow EEG activity in acute ischaemic stroke: delta/alpha ratio as an optimal QEEG index. Clin Neurophysiol. 2016; 127(2): 1452–1459. doi: 10.1016/j.clinph.2015.07.014. Epub 2015 Jul 22.

[18] Smith DJ, Howie MB. General anesthesia: intravenous and inhalational agents. In: Modern Pharmacology with Clinical Applications, 6th ed. Eds: Craig Ch R, Stitzel RE. Lippincott, Williams, Wilkins; Philadelphia; 2003; pp. 291–309.

[19] Vega-Zelaya L, Torres CV, Garnes-Camarena O, Ortega GJ, García-Navarrete E, Navas M, et al. Electrocorticographic evidence and surgical implications of different physiopathologic subtypes of temporal epilepsy. Clin Neurophysiol. 2014; 125: 2349–2357.

[20] Pastor J, Pulido P, Sola RG. Neurophysiological assisted transsulcal approach to a high grade glioma without affect neither motor nor somatosensory function. Rev Neurol. 2013; 56(7): 370–374.

[21] Van Drongelen W. Noise. In: Signal Processing for Neuroscientists. Amsterdam, Elsevier, 2004; pp. 34–53.

[22] Pastor J. Diagnóstico funcional: Neurofisiología. En: Cirugía raquimedular. Eds. C Botella, RG Sola, A Isla. Viguera Editores, Barcelona; pp. 99–114. ISBN 978-84-92931-26-2, 2014.

[23] Pastor J. Quirófano: Neurofisiología intraoperatoria. En: Cirugía raquimedular. Eds. C Botella, RG Sola, A Isla. Viguera Editores, Barcelona; pp. 157–170. ISBN 978-84-92931-26-2, 2014

[24] Pastor J, Reina MA. Fisiología del nervio periférico normal y patológico. In Wikinski JA, Reina MA, Bollini C, De Andrés JA, Salas X, Salgueiro C, et al, eds. Complicaciones neurológicas asociadas con la anestesia regional periférica y central. Buenos Aires: Ed. Panamericana; 2011. p. 87–103.

[25] Mauguière F. Somatosensory evoked potentials: normal responses, abnormal waveforms and clinical applications in neurological diseases. In: EEG, basic principles, clinical applications and related fields, Eds. Niedermeyer E, Lopes da Silva A.. Baltimore: Lippincott, Williams & Wilkins; 1993. pp. 1014–1058.

[26] Sala F, Lanteri P. Brain surgery in motor areas: the invaluable assistance of intraoperative neurophysiological monitoring. J Neurosurg Sci. 2003; 47: 79–88.

[27] Liégeois-Chauvel C, Trécuchon-Dafonseca A, Régis J, Marquis P, Chauvel P. Auditory evoked potentials in the definition of eloquent cortical areas. In: Presurgical Assessment of the Epilepsies with Clinical Neurophysiology and Functional Imaging. Eds: Rosenow F, Lüders HO. Elsevier, Amsterdam, 2004; 305–316.

[28] Wiedemayer H, Fauser B, Armbruster W, Gasser T, Stolke D. Visual evoked potentials for intraoperative neurophysiologic monitoring using total intravenous anesthesia. J Neurosurg Anesthesiol. 2003; 15: 19–24.

[29] Ota T, Kawai K, Kamada K, Kin T, Saito N. Intraoperative monitoring of cortically recorded visual response for posterior visual pathway. J Neurosurg. 2010; 112: 285–294.

[30] Kodama K, Goto T, Sato A, Sakai K, Tanaka Y, Hongo K. Standard and limitation of intraoperative monitoring of the visual evoked potential. Acta Neurochirurgica. 2010; 152: 643–648. doi:10.1007/s00701010-0600-2.

[31] Torres Díaz C, Pastor J, Rocio E, Sola RG. Continuous monitoring of cortical visual evoked potentials by means of subdural electrodes in surgery on the posterior optic pathway. A case report and review of the literature. Rev Neurol. 2012; 55(6): 343–348.

[32] Deletis, V. Intraoperative Neurophysiology and methodologies used to monitor the functional integrity of the motor system. In: Neurophysiology in Neurosurgery. Eds: Deletis V, Shils JL. Academic Press, London, 2002; pp: 25–54.

[33] Taniguchi M, Cedzich C, Schramm J. Modification of cortical stimulation for motor evoked potentials under general anesthesia: technical description. Neurosurgery. 1993; 32: 219–226.

[34] Rothwell J, Burke D, Hicks R, Stephen J, Woodforth I, Crawford M. Transcranial electrical stimulation of the motor cortex in man: further evidence for the site of activation. J Physiol. 1994; 481: 243–250.

[35] Szelényi A, Kothbauer KF, Deletis V. Transcranial electric stimulation for intraoperative motor evoked potential monitoring: stimulation parameters and electrode montages. Clin Neurophysiol. 2007; 118: 1586–1595.

[36] Pastor J, Perla-Perla P, Pulido-Rivas P, Sola RG. Hemispheric transcranial electrical stimulation: clinical results. Rev Neurol. 2010; 51: 65–71.

[37] Chang EF, Clark A, Smith JS, Polley MY, Chang SM, Barbaro NM, et al. Functional mapping-guided resection of low-grade gliomas in eloquent areas of the brain: improvement of long-term survival. Clinical article. J Neurosurg. 2011; 114(3): 566–573.

[38] De Witt Hamer PC, Robles SG, Zwinderman AH, Duffau H, Berger MS. Impact of intraoperative stimulation brain mapping on glioma surgery outcome: a meta-analysis. J Clin Oncol. 2012; 30: 2559–2565.

[39] Merrill DR, Bikson M, Jefferys JGR. Electrical stimulation of excitable tissue: design of efficacious and safe protocols. J Neurosci Methods. 2005; 141: 171–198.

[40] Peruzzi P, Puente E, Bergese S, Chiocca EA. Intraoperative MRI (ioMRI) in the setting of awake craniotomies for supratentorial glioma resection. Acta Neurochir. 2011; Suppl 109: 43–48.

[41] Duffau H, Capelle L, Sichez J, Faillot T, Abdennour L, Law Koune JD, et al. Intraoperative direct electrical stimulations of the central nervous system: the Salpetrier experience with 60 patients. Acta Neurochir (Wien). 1999; 141: 1157–1167.

[42] Boetto J, Bertram L, Moulinié G, Herbet G, Moritz-Gasser S, Duffau H. low rate of intraoperative seizures during awake craniotomy in a prospective cohort with 374

supratentorial brain lesions: electrocorticography is not mandatory. World Neurosurg. 2015 Dec; 84(6): 1838–1844. doi: 10.1016/j.wneu.2015.07.075.

[43] Li T, Bai H, Wang G, Wang W, Lin J, Gao H, et al. Glioma localization and excision using direct electrical stimulation for language mapping during awake surgery. Exp Ther Med. 2015 May; 9(5): 1962–1966.

[44] Hervey-Jumper SL, Li J, Lau D, Molinaro AM, Perry DW, Meng L, et al. Awake craniotomy to maximize glioma resection: methods and technical nuances over a 27-year period. J Neurosurg. 2015; 123(2): 325–339. doi: 10.3171/2014.10.JNS141520.

[45] Milian Ml, Tatagiba M, Feigl GC. Patient response to awake craniotomy— a summary overview. Acta Neurochir (Wien). 2014; 156(6): 1063–1070. doi: 10.1007/s00701-014-2038-4.

[46] Delion M, Terminassian A, Lehousse T, Aubin G, Malka J, N'Guyen S, et al. specificities of awake craniotomy and brain mapping in children for resection of supratentorial tumors in the language area. World Neurosurg. 2015; 84(6): 1645–1652. doi: 10.1016/j.wneu.2015.06.073.

[47] Bello L, Fava E, Cascaceli G, Bertani G, Carrabba G, Papagno C, et al. Intraoperative mapping for tumor resection. Neuroimag Clin N Am. 2009; 19: 597–614.

[48] Bertani G, Fava E, Casaceli G, Carrabba G, Casarotti A, Papagno C, et al. Intraoperative mapping and monitoring of brain functions for the resection of low-grade gliomas: technical considerations. Neurosurg Focus. 2009; 27(4): E4.

[49] Lwu S, Hamilton MG, Forsyth PA, Cairncross JG, Parney IF. Use of peri-operative anti-epileptic drugs in patients with newly diagnosed high grade malignant glioma: a single center experience. J Neurooncol. 2010 Feb; 96(3): 403–408.

[50] Simon MV, Sheth SA, Eckhardt CA, Kilbride RD, Braver D, Williams Z, et al. Phase reversal technique decreases cortical stimulation time during motor mapping. J Clin Neurosci. 2014; 21: 1011–1017.

[51] Porter R, Lemon R. Corticospinal function and voluntary movement. Oxford: Oxford University Press; 1993.

[52] Cuadrado ML, Arias JA, Palomar MA, Linares R. The pyramidal tract: new pathways. Rev Neurol. 2001; 32(12): 1151–1158.

[53] Schott GD. Penfield's homunculus: a note on cerebral cartography. J Neurol Neurosurg Psychiatry. 1993; 56: 329–333.

[54] Sanai N, Berger MS. Intraoperative stimulation techniques for functional pathway preservation and glioma resection. Neurosurg Focus. 2010; 28: E1.

[55] Krieg SM, Schäffner M, Shiban E, Droese D, Obermüller T, Gempt J, et al. Reliability of intraoperative neurophysiological monitoring using motor evoked potentials during

resection of metastases in motor-eloquent brain regions. J Neurosurg. 2013; 118: 1269–1278.

[56] Kamada K, Todo T, Ota T, Ino K, Masutani Y, Aoki S, et al. The motor-evoked potential threshold evaluated by tractography and electrical stimulation. J Neurosurg. 2009; 111(4): 785–795.

[57] Seidel K, Beck J, Stieglitz L, Schucht P, Raabe A. The warning-sign hierarchy between quantitative subcortical motor mapping and continuous motor evoked potential monitoring during resection of supratentorial brain tumors. J Neurosurg. 2013; 118(2): 287–296.

[58] Lang DA. Surgery of the cranial base. In: Surgery of Cranial Base Tumors, Eds.: Sekhar LN, Janecka IP. New York, Raven Press, 1993; pp. 93–121.

[59] Sala F, Manganotti P, Tramontano V, Bricolo A, Gerosa M. Monitoring of motor pathways during brain stem surgery: what we have achieved and what we still miss? Neurophysiol Clin. 2007; 37(6): 399–406.

[60] Schlake HP, Goldbrunner R, Siebert M, Behr R, Roosen K. Intra-Operative electromyographic monitoring of extra-ocular motor nerves (Nn. III, VI) in skull base surgery. Acta Neurochir (Wien). 2001; 143(3): 251–261.

[61] Alberti O, Sure U, Riegel T, Bertalanffy H. Image-guided placement of eye muscle electrodes for intraoperative cranial nerve monitoring. Neurosurgery. 2001; 49(3): 660–663; discussion 663–664.

[62] Dong CC, Macdonald DB, Akagami R, Westerberg B, Alkhani A, Kanaan I, et al. Intraoperative facial motor evoked potential monitoring with transcranial electrical stimulation during skull base surgery. Clin Neurophysiol. 2005; 116(3): 588–596.

[63] Simon MV. Neurophysiologic intraoperative monitoring of the vestibulocochlear nerve. J Clin Neurophysiol. 2011; 28(6): 566–581

[64] Bricolo A, Turazzi S. Surgery for gliomas and other mass lesions of the brainstem. Adv Tech Stand Neruosurg. 1995; 22: 261–341.

[65] Morota N, Deletis V, Epstein FJ, Kofler M, Abbott R, Lee M, et al. Brain stem mapping: neurophysiological localization of motor nuclei on the floor of the fourth ventricle. Neurosurgery. 1995; 37: 922–930.

[66] Sola RG, Pulido P, Pastor J, Ochoa M, Castedo J. Surgical treatment of symptomatic cavernous malformations of the brainstem. Acta Neurochir (Wien). 2007; 149(5): 463–470

[67] Wong AP, Dahdaleh NS, Fessler RG, Melkonian SC, Lin Y, Smith ZA, et al. Risk factors and long-term survival in adult patients with primary malignant spinal cord astrocytomas. J Neurooncol. 2003; 115(3): 493–503.

[68] Chamberlain MC, Tredway TL. Adult primary intradural spinal cord tumors: a review. Curr Neurol Neurosci Rep. 2011; 11(3): 320–328.

[69] Deletis V, Sala F. Intraoperative neurophysiological monitoring of the spinal cord during spinal cord and spine surgery: a review focus on the corticospinal tracts. Clin Neurophysiol. 2008; 119(2): 248–264.

[70] Sala F, Bricolo A, Faccioli F, Lanteri P, Gerosa M. Surgery for intramedullary spinal cord tumors: the role of intraoperative (neurophysiological) monitoring. Eur Spine J. 2007; 16 Suppl 2: S130–9.

[71] Kothbauer K, Deletis V, Epstein FJ. Intraoperative spinal cord monitoring for intramedullary surgery: an essential adjunct. Pediatr Neurosurg. 1997: 247–254.

[72] de Haan P, Kalkman CJ, Ubags LH, Jacobs MJ, Drummond JC. A comparison of the sensitivity of epidural and myogenic transcranial motor-evoked responses in the detection of acute spinal cord ischemia in the rabbit. Anesth Analg. 1996; 83: 1022–1027.

[73] Hyun SJ, Rhim SC. Combined motor and somatosensory evoked potential monitoring for intramedullary spinal cord tumor surgery: correlation of clinical and neurophysiological data in 17 consecutive procedures. Br J Neurosurg. 2009; 23(4): 393–400.

[74] Skinner SA, Nagib M, Bergman TA, Maxwell RE, Msangi G. The initial use of free-running electromyography to detect early motor tract injury during resection of intramedullary spinal cord lesions. Neurosurgery. 2005; 56 (2 Suppl): 299–314.

[75] Skinner SA, Transfeldt EE. Electromyography in the detection of mechanically induced spinal motor tract injury: observations in diverse porcine models. J Neurosurg Spine. 2009; 11(3): 369–374.

[76] Skinner SA, Hsu B, Transfeldt EE, Mehbod AA, Rippe DM, Wu C, et al. Spinal cord injury from electrocautery: observations in a porcine model using electromyography and motor evoked potentials. J Clin Monit Comput. 2013; 27(2): 195–201.

9

Advanced MR Imaging Techniques in the Diagnosis of Intra-axial Brain Tumors

Anastasia Zikou, George Alexiou and
Maria Argyropoulou

Abstract

Intracranial masses are a significant health problem and present several imaging challenges. The role of imaging is no longer limited to merely providing anatomic details but the advanced MR techniques permit the assessment of the freedom of water molecule movement, the microvascular structure and hemodynamic characteristics, and the chemical makeup of certain metabolites of lesions. In the current chapter, we will discuss the role of the advanced MR imaging techniques, namely perfusion, diffusion-weighted imaging, and MR spectroscopy in the diagnosis and classification of the most frequent brain tumors in adults. We provide a brief description of the advanced MR techniques that are currently used, and we discuss in detail the imaging findings for each lesion. These lesions include gliomas both high and low grade, metastatic lesions, lymphomas, and lesions that may mimic tumors such as tumefactive demyelinating lesions, abscesses, and encephalitis. Our goal is to summarize the diagnostic information that advanced MR imaging techniques offer for establishing a diagnosis and clinical decision making.

Keywords: MRI, brain tumors, perfusion, diffusion tensor imaging, spectroscopy

1. Introduction

Among primary brain and central nervous system tumors in adults, meningiomas are the most common, accounting for 36.4% of all, followed by pituitary tumors (15.5%) and glioblastoma (WHO Grade IV) (15.1%), which is the most malignant primary brain tumor. Other types are nerve sheath tumors (8.1%), all other astrocytomas (5.7%), lymphoma (2%), ependymal tumors

(1.9%), oligodendrogliomas (1.6%), embryonal tumors (1.1%), oligoastrocytic tumors (0.9%), and all other less frequent tumors (11.7%) [1].

Imaging has a fundamental role in intracranial tumor management. Magnetic resonance imaging (MRI) is the imaging modality of choice for establishing diagnosis, classification, surgical planning, and post-treatment follow-up. The latest MRI techniques, namely diffusion, perfusion, and spectroscopy, offer more than the anatomical information that conventional imaging provides. Diffusion allows the assessment of water displacement within tissue. Diffusion tensor imaging permits the mapping of axonal organization. Perfusion MRI is a technique for the assessment of cerebral perfusion. Dynamic susceptibility contrast imaging (DSC-MRI) perfusion technique is currently the most widely used and allows the calculation of relative cerebral blood volume (rCBV) and relative cerebral blood flow (rCBF). MR spectroscopy, with single-voxel or multi-voxel techniques, can detect metabolites within tissue such as N-acetyl aspartate (NAA), choline-containing compounds (Cho), myoinositol (mI), lactate (Lac), creatine (Cr), and other molecules. However, no tumor-specific metabolite has been recognized to date.

Although the discrimination between intra-axial and extra-axial lesions is relatively straightforward, for the accurate discrimination of the variety of intra-axial tumors of several difficulties exist. This is of paramount importance for timely and appropriate patients' management. Herewith, we provide an overview of the latest MR techniques for the differential diagnosis of intra-axial tumors.

2. Primary tumors

Gliomas are the most common primary brain tumors. Glioblastoma accounts for 55% of all cases followed by diffuse astrocytoma (8.6%), ependymal tumors (6.9%), anaplastic astrocytomas (6.1%), oligodenrogliomas (5.7%), pilocytic astrocytomas (5.2%), and other less frequent glioma types [1]. Incidence is higher in males and in whites than in blacks. For glioblastoma, the median age of diagnosis is 64 years but for low-grade gliomas (grades I and II), most often occur between 20 and 40 years. The major diagnostic goal in gliomas is the differentiation of low-grade from high-grade gliomas and from other pathologies that have similar imaging features.

2.1. Diffusion-weighted imaging

Apparent diffusion coefficient (ADC) maps alone cannot differentiate between glioma from another neoplasm or glioma type. Malignancy is usually associated with increased cellular density, resulting in decreased signal intensity on ADC images. High-grade gliomas usually have significant lower ADC values than low-grade gliomas. A lesion-to-normal (L/N) ADC ratio of 1.43 could differentiate low-grade from high-grade gliomas with 100% sensitivity and 94.4% specificity [2]. Evaluation of the perilesion area may aid the diagnosis of a primary tumor due to its infiltrative nature (**Figure 1**).

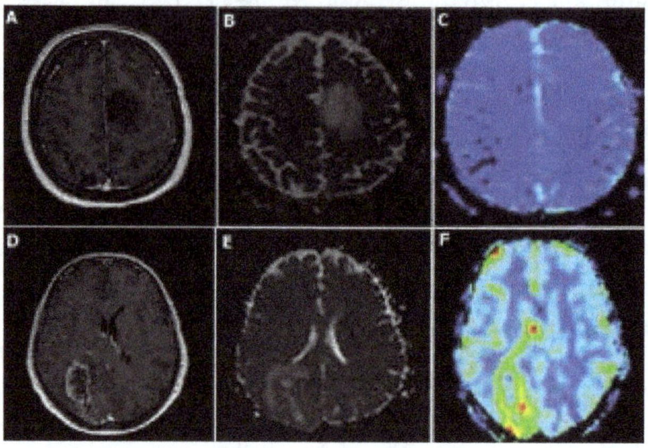

Figure 1. (A) A case of a grade II astrocytoma and of glioblastoma (D). There is a lower ADC value in astrocytoma (B) than glioblastoma (E). The rCBV map shows increased perfusion in glioblastoma (F) contrary to astrocytoma (C).

2.2. Perfusion imaging

Perfusion MRI can be performed using a variety of methods. The most common techniques are as follows: T2-weighted dynamic susceptibility contrast (DSC), T1-weighted dynamic contrast enhanced (DCE), and arterial spine labeling (ASL). The latter do not require contrast administration. The relative cerebral blood volume (rCBV) is the most frequent reported metric. This can be calculated by comparing the cerebral blood volume in a region of interest that is drawn over the tumor to the CBV of a mirror region of interest placed over the normal white matter in the contralateral side.

Gliomas are characterized by increased blood vessels formation for the transport of nutrients and oxygen which are essential for tumor growth. Furthermore, apart from glioma infiltration to parenchyma, malignant cells can also migrate using a perivascular route through microvasculature [3]. Recent reports showed that glioblastoma cells can even differentiate into endothelial cells and pericytes, thus aiding tumor vascularization [4]. High-grade gliomas have a significantly higher rCBV ratio than low-grade gliomas (**Figure 1**). A cut-off ratio of 0.63 has been suggested for the differentiation between them [2]. Furthermore, a significant linear correlation has been reported between rCBV ratio and glioma proliferation potentials as assessed by Ki-67 index and tumor's cell cycle analysis [5, 6]. High-grade tumors had higher Ki-67 index, higher percentage of cells in G2/M phase, and lower percentage of cells in G0/G1 phase.

Oligodendrogliomas contrary to other low-grade gliomas have significant higher rCBV values (mean 3.68 ± 2.39) [7], overlapping even with high-grade gliomas. A possible explanation to this is their increased vascular density and cortical localization [7]. Another important exception is pilocytic astrocytoma, the most common pediatric brain tumor with usually infratentorial localization [8]. The tumor's mural nodule may show increased rCBV ratio in comparison with other low-grade gliomas. Clinicians should also bear in mind that hemangioblastomas may also demonstrate high rCBV ratios.

2.3. MR spectroscopy

Initial studies with MR spectroscopy showed promise for the diagnosis of brain lesions and grading; however, recent evidences are controversial. Several metabolites can be measured that correlate with various pathological alterations within lesions. NAA is the acetylated form of the amino acid, aspartate, which is found in increased concentrations in viable neurons. Given that non-neuronal neoplasms destroy normal neurons there is a reduction in NAA signal. Choline is a marker of cell membrane and can be found elevated in tumors and inflammatory processes. Creatine is a measure of energy stores, whereas lactate increases in cases of ischemia, in which the cell switches to anaerobic glycolysis and lactates accumulates. Thus, lactate is more likely to be present in high-grade than low-grade gliomas. Lipids have been recognized as a marker of myelin breakdown. Several studies have evaluated both single-voxel and multi-voxel spectroscopy. Multi-voxel has the advantage of greater spatial resolution and extent of coverage, thus permits the evaluation of different components of heterogeneous masses. Within tumor, some areas may be more metabolically active than others. In brain tumors, there is usually an increased signal of Cho, whereas NAA and Cr are reduced. Cho/Cr ratio tends to increase as glioma malignancy progresses. In a recent meta-analysis, Cho/NAA ratio showed a sensitivity of 80% and specificity of 76%, higher than Cho/Cr ratio and NAA/Cr ratio for the differentiation of high-grade from low-grade gliomas [9]. However, both sensitivity and specificity do not enable an accurate diagnosis, thus additional imaging modalities may be needed. A CHO/NAA ratio >1, in voxels outside of the enhancement region, suggests tumor infiltration and is indicative of a high-grade glioma (**Figure 2**).

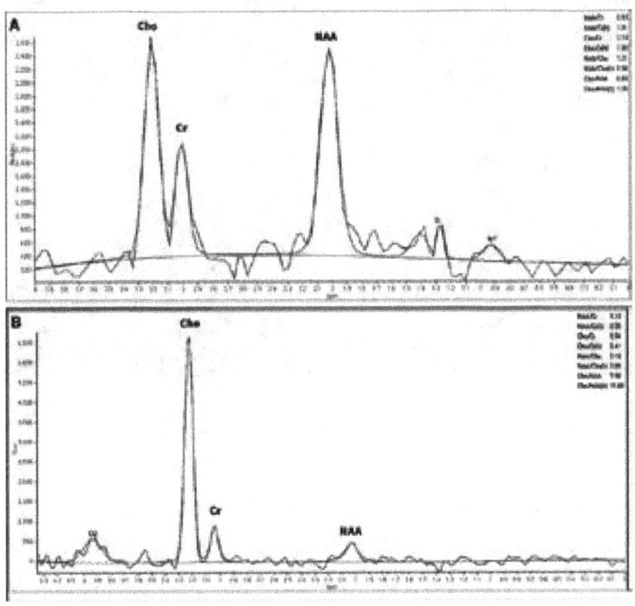

Figure 2. MR proton spectrum of a grade II astrocytoma (A) and of a glioblastoma (B). Contrary to low-grade glioma, glioblastoma exhibits depression of the NAA and creatine (Cr) peaks and elevation of the choline (Cho) peak.

3. Gliomatosis cerebri

Gliomatosis cerebri is a rare diffuse primary neoplastic process of glial origin with dismal prognosis. Based on WHO criteria, this diffusely infiltrating glial neoplasm involves at least three cerebral lobes. There is often bilateral involvement of the cerebral hemispheres and/or deep gray matter (**Figure 3**) [10]. Histopathologically, it is characterized by diffuse infiltration of brain parenchyma by small, immature glial cells that resembles astrocytes, oligodendroglia, or undifferentiated cells [10, 11]. The lesion can contain areas of WHO grades II or III tumors, and less frequent grade IV. Symptomatology is subtle and may involve changes in personality and mental status, headache, hemiparesis, ataxia, and seizures. Although it appears radiologically as extensive disease, clinical symptomatology may be silent. Diagnosis requires brain biopsy and histopathological examination.

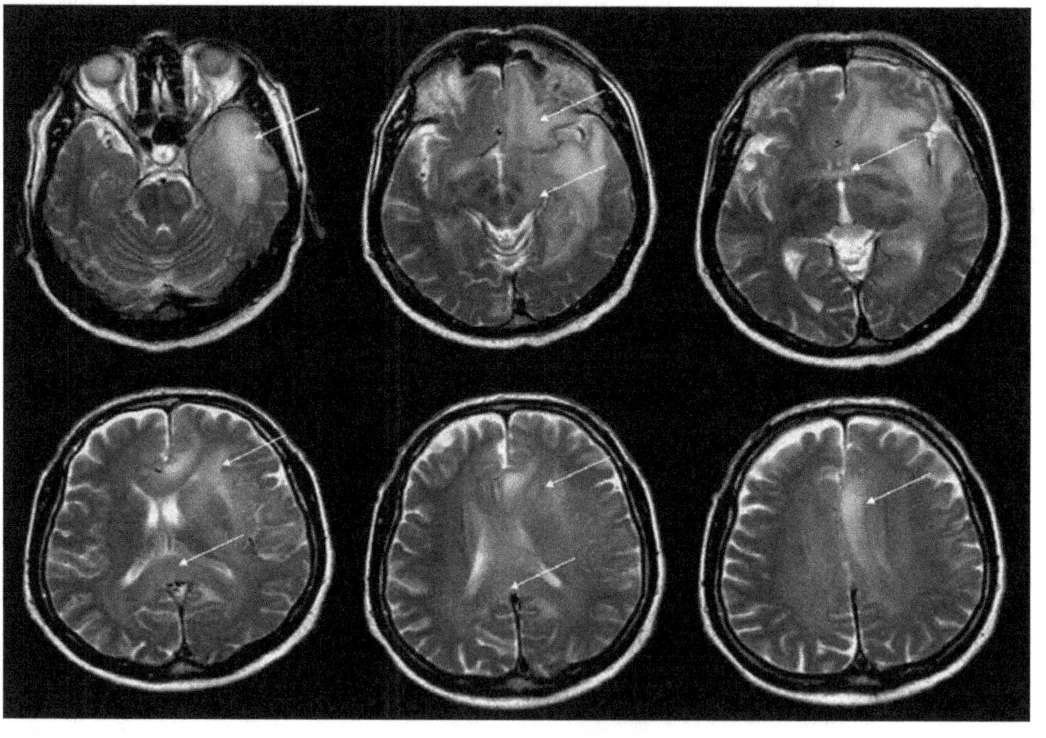

Figure 3. T2-W axial images show diffuse hyperintense lesions with enlargement of the involved structures and little mass effect (arrows).

Two subtypes can be identified radiologically: type 1 with no discrete component and type II with a solid component and diffuse CNS involvement. *IDH1* mutations have been reported more frequent in type II GC [12]. MRI findings are essential for establishing the correct diagnosis. Hypointensity in T1-weighted sequences and hyperintensity in T2-weighted and FLAIR sequences are the classical findings. Another usual MRI finding consists of diffuse infiltration of the cortex with an enlargement of the cortical sulci and the absence of clear delineation between white and gray. Contrast enhancement is absent [13]. In DWI, there is usually no restriction. Perfusion MR shows low or normal rCBV values correlating with the absence of vascular hyperplasia. MR spectroscopy reveals elevated Cho/NAA ratios and marked elevation of myoinositol [14] (**Figure 4**).

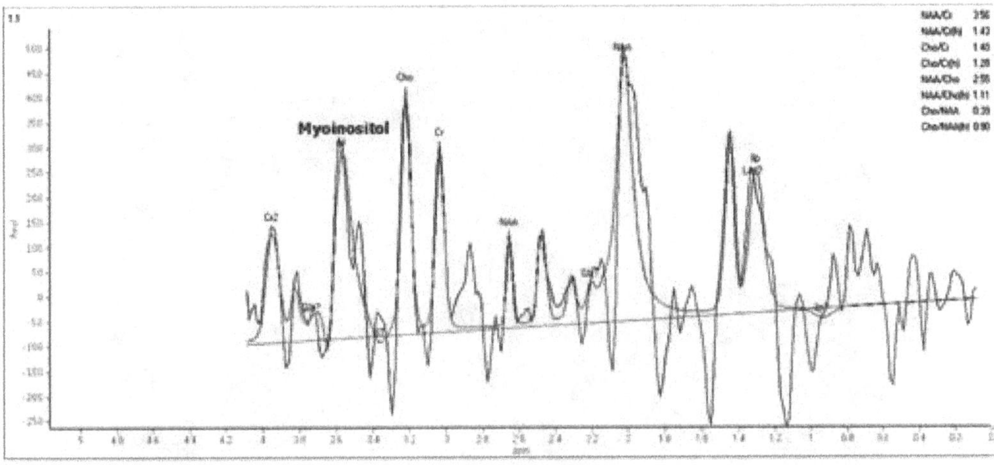

Figure 4. Short-echo MR proton spectrum shows an elevated myoinositol (mI) peak (at 3.55 ppm) in a case of gliomatosis cerebri.

4. Primary central nervous system lymphoma

Primary central nervous system lymphoma (PCNSL) is a rare variant of extranodal non-Hodgkin lymphoma and affects about 1,000 people in the United States each year. Non-invasive diagnosis of PCNSL is of paramount importance given the dramatic benefits of chemotherapy in this tumor. Typical MR imaging features of PCNSLs are frequent periventricular locations, perilesional edema, well-defined margin, and homogeneous and intense nodular enhancement.

4.1. Diffusion-weighted imaging

PCNSLs tend to have a low ADC value because of high cellularity (**Figure 5**). Brain abscess has higher ADC values than lymphomas; thus, this feature can help in differentiating these two entities [15].

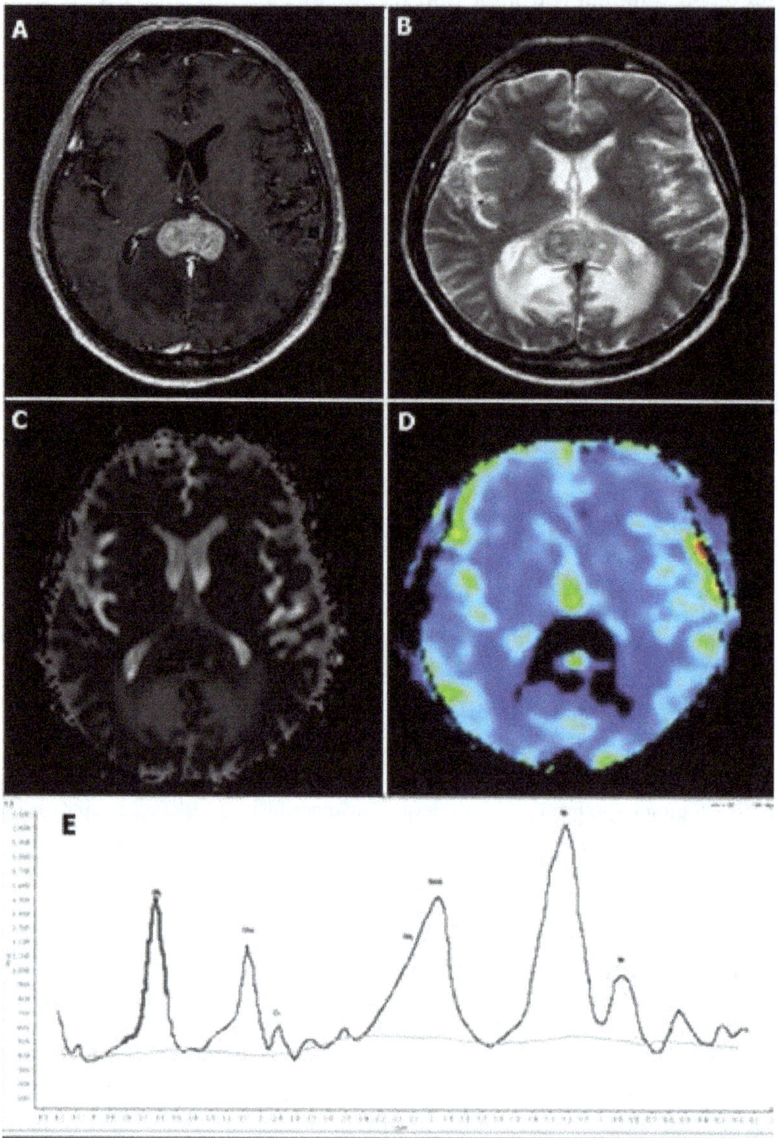

Figure 5. A case of lymphoma (A, B) revealing a low ADC value (C), low perfusion (D), and elevated levels of Lipids (E).

4.2. Perfusion imaging

PCNSL has low rCBV compared with that of high-grade gliomas and metastasis; however, overlapping values may exist (**Figure 5**). An important clue is that PCNSL demonstrates a significant increase in signal intensity above the baseline due to massive leakage of contrast media into the interstitial space contrary to high-grade gliomas [16]. Lymphoma tends to demonstrate higher rCBV compared with toxoplasmosis [15].

4.3. MR spectroscopy

Characteristic spectroscopic findings for PCNSL include elevated signals of lipid, choline, and lactate and reduced NAA signal **(Figure 5)**. Large lipid peaks on lesions without central necrosis are also strongly suggestive of PCNSL [17]. High lipid peak may be due to increased turnover of the membrane components in transformed lymphoid cells.

5. Differential diagnosis

5.1. Tumefactive demyelinating lesions

Tumefactive demyelinating lesions (TDLs) can be seen either during a relapse of a known multiple sclerosis or on acute onset. TDL can mimic high-grade gliomas on conventional MRI. In both conditions, there is contrast enhancement, perilesional edema, and central necrosis. Additional histopathology is not always straightforward since abnormal mitotic figures in reactive astrocytes can be present. In TDL, there is usually incomplete rim enhancement on MRI and little mass effect and edema (**Figure 6**).

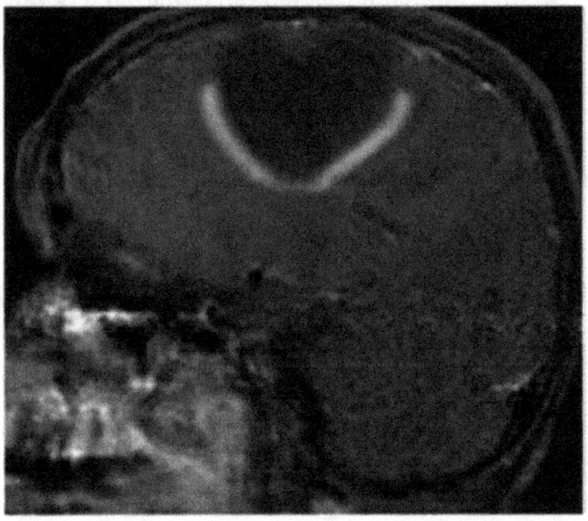

Figure 6. A case of TDL demonstarting incomplete rim enhancement on sagittal T1-weighted images after intravenous contrast administration.

5.1.1 Diffusion-weighted imaging

Min ADC values were higher in TDL than in PCNSLs or high-grade gliomas given that TDL is lesser cellular lesions than both PCNSLs and high-grade gliomas [18]. An important exception might be an acute demyelinating lesion which has areas of low ADC values (**Figure 7**). In acute phase in the TDL rim, there is peripheral restricted diffusion. The abnormal diffusion resolves within 1–3 weeks. Following restricted diffusion on initial MRI, subsequent Gd enhancement can be seen [19].

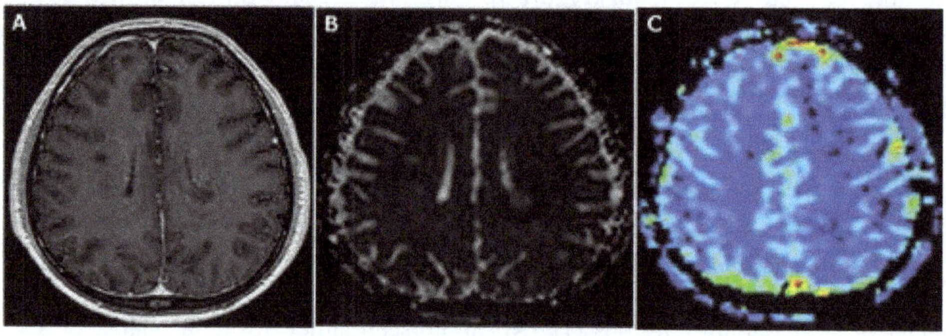

Figure 7. A case of TDL (A) demonstrating moderate ADC values (B). The rCBV maps show no elevation of Blood volume compared with contralateral normal white matter (C).

5.1.2. Perfusion imaging

TDL shows significant lower rCBV values (mean 0.88 ± 0.46) than high-grade gliomas (mean 6.47 ± 6.52), given the increased angiogenesis that the latter have (**Figure 7**). However, PCNSL had a less pronounced difference with a mean value of 2.11 ± 0.53 [20].

5.1.3. MR spectroscopy

TDL findings on spectroscopy are usually involve an elevated choline peak and reduced NAA signal. There may be also increased lactate and increased Cho/NAA that can reach high levels similar to that of high-grade gliomas; thus, differential diagnosis is problematic. The detection of glutamate and glutamine elevations has also been suggestive of TDL [21].

5.2. Brain abscess

Brain abscesses usually result from the extension of inflammation from the sinuses, the orbit, the mastoid cells, or the middle ear. As possible ways of spreading are either direct infection from a penetrating trauma, septic emboli, and contiguous or hematogenous spread. The most common pathogen is *Streptococcus pneumoniae*. Symptomatology is similar to any other mass lesions but tend to progress rapidly. Classical MRI findings of abscess in T2-weighted images are high-signal intensity with a thin rim of low intensity surrounded by edema. Furthermore, satellite lesions are more common in abscesses contrary to neoplastic lesions.

5.2.1. Diffusion-weighted imaging

The characteristic finding of brain abscess in DWI is a core of restricted diffusion due to pus consistency, whereas in neoplasms, there is usually low DWI signal (**Figure 8**). However, some necrotic brain metastasis may also display high signal intensity on DWI [22]. ADC values usually increase as treatment is successful even if cavity remains. Another finding in the rim of neoplastic lesions is a lower ADC value than that of an abscess.

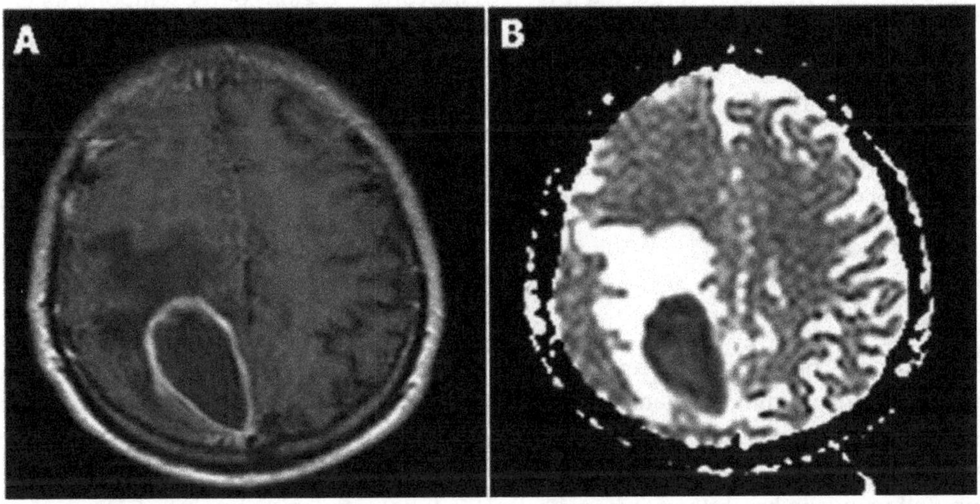

Figure 8. A case of an abscess (A) revealing low ADC values corresponding to the nonenhancing portion of the abscess (B).

5.2.2. Perfusion imaging

Contrary to glioblastomas and metastases, the enhancing rims of abscesses usually demonstrate lower rCBV values. The rCBV ratio of the enhancing portions of abscesses has be reported to be 0.79 ± 0.18, whereas in tumors was 1.40 ± 0.54 [23].

5.2.3. MR spectroscopy

Relative-specific MR spectroscopic feature of brain abscess is a succinate peak; however, it is not present in all cases. Apart from that elevated peaks of lactate, acetate, amino acids, alanine, valine, leucine, and isoleucine can be found. In abscesses reduced peaks of Cho/Crn and NAA are usually present [24]. Tuberculous abscesses typically have high lipid (mostly short-chain fatty acids such as butyric, isobutyric, caproic). Disappearance of metabolites of bacterial origin has been correlated with positive response to therapy [25].

5.3. Encephalitis

Encephalitis is an acute, usually diffuse, inflammatory process affecting the brain and may mimic mass lesions. Herpes simplex (HSV) encephalitis is the most common cause. Biopsy is helpful in some instances. Patients are usually confused and disoriented at the beginning and progress to coma within days. MRI demonstrates edema as high signal on T2, primarily within the temporal lobe, that may extend across sylvian fissure. Enhancement is usually present after the second week. Foci of hemorrhage occasionally can be found on MRI.

5.3.1. Diffusion-weighted imaging

Encephalitis typically demonstrates low ADC values due to cytotoxic edema. However, encephalitis may mimic an infarct that involves the cortical regions of the temporal lobe.

5.3.2. Perfusion imaging

Perfusion MRI has not been widely studied in encephalitis. At an early stage, there is an abnormal increase of blood flow in the affected area, followed by hypoperfusion at a later stage.

5.3.3. MR spectroscopy

On MR spectroscopy, finding encephalitis needs to be differentiated from a low-grade glioma which has similar findings. In general, there is a decrease in NAA peak usually 1–2 weeks after onset. After clinical recovery, there is a corresponding increase in NAA [26, 27]. Frequently, there is an increase in choline and myoinositol peak. An increased Cho/Cr ratio may be attributed to myelin breakdown. Sporadically, the lactate peak may be elevated.

5.4. Metastasis

Although the annual incidence of brain tumors is 17,000, for brain metastasis is 170,000 [28]. Thus, brain metastasis is the most common brain tumor seen clinically. The source of more than 50% of metastatic lesions is lung and breast cancer. When a single-brain lesion is found in a patient with a history of cancer, in 11% of these cases the lesion will not be metastatic. Four out of five of solitary metastases are located in the cerebral hemispheres. The majority tends to occur at the gray/white matter junction and is usually located posterior to the Sylvian fissure.

5.4.1. Diffusion-weighted imaging

The characteristic diffusion-weighted imaging feature for metastatic neoplasms is an elevated ADC. However, there is an overlap of the ADC values of metastatic lesions with those of primary neoplasms (**Figure 9**). Evaluation of ADC values in the non-enhancing T2-hyperintense areas surrounding the lesion may provide clues for the differentiation of high-grade gliomas from metastasis, given the lower ADC values in infiltrated areas of primary neoplasms compared with metastatic lesions. A threshold value of 1.302×10^{-3} mm^2/s for the minimum ADC value in the peritumoral regions had a sensitivity of 82.9% and specificity of 78.9% for distinguishing between glioblastoma and metastasis [29]. Although some studies have not found correlation between restricted diffusion or ADC values and various histologic types of metastases; however, a study reported that well-differentiated adenocarcinomas had lower DWI signal intensity compared with poorly differentiated carcinomas [30, 31].

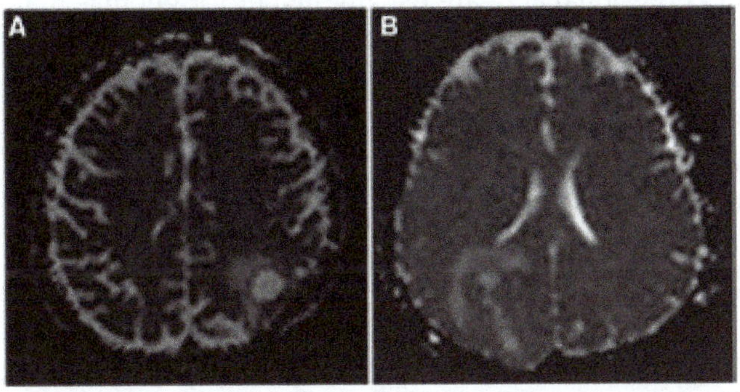

Figure 9. There is overlapping in the ADC values between a metastatic (A) and a primary brain tumor (B).

5.4.2. Perfusion imaging

Angiogenesis is essential for metastatic tumors growth. Thus, these lesions are associated with increased rCBV values compared with contralateral normal white matter. Thus, perfusion metrics tend to overlap between high-grade gliomas and metastatic lesions (**Figure 10**). The peak height and the percentage of signal intensity recovery derived from the T2* relaxivity curve on DSC MR has been reported to provide important clues [32]. Apart from that, metastasis from melanoma and renal cell carcinoma has been reported to have significant higher rCBV values than high-grade gliomas and metastases from lung cancer [33].

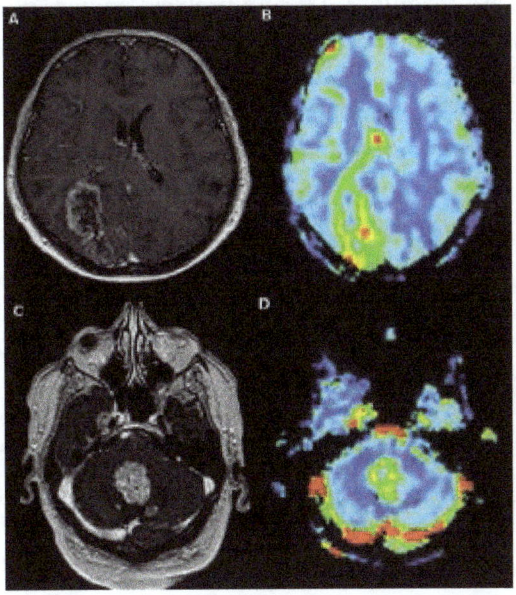

Figure 10. Both glioblastoma (A, B) and metastatic lesions (C, D) exhibits increased rCBV values, not permitting a differentiation based on perfusion imaging.

The rCBV values of perilesional area are usually higher for gliomas than metastatic lesions, due to glioma's infiltrative nature. In a study of 22 high-grade gliomas and 26 metastatic lesions, the rCBV ratios of peritumoural edema were 0.89 ± 0.51 in high-grade gliomas and 0.31 ± 0.12 in metastasis. A threshold rCBV value of 0.46 has been proposed, with a sensitivity of 77.3% and specificity of 96.2% for the differentiation of the two entities [34].

5.4.3. MR spectroscopy

Accurate differentiation between high-grade gliomas and metastatic lesion based on the enhancing part is problematic based on MR spectra. In metastatic lesions, there is no NAA peak, whereas necrosis results in a lipid peak. Lipid and lactate may be also elevated in primary brain tumors due to necrosis. Myoinosital peaks have not been reported to date in brain metastases, contrary to high-grade gliomas which tend to have elevated peaks [35, 36]. Given that primary tumors have a tendency to infiltrate, evaluation of the T2 hyperintense perilesional tissue provide more important information. Thus, although there is an intratumoral choline peak in both primary and metastatic lesions, there is no choline elevation in the peritumoural edema in metastatic lesions [37].

6. Conclusion

Intra-axial brain lesions are a significant health problem and are often a diagnostic imaging challenge. Advanced MRI techniques including proton spectroscopy, perfusion, and DWI have all been evaluated primarily in the context of distinguishing high-grade gliomas from metastases, abscess, and CNS lymphoma. Knowledge of the imaging characteristics of the most common intra-axial masses may allow the non-invasive diagnosis and classification of these masses.

Author details

Anastasia Zikou[1], George Alexiou[2*] and Maria Argyropoulou[1]

*Address all correspondence to: alexiougrg@yahoo.gr

1 Department of Radiology, School of Medicine, University of Ioannina, Ioannina, Greece

2 Department of Neurosurgery, School of Medicine, University of Ioannina, Ioannina, Greece

References

[1] Ostrom QT, Gittleman H, Fulop J, Liu M, Blanda R, Kromer C, Wolinsky Y, Kruchko C, Barnholtz-Sloan JS. CBTRUS statistical report: primary brain and central nervous system tumors diagnosed in the United States in 2008–2012. Neuro Oncol. 2015;14(Suppl 4):iv1–62.

[2] Alexiou GA, Zikou A, Tsiouris S, Goussia A, Kosta P, Papadopoulos A, Voulgaris S, Kyritsis AP, Fotopoulos AD, Argyropoulou MI. Correlation of diffusion tensor, dynamic susceptibility contrast MRI and (99m)Tc-Tetrofosmin brain SPECT with tumour grade and Ki-67 immunohistochemistry in glioma. Clin Neurol Neurosurg. 2014;116:41–5.

[3] Würdinger T, Tannous BA. Glioma angiogenesis: towards novel RNA therapeutics. Cell Adh Migr. 2009;3(2):230–5.

[4] Das S, Marsden PA. Angiogenesis in glioblastoma. N Engl J Med. 2013;369(16):1561–3.

[5] Zikou AK, Alexiou GA, Kosta P, Goussia A, Astrakas L, Tsekeris P, Voulgaris S, Malamou-Mitsi V, Kyritsis AP, Argyropoulou MI. Diffusion tensor and dynamic susceptibility contrast MRI in glioblastoma. Clin Neurol Neurosurg. 2012;114(6):607–12.

[6] Zikou A, Alexiou GA, Vartholomatos G, Goussia A, Xydis VG, Kosta P, Voulgaris S, Kyritsis AP, Argyropoulou MI. Correlation of diffusion tensor and dynamic susceptibility contrast MRI with DNA ploidy and cell cycle analysis of gliomas. Clin Neurol Neurosurg. 2015;139:119–24.

[7] Cha S, Tihan T, Crawford F, Fischbein NJ, Chang S, Bollen A, Nelson SJ, Prados M, Berger MS, Dillon WP. Differentiation of low-grade oligodendrogliomas from low-grade astrocytomas by using quantitative blood-volume measurements derived from dynamic susceptibility contrast-enhanced MR imaging. AJNR Am J Neuroradiol. 2005;26(2):266–73.

[8] Alexiou GA, Moschovi M, Stefanaki K, Sfakianos G, Prodromou N. Epidemiology of pediatric brain tumors in Greece (1991–2008). Experience from the Agia Sofia Children's Hospital. Cent Eur Neurosurg. 2011;72(1):1–4.

[9] Wang Q, Zhang H, Zhang J, Wu C, Zhu W, Li F, Chen X, Xu B. The diagnostic performance of magnetic resonance spectroscopy in differentiating high-from low-grade gliomas: a systematic review and meta-analysis. Eur Radiol. 2015 Oct 15 [Epub ahead of print].

[10] Chen S, Tanaka S, Giannini C, et al. Gliomatosis cerebri: clinical characteristics, management, and outcomes. J Neurooncol. 2013;112(2):267–75.

[11] Fuller GN, Scheithauer BW. The 2007 revised World Health Organization (WHO) classification of tumors of the central nervous system: newly codified entities. Brain Pathol. 2007;17:304–7.

[12] Chen S, Tanaka S, Giannini C et-al. Gliomatosis cerebri: clinical characteristics, management, and outcomes. J Neurooncol. 2013;112(2):267–75.

[13] Desclée P, Rommel D, Hernalsteen D, Godfraind C, de Coene B, Cosnard G. Gliomatosis cerebri, imaging findings of 12 cases. J Neuroradiol. 2010;37(3):148–58.

[14] Bendszus M, Warmuth-metz M, Klein R et-al. MR spectroscopy in gliomatosis cerebri. AJNR Am J Neuroradiol. 2000;21(2):375–80.

[15] Al-Okaili RN, Krejza J, Wang S, Woo JH, Melhem ER. Advanced MR imaging techniques in the diagnosis of intraaxial brain tumors in adults. Radiographics. 2006;26(Suppl 1):S173–89.

[16] Hartmann M, Heiland S, Harting I, Tronnier VM, Sommer C, Ludwig R, Sartor K. Distinguishing of primary cerebral lymphoma from high-grade glioma with perfusion-weighted magnetic resonance imaging. Neurosci Lett. 2003;338(2):119–22.

[17] Yamasaki F, Takayasu T, Nosaka R, Amatya VJ, Doskaliyev A, Akiyama Y, Tominaga A, Takeshima Y, Sugiyama K, Kurisu K. Magnetic resonance spectroscopy detection of high lipid levels in intraaxial tumors without central necrosis: a characteristic of malignant lymphoma. J Neurosurg. 2015;122(6):1370–9.

[18] Mabray MC, Cohen BA, Villanueva-Meyer JE, Valles FE, Barajas RF, Rubenstein JL, Cha S. Performance of apparent diffusion coefficient values and conventional MRI features in differentiating tumefactive demyelinating lesions from primary brain neoplasms. AJR Am J Roentgenol. 2015;205(5):1075–85.

[19] Hyland M, Bermel RA, Cohen JA. Restricted diffusion preceding gadolinium enhancement in large or tumefactive demyelinating lesions. Neurol Clin Pract. 2013;3(1):15–21.

[20] Cha S, Pierce S, Knopp EA, Johnson G, Yang C, Ton A, Litt AW, Zagzag D. Dynamic contrast-enhanced T2*-weighted MR imaging of tumefactive demyelinating lesions. AJNR Am J Neuroradiol. 2001;22(6):1109–16.

[21] Al-Okaili RN, Krejza J, Wang S, Woo JH, Melhem ER. Advanced MR imaging techniques in the diagnosis of intraaxial brain tumors in adults. Radiographics. 2006;26(Suppl 1):S173–89.

[22] Park SH, Chang KH, Song IC, Kim YJ, Kim SH, Han MH. Diffusion-weighted MRI in cystic or necrotic intracranial lesions. Neuroradiology. 2000;42:716–21.

[23] Holmes TM, Petrella JR, Provenzale JM. Distinction between cerebral abscesses and high-grade neoplasms by dynamic susceptibility contrast perfusion MRI. AJR Am J Roentgenol. 2004;183(5):1247–52.

[24] Pal D, Bhattacharyya A, Husain M, Prasad KN, Pandey CM, Gupta RK. In vivo proton MR spectroscopy evaluation of pyogenic brain abscesses: a report of 194 cases. AJNR Am J Neuroradiol. 2010;31(2):360–6.

[25] Lai PH, Weng HH, Chen CY, Hsu SS, Ding S, Ko CW, Fu JH, Liang HL, Chen KH. In vivo differentiation of aerobic brain abscesses and necrotic glioblastomas multiforme using proton MR spectroscopic imaging. AJNR Am J Neuroradiol. 2008;29(8):1511–8.

[26] Sämann PG, Schlegel J, Müller G, Prantl F, Emminger C, Auer DP. Serial proton MR spectroscopy and diffusion imaging findings in HIV-related herpes simplex encephalitis. AJNR Am J Neuroradiol. 2003;24(10):2015–9.

[27] Takanashi J, Sugita K, Ishii M, Aoyagi M, Niimi H. Longitudinal MR imaging and proton MR spectroscopy in herpes simplex encephalitis. J Neurol Sci. 1997;149(1):99–102.

[28] Johnson J D, Young B. Demographics of brain metastasis. Neurosurg Clin N Am. 1996;7(3):337–44.

[29] Lee EJ, terBrugge K, Mikulis D, Choi DS, Bae JM, Lee SK, Moon SY. Diagnostic value of peritumoral minimum apparent diffusion coefficient for differentiation of glioblastoma multiforme from solitary metastatic lesions. AJR Am J Roentgenol. 2011;196(1): 71–6.

[30] Hayashida Y, Hirai T, Morishita S, Kitajima M, Murakami R, Korogi Y, et al. Diffusion-weighted imaging of metastatic brain tumors: comparison with histologic type and tumor cellularity. AJNR Am J Neuroradiol. 2006;27:1419–25.

[31] Duygulu G, Ovali GY, Calli C, Kitis O, Yünten N, Akalin T, et al. Intracerebral metastasis showing restricted diffusion: correlation with histopathologic findings. Eur J Radiol. 2010;74:117–20.

[32] Cha S, Lupo JM, Chen MH, Lamborn KR, McDermott MW, Berger MS, Nelson SJ, Dillon WP. Differentiation of glioblastoma multiforme and single brain metastasis by peak height and percentage of signal intensity recovery derived from dynamic susceptibility-weighted contrast-enhanced perfusion MR imaging. AJNR Am J Neuroradiol. 2007;28(6):1078–84.

[33] Kremer S, Grand S, Berger F, Hoffmann D, Pasquier B, Rémy C, Benabid AL, Bas JF. Dynamic contrast-enhanced MRI: differentiating melanoma and renal carcinoma metastases from high-grade astrocytomas and other metastases. Neuroradiology. 2003;45(1):44–9.

[34] Hakyemez B, Erdogan C, Gokalp G, Dusak A, Parlak M. Solitary metastases and high-grade gliomas: radiological differentiation by morphometric analysis and perfusion-weighted MRI. Clin Radiol. 2010;65(1):15–20.

[35] Bendini M, Marton E, Feletti A, Rossi S, Curtolo S, Inches I, et al. Primary and metastatic intraaxial brain tumors: prospective comparison of multivoxel 2D chemical-shift imaging (CSI) proton MR spectroscopy, perfusion MRI, and histopathological findings in a group of 159 patients. Acta Neurochir (Wien). 2011;153:403–12.

[36] Fan G, Sun B, Wu Z, Guo Q, Guo Y. In vivo single-voxel proton MR spectroscopy in the differentiation of high-grade gliomas and solitary metastases. Clin Radiol. 2004;59:77–85.

[37] Fink KR, Fink JR. Imaging of brain metastases. Surg Neurol Int. 2013;4(Suppl 4):S209–19.

Permissions

All chapters in this book were first published by InTech Open; hereby published with permission under the Creative Commons Attribution License or equivalent. Every chapter published in this book has been scrutinized by our experts. Their significance has been extensively debated. The topics covered herein carry significant findings which will fuel the growth of the discipline. They may even be implemented as practical applications or may be referred to as a beginning point for another development.

The contributors of this book come from diverse backgrounds, making this book a truly international effort. This book will bring forth new frontiers with its revolutionizing research information and detailed analysis of the nascent developments around the world.

We would like to thank all the contributing authors for lending their expertise to make the book truly unique. They have played a crucial role in the development of this book. Without their invaluable contributions this book wouldn't have been possible. They have made vital efforts to compile up to date information on the varied aspects of this subject to make this book a valuable addition to the collection of many professionals and students.

This book was conceptualized with the vision of imparting up-to-date information and advanced data in this field. To ensure the same, a matchless editorial board was set up. Every individual on the board went through rigorous rounds of assessment to prove their worth. After which they invested a large part of their time researching and compiling the most relevant data for our readers.

The editorial board has been involved in producing this book since its inception. They have spent rigorous hours researching and exploring the diverse topics which have resulted in the successful publishing of this book. They have passed on their knowledge of decades through this book. To expedite this challenging task, the publisher supported the team at every step. A small team of assistant editors was also appointed to further simplify the editing procedure and attain best results for the readers.

Apart from the editorial board, the designing team has also invested a significant amount of their time in understanding the subject and creating the most relevant covers. They scrutinized every image to scout for the most suitable representation of the subject and create an appropriate cover for the book.

The publishing team has been an ardent support to the editorial, designing and production team. Their endless efforts to recruit the best for this project, has resulted in the accomplishment of this book. They are a veteran in the field of academics and their pool of knowledge is as vast as their experience in printing. Their expertise and guidance has proved useful at every step. Their uncompromising quality standards have made this book an exceptional effort. Their encouragement from time to time has been an inspiration for everyone.

The publisher and the editorial board hope that this book will prove to be a valuable piece of knowledge for researchers, students, practitioners and scholars across the globe.

List of Contributors

Judith Marcela Dueñas-Jiménez, Irene Aguilar-García, María de la Luz Galván-Ramírez, Sergio Horacio Dueñas-Jiménez, Jorge David Rivas-Carrillo and Erika Priscilla Domínguez-Rangel
University Center for Health Sciences, University of Guadalajara, Guadalajara, Jalisco, México

Anne Santerre
University Center for Biological and Agricultural Sciences, University of Guadalajara, Guadalajara, Jalisco, México

Ilhan Yaylim and Özlem Küçükhüseyin
Institute of Experimental Medicine, Department of Molecular Medicine, Istanbul University, Istanbul, Turkey

Sumeyya Azam
First Affiliated Hospital of Xinjiang Medical University, Xinjiang, Urumqi, PR China

Ammad Ahmad Farooqi and Muhammad Ismail
Institute of Biomedical and Genetic Engineering (IBGE), Islamabad, Pakistan

Ali Metin Kafadar
Department of Neurosurgery, Cerrahpaşa Medical Faculty, Istanbul University, Istanbul, Turkey

Jens Schittenhelm and Marco Skardelly
Department of Neuropathology, Institute of Pathology and Neuropathology, Germany
Department of Neurosurgery, University Medical Clinic, University of Tübingen, Germany

W. Phillip Law
Medical Imaging Department, Princess Alexandra Hospital, School of Medicine, University of Queensland, Brisbane, QLD, Australia

Romana Richterová and Branislav Kolarovszki
Department of Neurosurgery, Jessenius Faculty of Medicine in Martin, Comenius University in Bratislava, Martin, Slovakia

Takashi Sasayama, Kazuhiro Tanaka and Eiji Kohmura
Department of Neurosurgery, Kobe University Graduate School of Medicine, Kusunoki-cho, Chuo-ku, Kobe, Japan

Scott G. Turner, Maleeha Ahmad and Steven A. Toms
Departments of Neurology and Neurosurgery, Geisinger Medical Center, Danville, PA, USA

Lorena Vega-Zelaya and Jesús Pastor
Clinical Neurophysiology, Hospital Universitario de la Princesa, Madrid, Spain
Biomedical Research Institute, Hospital Universitario de la Princesa, Madrid, Spain

Rafael G. Sola
Neurosurgery, Hospital Universitario de la Princesa, Madrid, Spain

Anastasia Zikou and Maria Argyropoulou
Department of Radiology, School of Medicine, University of Ioannina, Ioannina, Greece

George Alexiou
Department of Neurosurgery, School of Medicine, University of Ioannina, Ioannina, Greece

Index

www.ingramcontent.com/pod-product-compliance
Lightning Source LLC
LaVergne TN
LVHW062234200926
848484LV00006B/1538

9798887400891